NURSING THE NEONATE

NURSING THE NEONATE

Edited by

Helen Yeo
RGN, ENB 904, WNB 998
Senior Sister
University Hospital of Wales,
Cardiff

b

**Blackwell
Science**

© 1998
Blackwell Science Ltd
Editorial Offices:
Osney Mead, Oxford OX2 0EL
25 John Street, London WC1N 2BL
23 Ainslie Place, Edinburgh EH3 6AJ
350 Main Street, Malden
  MA 02148 5018, USA
54 University Street, Carlton
  Victoria 3053, Australia
10, rue Casimir Delavigne
  75006 Paris, France

Other Editorial Offices:

Blackwell Wissenschafts-Verlag GmbH
Kurfürstendamm 57
10707 Berlin, Germany

Blackwell Science KK
MG Kodenmacho Building
7–10 Kodenmacho Nihombashi
Chuo-ku, Tokyo 104, Japan

First published 1998

Set in 10/13.5 pt Palatino
by DP Photosetting, Aylesbury, Bucks
Printed and bound in Great Britain by
MPG Books Ltd, Bodmin, Cornwall

DISTRIBUTORS

Marston Book Services Ltd
PO Box 269
Abingdon
Oxon OX14 4YN
(*Orders:* Tel: 01235 465500
            Fax: 01235 465555)

USA
Blackwell Science, Inc.
Commerce Place
350 Main Street
Malden, MA 02148 5018
(*Orders:* Tel: 800 759 6102
            781 388 8250
         Fax: 781 388 8255)

Canada
Login Brothers Book Company
324 Saulteaux Crescent
Winnipeg, Manitoba R3J 3T2
(*Orders:* Tel: 204 224-4068)

Australia
Blackwell Science Pty Ltd
54 University Street
Carlton, Victoria 3053
(*Orders:* Tel: 03 9347 0300
            Fax: 03 9347 5001)

A catalogue record for this title is available
from the British Library

ISBN 0-632-05049-7

Library of Congress
Cataloging-in-Publication Data
is available

The Editor, Contributors and Publishers have undertaken reasonable endeavours to check dosage and
nursing content for accuracy. Because the science of clinical pharmacology is continually advancing, our
knowledge base continues to expand. Therefore the reader should always check the manufacturer's
product information before administering any medication.

Contents

Preface

Neonatal nursing started at the beginning of this century and as the millennium approaches we can be justly proud of its achievements. The saving of smaller and sicker babies and the improvement in their quality of life has been achieved by technology, research and a high standard of medical and nursing care. To maintain this standard, continuing professional development and updating is essential. This book is written for students, nurses and midwives working on neonatal units. Its purpose is to inform, enlighten and guide people in this branch of nursing. The contributors are all experienced neonatal nurses, working and learning every day as they care for their small charges.

The book is written from a nursing perspective though it does of necessity include procedures and diagnoses that are the prerogative of other medical staff. To leave these matters out would make the text meaningless, as neonatology is a multidisciplinary speciality.

It would be impossible to cover comprehensively every condition encountered in the unit, so the chapters cover a spectrum of common diseases and their nursing management. Neonatal care is looked at through a series of life systems which cover most major neonatal problems. The chapter concerning the critically ill baby covers a number of conditions which often follow in sequence and examines nursing care and family involvement at all stages. Practical care of the baby is described and the rationale for carrying it out discussed. Meeting the psychological needs of parents is important for the continuing well-being of the family as a whole. This and the relevance of promoting family-centred care in the unit is examined in each chapter. Other nursing concerns such as ethics, transcultural nursing and stress are investigated.

The book is about the nursing management of new-born babies, whether in an intensive care situation or in the nursery; it looks at the long term results of that care which is intended to temper actions with caution.

Helen Yeo, 1998

ACKNOWLEDGEMENTS

I wish to acknowledge and thank Lynne Gunter, lecturer in midwifery, for her advice and guidance in the writing of this book; Julie Jessop, staff nurse on the Neonatal Unit, University Hospital of Wales for her drawing skills; Roger Yeo for his computer skills and for the patience, support and encouragement without which this work would not have been written.

'Surgical intervention for the repair of exompholos' in Chapter 5 is partially reprinted from *Professional Nurse* with kind permission of the Editor, Macmillan Magazines.

Mary Sheeran wrote chapter 16 while studying for the MSc in Health and Reproduction and wishes to acknowledge the financial support given by Smith and Nephew during this course.

Contributors

Carolyn Daniels
BN, RGN, Neonatal Modules 1 and 2
E Grade Staff Nurse
Neonatal Unit, University Hospital of Wales,
Cardiff
Contributed to Chapter 3

Lucy Gardner
RGN, RSCN, ENB 405, ENB 160, Teaching and
Assessing Modules
G Grade Sister
Neonatal Unit, University Hospital of Wales,
Cardiff
Contributed to Chapter 6

Angela Gorman
RGN, Neononatal Modules 1 and 2
F Grade Sister
Neonatal Unit, University Hospital of Wales,
Cardiff
Contributed to Chapter 11

Lynne Gunter
BA, SRN, SCM, ADM, MTD, Cert Ed., FEA,
ONC
Lecturer in Midwifery
University Hospital of Wales, College of
Medicine, School of Nursing Studies
Contributed to Chapter 1

Samantha Hallum
RGN, ENB 405, 998
E Grade Staff Nurse
Neonatal Unit, University Hospital of Wales,
Cardiff
Contributed to Chapter 10

Nicola Harvey
RGN, 405, 998
Neonatal Outreach Sister
Neonatal Unit, University Hospital of Wales,
Cardiff
Contributed to Chapter 13

Laura Hutchinson
RGN, 405, 998
E Grade Staff Nurse
Neonatal Unit, University Hospital of Wales,
Cardiff
Contributed to Chapter 3

Liv Lee
RGN, Neonatal Diploma Modules
Formerly D Grade Staff Nurse
Neonatal Unit, University Hospital of Wales,
Cardiff
Contributed the whole of Chapter 9

Antoinette Matthews
RGN, RGM, 405, 998, Paediatric Cardiac
Intensive Care Module
F Grade Sister
Neonatal Unit, University Hospital of Wales,
Cardiff
Contributed to Chapter 6

Terry Orford
MA, RGN, RM, NNEB, WNB998, ENB 904,
Diploma in Counselling, Certificate in
Pastoral Care, Guidance and Counselling
Parent/Staff Support Sister Counsellor
Paediatric/Neonatal Unit, University
Hospital of Wales, Cardiff
Contributed to Chapter 1

Alison Parry
BN, RGN, Neonatal Modules 1 and 2
E Grade Staff Nurse
Neonatal Unit, University Hospital of Wales,
Cardiff
Contributed to Chapter 4

Mary Pickard
RGN, SCM, Neonatal Modules 1 and 2,
Genetics Diploma Module
E Grade Staff Nurse
Neonatal Unit, University Hospital of Wales,
Cardiff
Contributed to Chapter 7

Jill Rainnie
RGN, 405, 998, Further Education Teaching
Certificate, Neonatal Certificate, Genetics
Diploma Module
Formerly G Grade Sister
Neonatal Unit, University Hospital of Wales,
Cardiff
Now in High Wycombe Hospital Neonatal
Unit
Contributed to Chapter 7

Mary Sheeran
RGN, RSCN, Neonatal Modules 1 and 2
Formerly F Grade Sister
Neonatal Unit, University Hospital of Wales,
Cardiff
Now studying in America
*Contributed to Chapter 4 and the whole of Chapter
16*

Susan Tester
RGN, 405, 998, Genetics Diploma Module
G Grade Sister
Neonatal Unit, University Hospital of Wales,
Cardiff
Contributed to Chapter 7

Jenny Webb
BN, RGN, Neonatal Modules 1 and 2
E Grade Staff Nurse
Neonatal Unit, University Hospital of Wales,
Cardiff
Contributed to Chapter 3

Helen Yeo
RGN, 998, 904, Genetics Module, Paediatric
Cardiac Intensive Care Module
G Grade Sister
Neonatal Unit, University Hospital of Wales,
Cardiff
*Contributed to chapters 1, 3, 4, 6, 7, 10, 11, 13 and
the whole of Chapters 2, 5, 8, 12, 14 and 15*

List of Abbreviations

AFP	Alpha-fetoprotein	DIC	Disseminated intravascular coagulation
AIDS	Acquired immune deficiency syndrome	DNA	Deoxyribonucleic acid
ANNP	Advanced neonatal nurse practitioner	EBM	Expressed breast milk
		EBV	Epstein–Barr virus
APH	Antepartum haemorrhage	ECG	Electrocardiogram
ARF	Acute renal failure	ECMO	Extra-corporeal membrane oxygenation
ASD	Atrial septal defect		
BP	Blood pressure	EDD	Estimated date of delivery
BPD	Bronchopulmonary dysplasia	ELBW	Extra-low birth weight
BW	Birth weight	ETT	Endotracheal tube
CAVH	Continuous arteriovenous haemofiltration	FBC	Full blood count
		FFP	Fresh frozen plasma
CCF	Congestive cardiac failure	FISH	Fluorescent *in situ* hybridisation
CF	Cystic fibrosis	FiO_2	Fractional inspired oxygen concentration
CHD	Congenital heart disease		
CLSE	Calf lung surfactant extract	$FiCO_2$	Fractional inspired carbon dioxide concentration
CMV	Cytomegalovirus		
CNS	Central nervous system	Fr	French gauge
CO_2	Carbon dioxide	G-6-PD	Glucose-6-phosphate dehydrogenase
CPAP	Continuous positive airway pressure		
		GBS	Group B streptococcus
CPB	Cardiopulmonary bypass	GFR	Glomerular filtration rate
CPD	Citrated phosphate dextrose	GI	Gastrointestinal
CPR	Cardiopulmonary rescusitation	GP	General practitioner
CRP	C-reactive protein	HBV	Hepatitis B virus
CSF	Cerebrospinal fluid	HFJV	High-frequency jet ventilation
CTG	Cardiotocograph	HFOV	High-frequency oscillatory ventilation
CVP	Central venous pressure		
CVS	Chorionic villus sampling	HLHS	Hypoplastic left heart syndrome
CXR	Chest X-ray	HIV	Human immunodeficiency virus

HMSO	Her Majesty's Stationery Office
HSV	Herpes simplex virus
HUGO	Human Genome Organisation
H_2O	Water
Hz	Hertz
IDM	Infant of diabetic mother
I:E	Inspiratory to expiratory ratio
IgA, IgM	Immunoglobulins A and M
IM	Intramuscular
IMV	Intermittent mandatory ventilation
IPPV	Intermittent positive pressure ventilation
IRT	Immune reactive trypsin
IUGR	Intrauterine growth retardation
IU/l	International units per litre
IV	Intravenous
IVC	Inferior vena cava
IVF	*In vitro* fertilisation
IVH	Intraventricular haemorrhage
kPa	Kilopascals
LA	Left atrium
LBW	Low birth weight
LCP	Long chain polyunsaturated fatty acids
LP	Lumbar puncture
LV	Left ventricle
MAP	Mean airway pressure
MCT	Medium chain triglycerides
$\mu mol/l$	Micromoles per litre
mmHg	Millimetres of mercury
mmH_2O	Millimetres of water
mmol/l	Millimoles per litre
MMR	Mumps measles and rubella (vaccine)
MRSA	Methicillin-resistant *Staphylococcus aureus*
NEC	Necrotising enterocolitis
NG	Nasogastric
NICU	Neonatal intensive care unit
NIDCAP	Neonatal individualised developmental care and assessment programme
NNU	Neonatal unit
NO	Nitric oxide
O_2	Oxygen
OI	Osteogenesis imperfecta
$PaCO_2$	Arterial partial pressure of carbon dioxide
PaO_2	Arterial partial pressure of oxygen
PCV	Packed cell volume
PD	Peritoneal dialysis
PDA	Patent ductus arteriosus
PEEP	Positive end expiratory pressure
PFC	Perfluorochemical
PIE	Pulmonary interstitial emphysema
PIP	Peak inspiratory pressure
pH	Hydrogen ion concentration
PKU	Phenylketonuria
PPHN	Persistent pulmonary hypertension of the newborn
PR	Per rectum
PVH	Periventricular haemorrhage
PVL	Periventricular leucomalacia
RA	Right atrium
RBC	Red blood cell
RE	Reticulo-endothelial
RDS	Respiratory distress syndrome
RFLPS	Refraction fragment length polymorphisms
RGN	Registered General Nurse
RM	Registered Midwife
ROP	Retinopathy of prematurity
RV	Right ventricle
SaO_2	Saturation oxygen level
SCBU	Special care baby unit
SG	Specific gravity
SGA	Small for gestational age
SIDS	Sudden infant death syndrome
SLE	Systemic lupus erythematosus
SVC	Superior vena cava
$TcPO_2$	Transcutaneous oxygen tension
T_e	Expiratory time
T_i	Inspiratory time
TGA	Transposition of great arteries
TOF	Tracheo-oesophageal fistula

TPN	Total parenteral nutrition	UTI	Urinary tract infection
TTN	Transient tachypnoea of the new-born	UVC	Umbilical venous catheter
		VLBW	Very low birth weight
UAC	Umbilical arterial catheter	VSD	Ventricular septal defect
UKCC	United Kingdom Central Council for Nursing, Midwifery and Health Visiting	WBC	White blood count

1 The Evolution of Neonatal Care

LEARNING OUTCOMES

When this chapter has been read and understood the reader should be able to:

- ◯ Compare mortality figures from 1970 to 1990.
- ◯ Discuss the findings of the Short Report 1979.
- ◯ List the steps in the history of neonatal nurse education.
- ◯ Identify the criteria for admission to the neonatal unit.
- ◯ Describe ways to foster family-centred care.

THE HISTORICAL PERSPECTIVE

In the last 35 years hospital provision for sick neonates has grown from a small area tacked on to the maternity ward to a giant, technical, scientifically based system of care.

From 1960 to 1980

During the 20 years from 1960 to 1980 there were only minor changes in neonatal care. There were few facilities or equipment for resuscitation, ventilation, nutrition, or monitoring sick new-born babies. Many babies with, what seem today, minor problems died soon after birth. Those who survived often had serious disabilities from the lack of knowledge of their needs at birth. Paediatricians had little or no training in neonatal medicine and learnt as they went along.

The premature baby unit

Most maternity hospitals had a 'prem' nursery where preterm babies were cared for. A weight of 2.5 kg (5lb 8oz) ensured a baby's admission to the unit regardless of gestation or condition (Vulliamy 1977). Babies who had a difficult instrumental delivery or a Caesarian section were admitted to the unit and the care given was ritualistic rather than researched. The nursing care was carried out by midwives. There was little input from doctors who saw the babies on admission and were subsequently called to the unit by the Sister, if she could not deal with a particular problem.

Milk feeds were given and diluted to half strength if the baby was under 2 kg (4½ lb) (Krollman *et al*. 1994). At one stage it was thought that these diluted feeds were easier for delicate babies to digest, though the benefit of early feeding with full strength milk was being recognised in the late seventies (Vulliamy 1977). Breast feeding was not greatly encouraged as parents were considered an infection risk in the unit. Expressed breast milk was given to some babies but not usually from their own mothers. This came from mothers on the maternity wards who had been persuaded to donate excess milk to 'help' these small babies. The milk was then steam 'sterilised' on the unit in bottles placed in a saucepan of boiling water over a heat ring. Mothers who produced large amounts of breast milk could sell their milk in some districts and this would be collected and pooled into milk banks. It was pasteurised and used to supply local hospitals who had premature or delicate babies in their care.

The dangers of unmonitored oxygen administration were becoming apparent during the 1960s and 1970s. Intravenous feeding was in its early infancy in larger centres in the middle of the 1970s (Vulliamy 1977) but most units were poorly equipped and underfunded. There were few research projects or equipment being developed in this area in the 1960s and 1970s.

High perinatal mortality rates

The perinatal mortality rate went from 33 deaths per 1000 births in 1960, to 25 deaths per 1000 in 1970 (House of Commons Social Services Committee Report 1979). This small improvement highlighted the fact that very little was being done for sick new-born babies at this time. There were to be no major changes until the result of perinatal surveys spurred governmental determination to bring down this mortality rate. There was public concern that babies were dying unnecessarily or suffering permanent damage during the latter part of pregnancy and the earliest part of infancy. The United Kingdom perinatal mortality rate was higher than that of other developed countries. In 1976 there were 18.8 deaths per 1000 births in England and Wales, compared with 12 deaths per 1000 in Sweden (Short Report 1979).

The Short Report

A report was commissioned by the government and in 1978 the Social Services Committee began an inquiry into the causes of perinatal and neonatal mortality. The name of the report was taken from the chairman Mrs Renée Short. This report found that the major causative factors of perinatal and neonatal mortality and handicap were:

- Socio-economic factors such as lack of education, poverty, poor housing, poor nutrition, unplanned pregnancy, smoking and alcohol abuse.
- Medical factors such as lack of antenatal care, low birth weight, asphyxia during delivery or after, congenital malformations, cerebral haemorrhage.

Among the many recommendations of this report were:

- That every region should have one or two referral/regional units equipped and staffed to provide the best possible intensive care for mother, fetus and new-born baby.

- That there should be sub-regional units dealing with problems that could not be dealt with in the delivering hospital.
- That every maternity hospital was to be equipped with the staff and facilities to cope with short term problems with new-born babies.
- That consultant paediatricians dealing with neonates should have had extra training in this speciality.
- That the training of pupil midwives should include greater emphasis on the physiology of fetal and neonatal life to give them further understanding of modern perinatal care.

These recommendations were implemented over the next few years and neonatal units were graded into regional, sub-regional and special care units.

CURRENT STRUCTURE OF NEONATAL CARE

Regional units

Regional units are based in large university hospitals and are equipped to provide care for the smallest and sickest babies. Mothers in premature labour, those who are likely to have a delivery complicated by their health, or that of the baby, should be referred to a maternity unit with a regional neonatal unit. There, they will be delivered and the baby will have expert treatment with the increased likelihood of a favourable outcome (Roper *et al.* 1988). The regional unit will have a consultant who has trained in neonatology, registrars who are specialising in the area and an experienced team of nurses. Nurses from other hospitals

and specialities undertaking relevant courses gain practical experience in these units.

Neonatal surgery is often undertaken in regional units and sometimes also neonatal cardiac surgery. There will be a rescue transport team who collect, stabilise and transfer sick babies safely from other hospitals to the regional one, where this is necessary.

Sub-regional units

Sub-regional units are subsidiary to the regional unit. They are attached to large maternity hospitals and each region should have three to five of them. They are placed at distances that are reasonably accessible to all pregnant women. These units are equipped to give full intensive care to very small and/or sick babies and babies with problems that cannot be dealt with in the district general hospitals. There may not be as many cots as in the regional unit, and there may not be facilities for neonatal surgery.

Special care units

Any hospital that has maternity services should have some emergency provision such as the facility to ventilate a sick baby until transfer to a larger unit is arranged. These units can care for a baby over 35 weeks who may need incubator warmth, phototherapy, or tube feeding.

REDUCING TODAY'S INFANT MORTALITY FIGURES

A report published in 1993, 'The 1993 Strategy to Reduce Infant Mortality', shows that the above measures have been reasonably successful. The Family Health Services

Authority (FHSA), who produced this report, found that the perinatal mortality was 6.5 deaths per 1000. This is still considered higher than acceptable so the report looked at further ways to reduce the figures. The recommendations of the FHSA Report included the following:

- That the effectiveness of health promotion should be reviewed.
- There should be increased application of already known successful interventions to help neonates such as:
  (a) giving antibiotics to mothers before a Caesarian section to reduce mortality and morbidity of the baby;
  (b) giving steroids to mothers before the delivery of a preterm baby to promote lung maturity;
  (c) skilled neonatal resuscitation for all infants who require it.

Health promotion

The emphasis is now on prevention of preterm births and the health of the fetus before delivery. Studies have shown a direct link between the social status of the mother and the health of the baby (Kogan 1995; Lumme *et al*. 1995; Wilcox *et al*. 1995). Low social status is commensurate with preterm labour, small babies and higher infant mortality rate. No one reason has been isolated and a number of factors have to be looked at to find out how these mothers can be helped. These factors encompass poverty, education, health promotion, and the education of midwifery staff.

Poverty

Those of low social status are often trapped in a cycle of poverty resulting in unemployment, poor housing, poor nutrition, little education,

and stress. Many of these mothers smoke heavily or may abuse alcohol or drugs. All these are known factors for preterm birth and high neonatal morbidity (Wilcox *et al*. 1995).

A high proportion are single mothers with little or no support except from the state. For many single mothers on social security benefits adequate nutrition is an unaffordable luxury (Davies 1995). A survey was taken in 1995 by NCH Action For Children based on impoverished families who used their family centres (NCH Action For Children 1995). It was found that two-thirds of babies born to such mothers had birth weight below the national average. Some 11% of babies are born to mothers under 20, who are the most likely to be on low income (Wynn 1995). Public resentment against hand-outs from public funds, which appear to reward and encourage girls to be single mothers, has led to governmental reductions in social benefits. This is seen, by some, as a welcome attempt to discourage young women without support from getting pregnant, but does not help those already in the situation.

Education of mothers

It has been found that increasing a mother's knowledge does not automatically lead to changes in attitudes, behaviour or diet (Anderson *et al*. 1995). A woman's pattern of life is influenced by social circumstances, class and educational level. This may mean that particular groups need different methods of advice and help from those currently given.

Smoking increases the risk of neonatal death. In a survey taken in Wales in 1992 it was found that the incidence of smoking in mothers whose babies died was 40% compared with the overall smoking rate of 30% in women of childbearing age (Cartlidge & Stewart 1996). This is an area that has been frequently targeted in attempts to eradicate smoking during pregnancy. As smoking and diet can have varying effects on pregnancy, advice given can appear contradictory. It has been found for instance that thin young women who smoke give birth to growth restricted preterm babies, and older obese multiparous mothers who smoke tend to deliver large babies who have a high morbidity rate (Lumme *et al.* 1995).

Trials of folate supplementation showed a 75% reduction in the incidence of neural tube defects among women considered at risk (Murphy *et al.* 1996). There is currently a campaign by the Department of Health Education to educate healthcare professionals, women and older school girls about the importance of folate supplementation before and during early pregnancy (Appendix 1). There has been media publicity about the dangers of eating soft cheeses and pâtés during pregnancy. These may contain bacteria that could be harmful to the baby and mothers need advice about these current anxieties.

Education of midwives

The knowledge of midwives, who are the main providers of health promotion to mothers, may need to be reviewed. A study looking at midwives' knowledge and education in nutrition during pregnancy found a lack of confidence among them about nutritional matters (Mulliner *et al.* 1995). This seems to be an area where improvements can be made. Midwives can be instrumental in communicating health promotion to families but they need up-to-date knowledge and the ability to give relevant advice (Anderson *et al.* 1995).

The United Kingdom Central Council for Nursing Midwifery and Health Visiting (UKCC) have issued several statements with policies for improved practice. Following these guidelines will ensure that all registered staff, continuously update knowledge and techniques to give good research-based care to their patients.

Known factors which help neonates

Midwives can ensure that mothers in premature labour are given antibiotics and steroids to lessen the effects of infection and respiratory distress in the baby (Crowley *et al.* 1990; Lewis & Mercer 1995). Resuscitation of the new-born must be swiftly and efficiently carried out by experienced doctors.

Recent mortality figures

In 1993 a change in the stillbirth definition caused an increase, on paper, of neonatal mortality figures. This was because babies that die between 24 and 27 weeks gestation now have to be registered as stillbirths rather than abortions. This put the mortality figures up to 8.5 per 1000 in 1993. In spite of this a survey in Wales in 1994 showed that infant mortality had dropped to 6.2 per 1000 births and that this was largely due to improvements in perinatal care and a reduced incidence of cot deaths (Cartlidge & Stewart 1996).

NEONATAL CARE TODAY

Neonatal units (NNUs) are now highly technical places alive with the noise of ventilators, monitors and equipment. Advances in technology are such that babies, who would have died a few years ago, are now surviving. The cost of this to the babies and their families is the lengthy period of hospitalisation that may be needed. Regional units can be as far as 100 miles from the homes of some parents. Sub-regional units too are often some distance away. This is an extra burden for parents already distressed by their baby's condition. The advantages of having the expertise in these centres are confirmed by the reduction of perinatal deaths, but the toll on family life is yet to be measured.

Transitional units

As neonatal units provide more care for the babies, midwives may become less expert at providing care for minor problems that could be treated without separating mother and baby. Klaus and Kennell wrote about maternal infant bonding in 1976, highlighting the emotional damage caused to parents by the separation. To minimise this problem, babies should be admitted to the neonatal unit only if the care they need cannot be given by the midwives on the postnatal ward. Some postnatal wards have better facilities and staff for caring for babies than others but ideally all postnatal wards should have enough staff who are suitably trained to care for these babies. Taking the baby to a neonatal unit immediately disempowers the parents. They see their parental roles assumed by the neonatal staff (Graham 1995) and may take time to recover their confidence to become primary carers.

Babies with conditions that could be cared for on postnatal wards include:

- Those needing blood glucose monitoring.
- Cold babies who can be warmly dressed and nursed in incubators, if necessary.
- Babies with cleft lip and palate, who can be seen by the dental team on the ward; this allows parents to manage the prosthetic plate at an early stage.
- Jaundiced babies who need phototherapy can be nursed on the postnatal ward.

- Any baby with a congenital abnormality that does not need immediate treatment or assessment in the neonatal period can stay on the postnatal ward.

Neonatal intensive care units (NICUs)

Most patients in the neonatal unit fall into the following categories:

- Preterm babies from 23 to 26 weeks gestation and small for gestational age babies.
- Babies with birth weight of less than 1.8 kg (4 lb).
- Any ill baby whatever gestational age.
- Babies needing emergency surgery for tracheo-oesophageal atresia, diaphragmatic hernia, intestinal obstruction, urethral valve obstruction.
- Babies with congenital abnormalities needing assessment and/or treatment in the neonatal period.
- Babies who have birth asphyxia, meconium aspiration, pneumonia or who have had severe fetal distress during labour.

Ethical considerations

The advent of technology has meant the saving of more babies' lives. It has also meant the saving of immature infants at the limits of accepted viability. Babies from 23 weeks gestational age are now being cared for in many units and often need prolonged hospitalisation. A significant proportion of extra-low birth weight (ELBW) babies have a poor outcome (Table 1.1).

The impact of very immature infants on neonatal services in the UK was examined using data from 1991 to 1993 in the Trent Health Region (Bohin *et al.* 1996). It was found that most infants of 24 weeks and under died within 48 hours, and consumed 2.14% of the

Table 1.1 Survival figures for extra-low birth weight neonates (Roberton 1993).

Birth weight (g)	Survival range* (%)
500–599	10–40
600–699	15–50
700–799	50–75

*The lower values are from national data and the higher values are from the results in a level three neonatal intensive care unit (Reprinted with kind permission of the BMJ Publishing Group.)

total ventilator days for the region. It concluded that, although each baby is considered individually and treatment should be given to all babies regardless of gestation, there was a general trend for operating a conservative policy towards infants born before 24 weeks gestation. Suggestions that neonatal intensive care should be given on the basis of gestational age or birth weight (Allen *et al.* 1993) could mean that babies of 25 weeks and over with a 50% chance of survival are aggressively treated, those with a gestational age of 22 weeks have no intervention and treatment of babies of 23 to 24 weeks gestation is discretionary.

Legally stillbirths must be registered at 24 weeks and above. A baby born at or beyond that time is capable of being born alive and surviving, however small, so the obligation for treatment is no different from that of a baby born at term.

Over 50% of babies now survive at weights of 700–800 g (1 lb 9 oz to 1 lb 12 oz) and just over 30% survive with weights of 600–699 g. Roberton (1993) found that 10% of sick babies had a significant handicap and that this figure had not increased, in spite of the numbers of low birth weight babies currently being saved, proving the efficacy of current neonatal care. Although the figure of 10% morbidity has remained constant, the improved survival of small babies has resulted in an increased number (but not percentage) of handicapped children. Although many of these babies are not 'handicapped' in the normal sense, studies have shown that very low birth weight babies have persistent growth problems which give them a smaller head circumference in comparison to their height than normal weight children. This may be associated with the poorer educational and cognitive outcomes of this group (McCarton *et al.* 1996; Powls *et al.* 1996).

Economic factors in saving very small babies

Neonatal intensive care is expensive and the issue of cost effectiveness emotive. When treatment results in healthy normal children there is no problem but treatment of very small babies may continue for weeks before being resolved or abandoned. Often the survivors are left with residual handicaps that will continue to burden the health authority and taxpayer. In the United Kingdom the current cost of running one cot in a neonatal intensive care unit is £1000 a day (Bohin *et al.* 1996). If the treatment improves long term survival then it is justified. But if it just puts off the mean age of death or results in a high incidence of morbidity then it does not mean that the money has been well spent (Williams 1993). The expertise and finance needed use valuable resources that could be used for babies who have a better prognosis. Care in the neonatal unit should not be affected by economics, but just because the technology is there does not mean it always has to be used.

STAFFING ON NEONATAL UNITS

The care for each baby in the neonatal unit has become more detailed and complicated. In

1992, a working group of the British Association of Perinatal Medicine and the Neonatal Nurses Association made recommendations for staffing the units. They recommended that for an intensive care bed, 5.5 whole time equivalent nurses were needed, for a high dependency cot 3.5 whole time equivalents, and for a special care cot one whole time equivalent. This is the ideal but in most hospitals it is not the case. A report in 1993 commissioned by the Department of Health found that in most units there was a discrepancy between establishment operation and that recommended (Redshaw *et al.* 1996). This means that nurse staffing levels in many units do not meet the standard required.

Education of the neonatal nurse

Improvements in prenatal diagnosis, fetal medicine, genetics and technological monitoring mean that the neonatal nurse is now caring for babies with diseases that could not have been actively treated in the recent past. This has created incentives to learn more skills, acquire in-depth theoretical knowledge and to base practice on researched evidence. This has led to nurses becoming more aware of their accountability, professional liability and duty of care and has been the impetus for the development of specialist educational programmes.

The need for professional awareness and understanding is essential in all nursing roles and the UKCC has laid down specific guidelines for this purpose (UKCC 1996) making each nurse accountable for their own practice.

Nurses working in neonatal units are required to have a professional qualification in the speciality. The educational establishments linked to regional and sub-regional units, produce and run courses to advance knowledge and skills. The neonatal units provide the students of such courses with clinical experience and expert supervision.

Some experienced nurses, after suitable training, become advanced nurse practitioners enabling them to assume a leading role in the clinical care of the sick neonate. This role is medically orientated and encompasses such tasks as attending deliveries, intubation, insertion of intravenous lines, lumbar puncture and other activities usually performed by senior house officers (Dillon & George 1997). Advanced nurse practitioners use their nursing experience and skills to provide optimum care to the baby and the family.

The neonatal team

On regional units the medical staff comprises one or two consultants trained in neonatology, with senior and junior registrars. These will be attended by house doctors, the number depending on the size of the unit. Neonatal medicine requires a multidisciplinary team approach which will involve many other specialities and services.

FAMILY-CENTRED CARE

The improvements in technology and mortality rates on neonatal units are not the only changes in neonatal care. There has been a significant change in the way families are involved. The days are gone when parents were allowed to visit at set hours and given little information on care or treatment. Psychological studies have proved the benefits of giving parents information, access and above all acceptance into the units (Klaus & Kennell 1976; Harvey 1987; Farrell & Frost 1992). The birth of a sick baby is a major upheaval for the parents. They have to come to terms with the loss of their dreams and expectations for their baby and face the reality of the NICU. They go through a variety of emotions akin to grieving as they come to terms with having a sick baby (Jupp 1992).

Before birth

Family care should start when the mother is in preterm labour or has a baby that is likely to need care on the neonatal unit. A neonatal nurse should visit the parents, forming a link with the unit, giving written information if available and helping to relieve some of their anxiety. If appropriate and the attending midwife agrees, the parents can be shown the neonatal unit. Most parents worry that their baby will be too small to survive and they often adopt a more positive outlook after seeing the unit. Many mothers in early labour will not have seen the neonatal unit as part of their antenatal induction. This could be a reason to show antenatal classes round the unit earlier in pregnancy, so that parents will have at least an idea of what can be done for their baby.

Admission of the baby

When parents first visit their baby they may be disorientated by the equipment, monitors and bleeping alarms. The stress of having a sick baby can mean that their normal reactions are blunted so that any information and explanations given at this stage need to be simplified and may need to be repeated. A nurse should be present during interviews with medical staff to facilitate further discussion later with parents. Good communications from medical and nursing staff, with consistent explanations, help to ensure and acknowledge parents' contribution to their baby's care.

Parents' problems

Parents may have problems with accommodation, finance, with each other and with the rest of their family members. Open communication is encouraged so that appropriate help can be offered. Many of the families in the neonatal unit come from the lower socio-economic groups and as such, often lack the resources, emotionally, educationally and financially to cope with their sick/small baby. Social workers can be used to help and these may know the family, thus providing a link. Many units have a family counsellor who will have had training in assisting with emotional problems.

When parents produce a small baby who needs care on the neonatal unit they lose the role as primary carers that they expected to have. Empowerment for this role should begin as soon as possible with involvement in the baby's treatment and daily physical care. Parents must be kept up to date and have daily access to medical staff if they wish. Every effort must be made to ensure that they play an important role in the care and recovery of their baby.

Making the family welcome

There has been much emphasis in recent years on trying to make the neonatal environment less stressful for babies and their families (Horsley 1988). Creating a home-like environment in which to nurse the sick neonate and support the family seems almost a contradiction: on the one hand a technically sophisticated special unit, staffed by nursing and medical personnel who by the very nature of their work are under stress; on the other, attempts to relieve parental anxiety through the creation of a welcoming environment. The layout of most neonatal units is not conducive to a privacy that helps parents relax with their baby. The aim is to make the unit less like a sterile hospital environment and appear a more welcoming place. In the intensive area this is difficult to achieve but even here toys and colourful curtains can make it less forbidding.

In the nursery areas colour schemes with nursery pictures improve the design. Nursery furniture and comfortable chairs will help parents appreciate that efforts are being made for their comfort. The use of attractive curtains, bedding and the use of baby clothes also helps to create a more home-like environment.

A parents' sitting room with facilities for making refreshments and a play area for siblings should be provided. Siblings need to be included in the parents' experience of the neonatal unit. They are an important part of the baby's family and having them in the unit helps the parents to see the family as a whole. But attention to the unit design is not all that is needed. It is not the colour of the wallpaper or the comfort of armchairs, so much as the fostering of an accepting atmosphere in which the family can work together with the staff toward a common purpose – the discharge home of a well baby.

Access for the family

In the 1960s parents could visit at strictly adhered-to times and even then were not allowed to touch their babies. The mother was given no opportunity to care for the baby during the hospital stay. If she was a first time mother, no help was given to feed or get to know her baby. She had no idea of the baby's habits, likes or dislikes, or temperament. Nowadays nurses are aware of the problems of separation and can do much to help. Photographs of the baby should be taken on admission and given to the parents. Booklets

are helpful, giving details of the unit facilities and explaining some of the equipment. Ideally parents should be allowed to stay with their sick baby and be accommodated near the neonatal unit. Free visiting helps the family get to know the baby. As early as 1959 the Platt report recommended this and most units have now implemented it.

Siblings

Quite drastic adjustments have to be made by a child whose mother delivers a healthy term baby with all the attendant excitement and attention. If the new baby is small or sick the effects upon the siblings may cause long standing problems from the anxiety and stress in the family (Burton 1975). Allowing siblings to visit and making them feel welcome on the unit will relieve some of their anxiety about the situation (Redshaw *et al.* 1985). Parents will be able to visit more often if their children come with them, not having the worry of finding a childminder. Siblings will not feel left out and can be involved in and watch the baby's progress. When the baby finally goes home they can join in the pleasure of their parents.

The extended family

The extended family can be important and excellent providers of support to the family. Grandparents are often involved with the practical care of older children and feel a close link with the parents. When the baby is well enough it is natural that grandparents should want to touch and cuddle if the parents so wish. This may cause a problem to the unit staff who may want to protect the baby from what they see as overhandling. A single mother may have a brother or close friend who will support her on going home. This special relationship should be encouraged by staff.

Conclusion

Many neonatal units employ a family care sister who is trained in psychological support. She will contact parents on the unit and keep a link with them during their stay. Often the link is kept after discharge, especially if the baby dies and bereavement counselling is needed.

It is up to the staff, nurses in particular, to make sure that these units are as welcoming as they can be. A family system of care is the ideal which should be aimed at for all units.

REFERENCES

Allen M, Donohue P, Dusman A. (1993) The limit of viability: neonatal outcome of infants born at 22–25 weeks gestation. *New England Journal of Medicine*, **329**, 1597–1601.

Anderson AS, Campbell DM, Shepherd R. (1995) The influence of dietary advice on nutrient intake during pregnancy. *British Journal of Nutrition*, **73** (2), 163–177.

Bohin S, Draper E, Field D. (1996) Impact of extremely immature infants in neonatal services. *Archives of Disease in Childhood, Fetal and Neonatal Edition*, **74**, 10–17.

Burton J. (1975) *The Family Life of Sick Children.* Routledge and Kegan Paul, London, Boston.

Cartlidge PHT, Stewart J. (1996) All Wales perinatal survey and confidential enquiry into stillbirths and deaths in infancy. *Journal of Neonatal Nursing*, **2** (2), 14–17.

Crowley P, Chalmers I, Keirse MJN. (1990) The effects of corticosteroid administration before pre-term delivery. An overview of evidence from controlled trials. *British Journal of Obstetrics and Gynaecology*, **97** (1), 11–25.

Davies RW. (1995) Hungry fears. *Nursing Times* 91 (48), 20–21.

Dillon A, George S. (1997) Advanced Neonatal Nurse Practitioners in the United Kingdom: Where are they and what do they do. *Journal of Advanced Nursing*, **25**, 257–264.

Family Health Services Authority (1993) *Strategy to Reduce Infant Mortality.* South East London Health Authority.

Farrell M, Frost C. (1992) The most important needs of parents of critically ill children – A parent's perception. *Intensive and Critical Care Nursing*, **8**, 130–139.

Graham S. (1995) Psychological needs of families with babies in the neonatal unit. *Journal of Neonatal Nursing* **1** (5), 15–18.

Harvey D. (1987) *Parent Infant Relationships.* John Wiley, Chichester.

Horsley A. (1988) The neonatal environment. *Paediatric Nursing*, February, 17–19.

House of Commons Social Services Committee (1979–1980) *Perinatal and Neonatal Mortality.* (The Short Report) HMSO, London.

Jupp S. (1992) *Making the Right Start.* Opened Eye Publications, Hyde, Cheshire.

Klaus MH, Kennell JH. (1976) *Maternal Infant Bonding.* Mosby, St Louis.

Kogan MD. (1995) Social causes of low birth weight. *Journal of the Royal Society of Medicine*, **88** (11), 611–615.

Krollman B, Brock DA, Nader PM, Neiheisel PW, Wissman CS. (1994) Neonatal transformation: 30 years. *Neonatal Network*, **13** (6), 17–20.

Lewis R, Mercer B. (1995) Adjunctive care of preterm labour – the use of antibiotics. *Clinical Obstetrics and Gynaecology*, **38** (4), 755–770.

Lumme R, Rantakallio P, Hartikainen AL *et al.* (1995) Pregnancy weight in relation to pregnancy outcome. *Journal of Obstetrics and Gynaecology*, **15** (2), 65–75.

McCarton CM, Wallace IF, Divon M, Vaughan HG. (1996) Cognitive and neurologic development of the premature, small for gestational age infant through age 6. *Pediatrics*, **98** (6), 1167–1177.

Mulliner CM, Spiby H, Fraser RB. (1995) A study exploring midwives education in, knowledge of and attitudes to nutrition in pregnancy. *Midwifery*, **11** (1), 37–41.

Murphy M, Seagroatt V, Hey K, *et al.* (1996) Neural tube defects 1974–1994 – down but not out. *Archives of Disease in Childhood, Fetal and Neonatal Edition*, **75**, 133–134.

NCH Action For Children. (1995) Poor Expectations: Poverty and Undernourishment in Pregnancy. NCH Action For Children, London.

Platt H. (1959) *Report on the Committee of the Welfare of Children in Hospital.* HMSO, London.

Powls A, Botting N, Cooke R, Piling D, Marlow N. (1996) Growth impairment in very low birth weight children at 12 years. *Archives of Disease in Childhood, Fetal and Neonatal Edition*, **75**, 152–156.

Redshaw M, Rivers R, Rosenblatt D. (1985) *Born Too Early.* Oxford University Press, Oxford.

Redshaw ME, Harris A, Ingram JC. (1996) *Delivering Neonatal Care. A Survey of Neonatal Nursing Commissioned by the Department of Health.* HMSO London.

Roberton NCR. (1993) Should we look after babies less than 800 gms? *Archives of Disease in Childhood,* **68**, 326–329.

Roper LP, Chiswick MI, Sims DG. (1988) Referrals to a regional neonatal unit. *Archives of Disease in Childhood,* **63**, 403–407.

UKCC (1996) *Guidelines For Professional Practice.* United Kingdom Central Council for Midwifery and Health Visiting, London.

Vulliamy DG (1977) *The Newborn Child.* Fourth Edition. Churchill Livingstone, Edinburgh.

Wilcox MA, Smith SJ, Johnson IR, *et al.* (1995) The effect of social deprivation on birthweight excluding physiological and pathological effects. *British Journal of Obstetrics and Gynaecology*, **102** (11), 918–924.

Williams L. (1993) Is the money well spent? *Child Health*, **3** (2), 68–72.

Wynn M. (1995) Has there ever been a better time to have a baby? *Modern Midwife* **5** (2), 37–38.

2 | Preterm Labour and the Birth of a Small Baby

LEARNING OUTCOMES

When this chapter has been read and understood the reader should be able to:

○ Discuss the causes of preterm delivery.
○ List the interventions in preterm labour to improve outcome.
○ Compare characteristics of preterm baby and small for gestational age baby.
○ Identify measures to prevent hypothermia/hypoxaemia at birth.
○ Discuss ways to support parents of a small/sick baby.
○ Describe the steps taken to stabilise a sick baby for transfer.

THE LOW BIRTHWEIGHT BABY

Neonatal research, which has made advances in ventilation, nutrition, haematology and psychosocial outcomes, continues to develop as more very low birth weight babies are born. In spite of such improvements low birth weight is a major factor in death in the first year of life, a figure of 20 times greater than infants with a normal birth weight was quoted in Cartlidge & Stewart 1996. The residual handicap figure for survivors remains at 10% (Roberton 1993a).

In 1991 the percentage of very low birth weight (VLBW) infants with weights less than 1500 g (3 lb 5 oz) was the highest since 1965 (Lewis & Mercer 1995). One of the reasons for this is the advances in antenatal care, such as the use of prenatal scanning and blood test screening. These have enabled doctors and parents to make decisions about early delivery if the baby is not growing adequately or has a life-threatening disorder (Proud 1994). Obstetricians are increasingly aware of the skills of neonatology and many now electively deliver preterm babies who would otherwise have died *in utero* or been stillborn. Medical, nursing and technical expertise in the care of these babies has ensured an increasing survival rate. Figures for neonatal survival per 1000 live births in England and Wales showed, in one study quoted by Roberton 1993a, figures for birth weights of 500–599 g (1 lb 2 oz to 1 lb 5 oz) had improved from 78 per 1000 in 1983 to 215 in 1989.

Causes of low birth weight

There are a number of reasons why a baby is born with low birth weight.

Preterm labour

There are thought to be many causes for preterm labour – infection, stress, multiple fetuses, placental ischaemia, haemorrhage (Lockwood 1995). In spite of extensive research there is to date, no reliable way of finding out which mothers will be affected or which known causative factor will precipitate the labour.

Preterm delivery

Preterm delivery is described as before 37 weeks. A survey in the USA found 8–10% of births came under this heading (Lockwood 1995). It is seen as a leading cause of neonatal morbidity and mortality, 85% of neonatal deaths are caused by preterm delivery (Fleming *et al.* 1991). Preterm delivery may occur spontaneously or may follow premature rupture of membranes or medical induction for maternal complications.

Premature rupture of membranes

The amniotic sac which holds the fetus, placenta and amniotic fluid normally ruptures during labour or delivery and helps precipitate the baby into the birth canal. If rupture happens more than 24 hours before the birth the fetus is at risk of infection from bacteria entering the uterus through the vagina. It is not known why membranes rupture prematurely but usually this precipitates labour or may cause a maternal infection that will lead to preterm labour (Lewis & Mercer 1995).

Maternal factors

Eclampsia is the occurrence of a seizure associated with pre-eclampsia, a condition that causes high blood pressure and renal problems during pregnancy. Treatment is aimed at reducing the mother's blood pressure to a safe level so that the pregnancy can continue. Eclampsia remains a major cause of maternal mortality from thrombosis and renal failure and emergency Caesarian section is often essential.

Placental abruption occurs when the placenta starts to separate from the uterine wall. It results in sudden disastrous bleeding which can only be stemmed by immediate Caesarian section whatever the gestation of the fetus. A serious accident to the mother may mean the baby has to be delivered urgently to save both lives. The pregnancy in a mother with cervical incompetence can be safeguarded by suturing the os and then removing the suture after the 37th week of gestation to allow normal labour and delivery. Mothers carrying more than one fetus are likely to deliver early, as are diabetic mothers, because of uterine over-distension.

It is a well known fact that women in the lower socio-economic band are more likely to go into preterm labour (Wilcox *et al.* 1995). Factors such as smoking, drug or alcohol abuse, educational and economic deprivation and stress are known causes of low birth weight and preterm labour. The causative factor may be one or a combination of these problems and research so far has concentrated on antenatal help and maternal health education (Kogan 1995; Lumme *et al.* 1995; Wilcox *et al.* 1995).

Fetal complications

Poor fetal growth may indicate placental failure and without intervention the baby may die. Elective Caesarian section may be carried out when the baby reaches a viable age. Babies with congenital malformations such as exomphalos or gastroschisis need to be delivered between 34 and 36 weeks to prevent further damage to their intestines. Babies who have severe haemolytic diseases are often delivered early to prevent fatal complications.

CARE OF A WOMAN IN PRETERM LABOUR

A woman with a history of preterm birth will be carefully monitored during her pregnancy. If she shows signs of preterm labour she will be admitted to hospital for observation and treatment. Any pregnant woman of 35 weeks gestation or less, having abdominal pain, rupture of membranes, contractions, blood loss will be treated for preterm labour.

The mother in suspected preterm labour will be scanned so that a decision can be made about whether to suppress the labour or not. If the fetus is at least 2.2 kg (4 lb 14 oz) it is usual to let the labour proceed (Proud 1994). If the baby is very small the mother will be transferred, if necessary, for delivery at a hospital with a neonatal intensive care unit. The risks associated with the transfer of a sick baby can then be avoided.

If the gestation is under 23 weeks every effort will be made to delay the birth as survival rate improves by 2% a day at this stage (Rennie 1996). Betamimetics, such as ritodrine, calm uterine action and are commonly used to arrest premature labour (CPLG 1992). Prostaglandin synthetase inhibitors, such as indomethacin, which delay the delivery, have given rise to conflicting reports on fetal and neonatal safety (Gordon & Samuels 1995). There has been an increased incidence of babies developing necrotising enterocolitis, intracranial haemorrhage or patent ductus arteriosus in the neonatal period.

Antibiotics

The administration of antibiotics to the mother to eliminate infection after rupture of membranes can prevent ascending infection from vaginal flora and possibly prevent the development of preterm labour (Lewis & Mercer 1995). At the time of writing, Oracle (Overview of the Role of Antibiotics in Curtailing Labour and Early delivery) is ending a 3-year trial to determine if the antibiotic treatment of all women in preterm labour, or with premature rupture of membranes, reduces neonatal mortality and morbidity due to preterm birth (Kenyon 1995).

Steroids

Corticosteroids given to the mother before a preterm delivery have improved the morbidity and survival rate for babies. Corticosteroids encourage maturation of fetal lungs and production of surfactant, reducing the severity of respiratory distress syndrome. They have also been found to reduce the risk of intraventricular haemorrhage, necrotising enterocolitis and neonatal death. All preterm labour should be delayed by 24–48 hours if possible to allow the baby maximum benefit from the steroids. The risks of infection to the fetus may be increased if the steroids are given after prolonged rupture of membranes (Crowley *et al.* 1990).

Viability

In 1990 the Human Fertilisation and Embryology Act stated that beyond the 24th week of pregnancy a baby is capable of surviving (Roberton 1993a). Viable gestational age is by law considered to be 24 weeks and over, whatever the baby's weight.

Psychologically it is important to give the mother realistic expectations as to the outcome of preterm labour. If she is likely to deliver at 23–26 weeks gestation, she and her partner should be aware that there may be a poor outcome. There are arguments that intensive care should be an optional choice for parents of babies born at 23–24 weeks (Rennie 1996). Ideally, at this gestation, a senior neonatologist should discuss the parents' wishes beforehand and formulate a plan with them and the delivering midwife, about intensive treatment of their baby.

This type of counselling has to be carried out with great care as difficult choices are involved on both sides. Current knowledge permits only assessment of prognosis and is insufficient to deny all babies at this gestation access to intensive care. The delivery plan should allow for changes if the baby is larger than expected and vigorous at birth. Any decision made at this point should consider the baby's future. If there is the likelihood of severe handicaps resulting in a poor quality of life then aggressive resuscitation measures should not be pursued.

Gestational age

Gestational age can be calculated by ultrasound scanning. Parameters of the baby's skull and femur are measured and compared. The age in days as well as size and weight can be accurately forecast (Proud 1994). Scanning can also determine whether the baby is the correct size for gestational age, growth restricted, or larger than expected. This may influence antenatal treatment and the decision as to when delivery will take place. Low birth weight (LBW) babies are less than 2.5 kg (5 lb 8 oz) at birth. Very low birth weight (VLBW) is less than 1.5 kg (3 lb 5 oz) and extremely low birth weight (ELBW) is under 1 kg (2 lb 3 oz).

Preterm babies

A preterm baby may be the expected weight for gestational age but it has been found that many mothers who go into spontaneous preterm labour deliver babies with significant fetal growth restriction. The reasons for this are not clear (Hediger *et al.* 1995). Preterm babies are often born before lungs, brain, eyes, skin, digestive, muscular, skeletal, nervous and immune systems are fully mature. They will look very different from full term or even growth restricted babies (Table 2.1).

Growth restricted babies

These babies can be termed growth retarded or small for gestational age. These types of growth restriction are sometimes referred to as asymmetrical and symmetrical.

Asymmetrical babies have a normal size head and brain for the gestational age but the abdominal circumference is small in comparison. These are growth retarded babies with depleted fat and glycogen stores. The brain has received sufficient nutrients and these babies usually make up their growth in the first year or two.

The small for gestational age baby is symmetrically small from insufficient nutrition which affects the brain and other organs. The fetus is small from the first scan. This is a more serious condition and can be associated with

Table 2.1 Physiological differences between the preterm baby and the growth restricted one.

Characteristic	Preterm baby	Growth restricted
Vernix	Copious	Little or more
Skin	Red and shiny	Dry and baggy
Face	Smooth, doll-like	Wizened, mature
Abdomen	Protruding	Flat
Posture	Hypotonic	Active
Skull	Soft, bones movable	Firmer
Cord	Thick and fleshy	Thin
Cry	Feeble	Normal

chromosomal abnormalities and delayed developmental outcome (Proud 1994).

The growth restricted baby has been deprived of nutrients in the uterus from poor placental supplies though the causes are not always clear. It is known that maternal health and habits such as smoking contribute and that poorly nourished mothers are liable to produce small babies. Sometimes mothers who have given birth to well nourished babies in the past may have a growth restricted baby with no apparent cause.

Although the growth restricted baby may be very small and sometimes weigh under 1 kg (2 lb 3 oz), the physiology will be different from that of a preterm baby the same weight, but of earlier gestation. All systems will be more mature and there is less likelihood of developing respiratory distress syndrome (Table 2.1). At birth the growth restricted baby may develop hypoglycaemia as nutritional reserves will have been used surviving *in utero*.

Babies who weigh more than expected

Heavy-for-dates babies weigh more than expected for their gestational age due to an over-rich supply of nutrients from the placenta. A baby weighing 4000 g (8 lb 13 oz) or over will be in this category. The mothers of these large babies are often diabetic or develop diabetic symptoms while they are pregnant. The extra glucose goes to the baby through the placenta allowing excessive growth.

The baby may have a difficult delivery because of size. There may be shoulder dystocia, where the shoulder gets jammed in the vaginal entrance. This may cause injury to the baby's shoulder, neck and facial nerve. Lacerations to the mother's vagina and perineum may occur in the attempt to deliver. Uterine over-distension from such a large baby increases the risk of preterm labour and delivery so that these babies may suffer from respiratory diseases and other problems that beset small preterm infants.

Babies of diabetic mothers are prone to congenital problems such as cardiomyopathy, a thickening of the heart muscle, hypoglycaemia and polycythaemia. Hypoglycaemia is a common problem in the first hours/days after birth because the blood sugar levels plummet without the generous supply of glucose from the placenta. Polycythaemia is caused by red blood cell overproduction. This makes the blood thick and the flow sluggish and may cause thrombolytic emboli. A plasma dilution exchange may be needed to dilute the blood.

LABOUR AND DELIVERY OF A MOTHER WITH A PRETERM BABY

The neonatal unit will be alerted when any woman with a pregnancy of 35 weeks or less is admitted to the labour ward. If possible the member of the neonatal unit staff who is taking the admission will meet the parents to provide a link with the unit for them. They may want to come and see the unit if the labour has not progressed too far, or if it is a planned induction or Caesarian section.

Parents are very anxious at the thought of having a preterm baby and worry about the survival. When they visit the unit, seeing the babies, equipment and the incubator that their baby may occupy helps them prepare psychologically (Graham 1995). There may be photos of babies who have graduated from the unit that they can see.

Type of delivery

The route of delivery depends on the reason for the preterm labour and the health of the fetus. If the fetal heart rate is steady at 120 or above, beats per minute, and blood gas is within normal limits (see Appendix 2) then the mother can deliver vaginally. Elective or non-emergency Caesarian deliveries are often performed using epidural analgesia as this is considered safer than using a general anaesthetic. The maternal and perinatal morbidity associated with Caesarian section is higher than for normal delivery.

Emergency Caesarian section

Emergency operations may be carried out when the mother or baby have a sudden deterioration or when complications occur during labour. The causes include:

- Placental abruption.
- Antepartum haemorrhage.
- Cord prolapse in the first stage of labour.
- Mother having or threatening an eclamptic convulsion.
- Fetal distress.
- Deep transverse arrest during labour when the baby gets 'stuck' in a sideways position.

Planned Caesarian section

A planned Caesarian section is carried out because of a number of problems that make vaginal delivery unsafe. A Caesarian section is usually carried out at 38–40 weeks gestation before the mother goes into labour. The causes may include:

- Poor fetal growth.
- Falling placental oestriol levels measured from blood tests.
- Breech presentation.
- Mother's pelvic insufficiency.
- Fetal malformation, such as hydrocephalus.
- With multiple fetuses such as quads, mother and babies are closely monitored by scan and a Caesarian section is carried out after a joint decision by the obstetrician and neonatologist.

Inductions

Mothers with preterm babies may have labour induced if the baby has a condition that could worsen with the continuance of pregnancy.

Delivery

A paediatrician and a neonatal nurse attend deliveries of all preterm babies. Rooms used to deliver a preterm mother should be pre-warmed to 30–32°C to prevent cooling of the baby during delivery and resuscitation.

Neonatal equipment needed in labour ward

Equipment for the resuscitation of the baby should be gathered and checked by the neonatal nurse attending the delivery. Neonatal equipment for a preterm/sick baby's delivery should include:

- Endotracheal tubes cut to the estimated size.
- Means for securing tubes – holders, hat, ribbons, tape.
- Endotracheal introducers.
- Laryngoscope with small blade.
- Bag and mask for resuscitation, attached to oxygen.
- Suction and oxygen checked, connected and switched on.
- Overhead heater switched on at the Resuscitaire.
- Warm towels on the Resuscitaire.
- Portable incubator heated to 35–36°C with a ventilator facility should be nearby, plugged in to save the battery.

The Apgar scoring system is used on every baby to assess the condition of the baby at birth. The top score is ten and the baby is assessed at 1 min, 5 min and 10 min of age. Although this system has been in use since 1953 it is still useful as a record of the condition at birth. There have been attempts to improve on these assessments at birth as resuscitation techniques have changed since it was first introduced but so far there have been no viable alternatives (Marlow 1992).

The time of birth will be noted and the clock started. Apgar scores are assessed and recorded in the notes. The baby will be wrapped in a warm towel and taken by the paediatrician to the Resuscitaire. Oral suction and oxygen are given if necessary and when respiration is established the baby will be briefly examined for defects. The presence of a major defect should not influence the resuscitation of the baby. No decision can be made about the treatment of the baby until a full medical assessment is made.

Establishment of respiration

It will be necessary to pass an endotracheal tube immediately if the baby is making poor or no respiratory efforts after oral suction and hand bagging has been unsuccessful. Failure to establish adequate oxygenation during the first few minutes of life can result in hypoxia, which damages vital organs such as the brain, nervous system, gut and lungs. The longer the hypoxia lasts the more severe the insult to the baby's organs and the higher the risk of adverse neurological effects. Once the endotracheal tube is passed and secured the baby should either be 'bagged' continuously or linked up to the ventilator in the transport incubator.

Babies under 1 kg (2 lb 3 oz) in weight and under 26 weeks gestation may be electively intubated to prevent exhaustion from efforts needed to maintain respiration. Future treatment will depend on blood gas and monitoring assessment on the neonatal unit.

Warmth

In utero the baby has been dependent on the maternal environment to maintain body heat, so he or she has a poor self-regulating temperature control at birth. Body temperature can drop 4.5°C in the first minute after birth if immediate attention is not given to prevention of heat loss (Thomas 1994). Cold stress causes worsening of any respiratory problems by slowing surfactant production and if the baby uses nutritional reserves to keep warm, hypoglycaemia may result. These two factors contribute to hypoxia which may need ventilatory treatment and must be prevented.

When the baby is born and taken to the Resuscitaire for assessment, liquor and blood should be quickly wiped off and a warm dry towel used as a wrap. During resuscitation, exposure to room temperature causing heat loss must be avoided.

The parents

Parents are usually shocked at the preterm birth of their baby and will have many worries and doubts about their baby's ability to survive. They will be shown the baby and can cuddle him or her if the condition permits. Before the baby is transferred, parents are given directions to the unit and brief information about seeing the baby there and speaking to a doctor about the treatment (Farrell & Frost 1992). If the birth was by Caesarian section under general anaesthetic, the father can accompany the baby to the neonatal unit, if he wishes, and be given a photograph and unit booklet to show the mother when she wakes up.

ADMISSION TO THE UNIT

If a neonatal nurse could not attend the delivery, one will now admit the baby and assume responsibility for nursing care and family needs. The first hour of the small

baby's life is vital to the long term well being and neurological outcome (Roberton 1993b). The aim is to increase the chances of a neurologically intact survival. This is done by:

- Controlling respiratory distress.
- Preventing hypoglycaemia and cold injury.
- Averting intraventricular haemorrhage.

Assessment

Preterm babies are usually admitted to the intensive care room in an incubator for assessment. Monitoring of heart, respiratory rate, blood pressure, and oxygen saturation levels will be started for continual assessment of vital signs. In order to warn of any changes in vital signs, monitors need to have set alarms. A preterm baby's heart will normally beat at a rate of 100–180 a minute. Normal respiratory rate for a preterm baby is 40–50 breaths a minute but there is frequently tachypnoea or the respiratory rate may be dependent on ventilator rates. Oxygen saturation monitors measure the level of oxygen concentration in the blood. The reading should be around 95%, as this level is considered sufficient to prevent hypoxia without damaging the retina and causing retinopathy of prematurity (Greenough 1994). For this reason it is important to set alarm levels at 88% for low alarm and 95% high. Blood pressure alarms must be set according to the baby's gestational age, that is a 26 week baby will have a mean of approximately 26 mmHg. A monitoring alarm on an arterial line is essential to warn of bleeding if the line disconnects or becomes dislodged.

Bloods for culture to eliminate/diagnose infection and to assess glucose, electrolytes, haemoglobin levels and gases are taken and an intravenous infusion of dextrose is started as soon as a vein is cannulated.

Stabilising the baby

The most important needs of the baby immediately after admission will be:

- Adequate respiratory maintenance
- Warmth
- Nutrition
- Haematological stability

Adequate respiratory maintenance

Respiratory difficulties are the most common problem affecting neonates and all babies are carefully monitored to enable early treatment and control. On admission, an oxygen saturation probe is attached to a hand or foot which gives a continuous measurement of the percentage of oxygen in the blood. Oxygen saturations should be maintained around 95% and if the baby is not ventilated, incubator oxygen is given to maintain this level. Observation and recording of oxygen needs is essential as increasing oxygen requirements may mean that mechanical help is needed to assist respiration.

Blood gases will be taken on all babies to assess their respiratory status, and treatment given if necessary. Surfactant is given to those babies who meet the unit's protocol (ventilatory support is discussed in Chapter 4).

Temperature control

The baby should be nursed in a neutral thermal environment. That is the temperature needed to keep peripheral temperature over 36.5°C with the minimum oxygen usage and energy expenditure. Keeping the baby warm is vital to prevent worsening of problems likely to develop at birth. Even mild cold stress results in significantly reduced survival (Fleming *et al.* 1991). The effects of cooling are:

- Peripheral vasoconstriction.
- Increasing acidosis.
- Hypoxia.
- Increased calorific expenditure leading to hypoglycaemia.
- Decreased surfactant production so worsening of respiratory distress.
- Metabolism of brown fat leading to reduction in glucose (hypoglycaemia) and interference with bilirubin binding (hyperbilirubinaemia).

Cooling results in increased oxygen consumption, hypoglycaemia and hypotension, all of which worsen respiratory distress and contribute to intraventricular haemorrhage with possible poor neurological outcome.

It is important to be aware that the baby will lose heat (Fig. 2.1):

- By radiation from the body.
- By conduction from lying on a cold surface.
- By convection from currents of cold air.
- By evaporation from the skin.

The incubator

Babies are always admitted into an incubator and the incubator temperature is vital in the regulation of the baby's temperature. For admission it should be heated to its maximum which is usually about 38°C. Temperature must be monitored closely as overheating causes fluid and weight loss, hypernatraemia and hyperbilirubinaemia leading to increased mortality.

Incubator doors should be kept closed to prevent draughts until the baby's temperature reads at least 36.8°C. Small babies who need incubator care should not be washed or bathed. When treatment or procedures are taking place, temperature should be monitored and all but emergency treatment stopped if it falls below 36.4°C.

Heat can be conserved by using an incubator

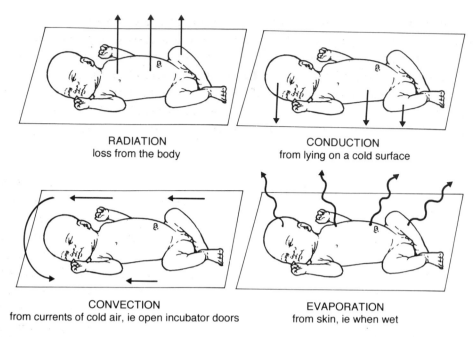

RADIATION
loss from the body

CONDUCTION
from lying on a cold surface

CONVECTION
from currents of cold air, ie open incubator doors

EVAPORATION
from skin, ie when wet

Fig. 2.1 Ways in which heat is lost.

with a heat shield to prevent heat loss from draughts and radiation. Harpin and Rutter (1985) showed that nursing preterm babies of less than 30 weeks gestation in incubators with a relative humidity of 85–90% reduced the evaporative water loss and improved control of body temperature. Care has to be taken that bedding does not get wet and cause cooling as a result of evaporation. A quilt of bubble plastic, if using humidity, helps prevent heat loss. Heat can be conserved by using a woolly hat and a baby who does not need humidity can be dressed in warm clothes.

Monitoring temperature

Babies with a rectal temperature of 37°C can still have significant cold stress as this falls only when compensatory mechanisms fail (Fleming *et al.* 1991). Because of this, temperature should be monitored peripherally by probe attached to the abdomen or a toe. Axilla readings can be used – the thermometer should be left in place for 3 min to give an accurate reading. The drawback of this is that the baby has to be disturbed and possibly undressed. Many modern incubators have a servo control temperature regulator. By attaching a probe to the baby's abdomen the incubator can be set at the temperature desired for the baby, about 36.8–37°C. The incubator will then heat until this temperature is reached.

While the baby is ill temperature is monitored continuously. When the baby is stable it can be taken when hygiene needs are carried out and later temperature can be taken once or twice a day. It is important that temperature is monitored during the whole of the baby's stay in the neonatal unit as fluctuations in temperature may mean the baby has an infection or is using energy to keep warm instead of to grow.

Nutrition

The low birth weight baby has a high metabolic rate to meet the energy demands of the large body surface area and increased energy demands of growth and maintenance. There are also deficient glycogen stores and any stressful event such as respiratory distress or cold stress, will deplete these stores and cause hypoglycaemia.

Intravenous fluids must be commenced urgently soon after admission. A solution of 10% dextrose and electrolytes at 80 ml per kg is usually given on the first day if the baby is under 1500 g (3 lb 5 oz). This should prevent hypoglycaemia but blood sugar levels should be checked 3–4 hourly for the first 6–12 hours after birth and for longer if unstable. Hypoglycaemia is diagnosed when the blood glucose levels fall to 2 mmol/l or under. Fluids can then be increased or strengthened to 12.5% glucose. There may be symptoms which include apnoea, bradycardia, irritability or none at all. Untreated or prolonged hypoglycaemia can cause central nervous system damage with spastic quadriplegia. Severe intellectual retardation has been noted, on follow-up, in 30% of such cases (Roberton 1993b).

Haematological stability

Blood pressure
Blood pressure should be monitored continuously at first. Fluctuating blood pressure is implicated in ventricular haemorrhage (Emery 1996). The mean blood pressure of a baby should approximate at least the number of weeks gestation. So that a 26 week baby will have a mean blood pressure of at least 26 mmHg. Below this is hypotension caused by hypovolaemia, severe metabolic disturbance or hypoxaemia requiring urgent correction with fresh frozen plasma or drugs before the baby has further deterioration. Human albumin is used in an emergency and this is often kept on the unit.

Blood pressure is most accurately assessed by arterial line monitoring, but if this is not possible then cuff monitoring is reasonably accurate. The size of the cuff is important and should be large enough to cover three-quarters of the arm in order to give an accurate reading (Gunderson & Cusson 1994).

Anaemia
Anaemia from twin to twin transfusion or bleeding into the cord causes increased oxygen requirements and low blood pressure. This will be corrected by blood transfusion. Polycythaemia, with a high haemoglobin and packed cell volume, could be caused by receiving blood from a twin or the placenta and is often seen in babies of diabetic mothers. The blood is thick and sluggish and may throw off emboli causing thrombosis of cerebral or heart vessels. Treatment is by dilution exchange transfusion where blood is removed and replaced by plasma in suitable aliquots.

Blood products must be treated for HIV, hepatitis B and cytomegalovirus before use. A blood transfusion to correct anaemia should be given over 2 or 3 hours with a diuretic given half way through so that the baby's system does not get overloaded with fluid. Careful monitoring of vital signs is needed as any changes in heart or respiratory rate could mean an adverse reaction to the transfusion which should then be stopped and the doctor informed. The site of the intravenous cannula must be closely observed for blood extravasating into the tissues. Blood should not be given through a peristaltic infusion pump, which damages the blood cells, so a continuous syringe driver is commonly used.

Infection
Any baby who has clinical signs of respiratory distress or whose mother had rupture of the amniotic membranes for more than 24 hours

will need antibiotic cover until the results of the blood cultures are obtained. This is to treat potentially lethal congenital infections.

Parents

The parents should be allowed to see their baby as soon as they wish. It is usually the father who will make this first visit as the mother may be still incapacitated by the birth. The father will talk to the nurse looking after the baby and be given a photograph and written information about the unit. A brief resume of the unit's routine, information on visiting and relatives' access is useful at this stage. It needs to be kept brief as the father is unlikely to retain very much information at this time due to the tension and excitement of labour and delivery. A doctor should speak to him about the baby's condition, treatment and possible prognosis. The father should be encouraged to touch the baby, but may not wish to at this stage, being too nervous or wanting to wait for his wife so that they can make the first contact with the baby as a couple.

There are times when there is no partner around at the time of the baby's birth and the mother's parents may be her main support. This may be particularly relevant if the mother is ill after the birth and unable to visit. The grandparents, by arrangement with her, should be allowed to see the baby. Neonatal staff can visit the mother and keep her informed of treatment and progress. It is sometimes helpful to start a diary for the baby if the mother cannot visit for days or is ill in another hospital. The diary can be given to the mother later for her to continue if she wishes. It can contain events, written by staff or father, such as discontinuing oxygen or ventilation, or simpler items such as colour of clothes.

When the mother visits she will meet the baby's nurse and speak to a doctor about the baby. There may be questions and worries arising from the father's visit that need reassurance. She will be encouraged to touch and stroke the baby and asked about her plans for feeding. Most mothers decide this in pregnancy and if she is not planning to breast feed she will be asked to consider expressing her milk for a few weeks. Most mothers are happy to do this as milk feeding can usually begin earlier if breast milk is available. There is less likelihood of gut and digestive problems and the immune status of the baby is improved. Assistance with expressing breast milk will be given on the maternity ward initially and later on the unit.

Often parents will have a name for the baby but many may have not decided. In some cultures the naming is delayed while parents consult the family. If the baby is ill at birth the parents may wish to have a religious ceremony which can be arranged on the unit with either the hospital chaplain or representative of their own religion officiating.

Parents need to feel that they and their family are welcome in the unit and are able to ask questions and have treatment explained clearly. For those parents who do not communicate well, treatment and care of the baby should be explained even when they do not ask (Farrell & Frost 1992). Nurses aim to build a relationship of trust so that parents have their needs and those of their baby met.

TRANSPORT OF A SICK BABY TO A SPECIALIST UNIT

Wherever possible the mother will be delivered in a hospital that has facilities to cope with her small/sick baby. It has been shown that it is safer for the baby to be transferred *in utero* than after birth (Nicholls *et al.* 1993). Emergencies, however, do occur and women arrive in preterm labour at hospitals without neonatal intensive care facilities or deliver at home. Sometimes there is no safer course than to deliver the woman at the nearest hospital and transfer the baby later. Transfer to another unit will occur if the baby has an unforseen problem that cannot be dealt with in the delivering hospital.

Transport team

Transporting babies between neonatal units is an important part of neonatal intensive care. A regional unit will have a rescue team which can be sent to pick up a sick baby. The team will consist of an experienced neonatal nurse or neonatal practitioner and doctor, usually of registrar status. They will have a transport incubator with ventilation and monitoring facilities that will work on battery or mains electricity. There will also be a bag or box containing resuscitation equipment, intravenous cannulae, fluids and drugs.

When the unit is contacted about a baby a decision will be made as to whether the rescue team will go to collect the baby or the referring hospital will bring it. This may depend on staffing levels, how sick the baby is and how quickly an ambulance can be arranged. It is usual for the regional unit team to go to collect the baby and to make all the arrangements for the pick-up. The rescue team should ascertain the condition of the baby before they set out and give any advice as to management. They should give an estimated time of arrival at the referring hospital or phone when they are leaving the specialist unit after checking their equipment and the arrival of the ambulance.

There are often psychological as well as technical problems in the transport of babies between units (Scheans 1994). Poor inter-

hospital communication, equipment failure, lack of communication about times of arrival and attitudes of staff make for bad relations between units and uneasy working relationships. A formation of a policy for transferring babies between hospitals is helpful. A copy can be given to the hospitals likely to be involved. The transfer policy should include instructions for the rescue team as well as the transferring hospital.

Arrival of rescue team

When the team arrive at the specialist unit they should not pounce on the baby and start work. Before starting they should identify the senior nurse on the shift and the person looking after the baby. After receiving a handover report and conferring with local staff they should take into account the recent interventions the baby has had before starting the stabilising process for the journey. Failure to do this results in a climate of hostility, which does not facilitate the work of the transport team (Leslie & Middleton 1995).

Care should be taken by the transport team not to criticise implicitly or explicitly the care of the baby. They should remember that the staff may have been striving desperately with facilities that are not meant for intensive care (Leslie & Middleton 1995). The local hospital should help matters by contacting the regional hospital as early as possible in the baby's illness, giving specific information about the condition and following any advice given.

Stabilising for transport

When the team has had the handover briefing, they will take time to stabilise the baby before taking him or her back to their hospital. This should not imply that they are making good what has already been done (Leslie &

Middleton 1995). The aim is to get ready for the journey and it may take a few hours for the baby to be in a stable enough condition for transport.

First of all the airway must be secure and patent. Re-intubation may be necessary to ensure that the tube can be fastened more securely for the journey. If the baby needs high rates and pressures, paralysis treatment and pain relief are given. The baby's blood pressure should be stabilised with plasma or inotropic drugs. Intravenous sites should be patent and maintenance fluids such as dextrose running through them at the appropriate rate for the weight of the baby. Time must be taken to warm the baby as cold stress will lead to low blood sugar and an increased need for oxygen. Temperature will be monitored on the return journey and ideally the baby should be wrapped in a silver foil swaddler. If the baby has a problem such as gastroschisis, exomphalos or a leaking spinal lesion that is causing heat and fluid loss, a plastic wrap such as cling film around the lower trunk will act as efficient first aid for the journey. This can be placed over the lesion before wrapping the baby in the silver swaddler. A nasogastric tube should be passed to empty the stomach of air and fluid. The action of the ambulance may trigger off 'travel sickness' and make the baby vomit.

Before leaving, the baby is placed in the heated portable incubator, stabilised on the ventilator and the endotracheal tube sucked out. Syringe pump drivers with fluids appropriately labelled should be in place. The team will talk to the parents before they leave, showing them the baby and giving information about their unit. They can also let parents know the likely course of treatment the baby will need. If possible the transport nurse will spend the last few minutes, after settling the baby and before leaving, talking to the parents

and answering their questions. If the parents are to follow they may need directions and the telephone number.

It may be the case that the mother will still be recovering from the birth and unable to accompany her baby. The father then has to make the difficult decision as to whether to go with the baby or stay with his partner. If neither parent is going and the baby has a problem that may need emergency surgery, a consent for surgery will be discussed and a form signed before leaving.

The journey

When the baby is settled in the transport incubator, fully monitored, with all intravenous lines checked and working and as stable as possible the team will leave. Notes and X-rays should be collected. The ambulance crew will have been asked to warm the ambulance and proceed as smoothly as possible. If the transfer takes place during busy times in a town or city a police escort helps to hasten the journey. A 'blue light', very fast journey is not always essential and may jolt and bump the baby and equipment. It is very difficult with all the noise and vibrations in the ambulance to keep the monitors working accurately so the team may have to rely on observing vital signs (Crawford & Morris 1994).

Air transport

Some hospitals have air facilities, either helicopter or fixed wing aircraft, to transport babies more swiftly to regional centres. This poses a new set of problems for the rescue team. Pressure falls at high altitudes causing difficulties with oxygenation as there is less pressure to push oxygen into the lungs (Miller 1994). Gas expands at high altitude increasing the risk of pneumothorax, pneumomediastinum, pnuemopericardium and pulmonary interstitial emphysema. These can be devastating to an already compromised baby. The gas expansion also causes abdominal distension in babies with gases trapped in the gastrointestinal tract.

To counteract these problems the baby should be paralysed and given pain relief before leaving, if ventilated, ventilator pressures should be kept as low as safely possible while maintaining reasonable gases. A chest drain pack and portable transilluminating device for emergency location of a pneumothorax needs to be part of the equipment. This type of transport is much quicker than road transport especially in busy congested sites or where there is a great distance to travel.

Returning the baby

When the baby has had the treatment at the regional hospital and can be managed by the referring hospital, transfer back is arranged. This is done so that the family of the baby will find visiting easier and also to release bed space in the regional unit.

Some hospitals come to an arrangement whereby if the transport team collects the baby then the referring hospital will arrange transport back. The regional unit should make sure that all the baby's documentation is up-to-date and ready and that the baby is in good condition for the transfer. This will ensure continuity of care and continuing good relations with the other unit.

Parents' attitude to transfer

Parents should be informed soon after the baby's admission that there will be a transfer back when the baby is well enough. When the time comes the parents may be anxious about the transfer, thinking that their baby will not now get the best care. They will have been through the worse days of their baby's illness with the staff of the regional unit and may feel a close bond. They may also feel that their own hospital did not do its best for their baby especially if they picked up adverse comments from the transport team at the time. Research in America showed that parents took about 3 days to accept that their baby was to be moved and a further 5–7 days to fully accept and relax after their baby's transfer back (Kuhnly & Freston 1993).

Staff need to give as much information as possible to the parents about the care the baby will have in that hospital. Parents will want to know who will accompany the baby and the transport arrangements. They will be worried about infusion needles falling out on the journey or feeding tubes being dislodged, even about traffic jams holding up the ambulance (Kuhnly & Freston 1993). When the benefits and changes that they will encounter in the home hospital are discussed parents usually see the move as a positive manoeuvre.

Good communications between hospitals mean that the nurses are able to obtain more information about other units to give to the parents. If interhospital relationships are good the parents will get a positive view of the home hospital and this will help them through the often emotionally traumatic experience of back transport (Kuhnly & Freston 1993).

REFERENCES

CPLG – The Canadian Preterm Labor Investigators' Group. (1992) Treatment of preterm labor with the beta-adrenergic agonist ritodrine. *New England Journal of Medicine*, **327** (5), 308–312.

Cartlidge PHT, Stewart J. (1996) All Wales perinatal survey and confidential enquiry into stillbirths and deaths in infancy. *Journal of Neonatal Nursing,* **2** (2), 14–17.

Crawford D, Morris M. (1994) *Neonatal Nursing.* Chapman and Hall, London.

Crowley P, Chalmers I, Keirse MJN. (1990) The effects of corticosteroid administration before preterm delivery. An overview of evidence from controlled trials. *British Journal of Obstetrics and Gynaecology,* **97** (1), 11–25.

Emery M. (1996) Periventricular/ventricular haemorrhage in the preterm infant. *Journal of Neonatal Nursing,* **2** (1), 16–18.

Farrell MF, Frost C. (1992) The most important needs of parents of critically ill children. *Intensive and Critical Care Nursing,* **8**, 130–139.

Fleming PJ, Speidel BD, Marlow N, Dunn PM. (1991) *A Neonatal Vade Mecum,* Second Edition. Edward Arnold, London.

Gordon MC, Samuels P. (1995) Indomethacin. *Clinical Obstetrics and Gynaecology,* **38** (4), 697–705.

Graham S. (1995) Psychological needs of families with babies in the neonatal unit. *Journal of Neonatal Nursing,* **1** (5), 15–18.

Greenough A. (1994) Pulse oximetry. *Current Paediatrics* **4**, 96–99.

Gunderson LP, Cusson RM. (1994) Instrumentation in neonatal reseach, arterial blood pressure monitoring. *Neonatal Network,* **13** (4), 51–53.

Harpin VA, Rutter N. (1985) Humidificants in incubators. *Archives of Disease in Childhood,* **60**, 219–224.

Hediger ML, Scholl TO, Scholl JL (1995) Fetal growth and the etiology of preterm delivery. *Obstetrics and Gynaecology,* **85** (2), 175–182.

Kenyon S. (1995) Oracle – an overview of the evidence. *MIDIRS Midwifery Digest,* **5** (1), 14–16.

Kogan MD. (1995) Social causes of low birth weight. *Journal of the Royal Society of Medicine,* **88** (11), 611–615.

Kuhnly JE, Freston MS. (1993) Back transport: exploration of parents feelings regarding the transition. *Neonatal Network,* **12** (1), 49–56.

Leslie A, Middleton D. (1995) Give and take in neonatal transport. *Journal of Neonatal Nursing,* **1** (5), 27–31.

Lewis R, Mercer B. (1995) Adjunctive care of preterm labour – the use of antibiotics. *Clinical Obstetrics and Gynaecology,* **38** (4), 755–770.

Lockwood C. (1995) The diagnosis of pre-term labour and the prediction of preterm delivery. *Clinical Obstetrics and Gynaecology,* **38** (4), 675–687.

Lumme R, Rantakallio P, Hartikainen AL *et al.* (1995) Pregnancy weight in relation to pregnancy outcome. *Journal of Obstetrics and Gynaecology,* **15** (2), 65–75.

Marlow N. (1992) Do we need an Apgar score? *Archives of Disease in Childhood, Fetal and Neonatal Edition,* **67**, 765–769.

Miller C. (1994) The physiologic effects of air transport on the neonate. *Neonatal Network,* **13** (7), 7–10.

Nicholls G, Upadhyaya V, Gornall P, Buick RG, Corkery JJ. (1993) Is specialist centre delivery of gastroschisis beneficial? *Archives of Disease in Childhood,* **69**, 71–73.

Proud J. (1994) *Understanding Obstetric Ultrasound.* Books for Midwives, Hale, Cheshire.

Rennie JM (1996) Perinatal management at the lower margin of viability. *Archives of Disease in Childhood, Fetal and Neonatal Edition,* **74**, 214–218.

Roberton NCR. (1993a) Should we look after babies of less than 800 gm. *Archives of Disease in Childhood,* **68**, 326–329.

Roberton NCR. (1993b) *A Manual of Neonatal Care,* Third Edition. Edward Arnold, London.

Scheans P. (1994) Transport pitfalls. *Neonatal Network,* **13** (7), 5–6.

Thomas K. (1994) Thermoregulation in neonates. *Neonatal Network,* **13** (2), 15–22.

Wilcox MA, Smith SJ, Johnson IR, *et al.* (1995) The effect of social deprivation on birthweight excluding physiological and pathological effects. *British Journal of Obstetrics and Gynaecology,* **102** (11), 918–924.

3 | Nursing Care of the Small Baby

LEARNING OUTCOMES

When this chapter has been read and understood the reader should be able to:

○ Identify the nursing needs of a preterm baby.
○ Discuss the importance of thermoregulation.
○ List the complications of prematurity.
○ Describe ways of positioning babies and their relative advantages.
○ Describe ways in which babies are given good experiences in the NICU.

NURSING MANAGEMENT OF THE SMALL BABY

Immediately after delivery the baby has to adapt to extrauterine life. The first 24 hours are the transitional period during which physiological changes take place in response to the new environment. The placental tasks of breathing, nutrition, blood circulation and waste disposal now have to be performed by the baby's body. The normal full term baby is equipped to accomplish these changes naturally. The preterm baby needs specialised help from the neonatal unit to survive.

The needs of small babies require careful management in order to maximise their potential, both in the present and the future. These needs encompass:

- Respiratory status
- Thermal environment
- Nutrition and growth (see Chapter 10)
- Observation and assessment
- Drug administration
- Pain relief
- Skin integrity
- Positioning
- Parental involvement

RESPIRATORY STATUS

The most common problem affecting preterm babies is inadequate lung function. This causes respiratory distress syndrome (RDS) which affects many babies born before 36 weeks and is the commonest cause of neonatal mortality in the United Kingdom (Roberton 1993). The disease is caused by lack of surfactant, a natural substance in the lungs which lowers surface tension to assist efficient expansion and contraction of the alveoli. Babies born early miss the surge of surfactant production that occurs in the last few fetal weeks.

Preventative measures in the last decade have greatly reduced mortality and morbidity from the disease (Schwartz *et al.* 1994). Measures such as giving the mother steroids before a preterm birth help mature lungs and encourage surfactant production in the baby. After delivery pharmaceutically produced surfactant can be introduced into the lungs of babies who have symptoms of RDS or given as a preventative measure in the labour ward to those at risk (Polak 1992).

Babies with RDS will usually need ventilating and are often very ill. If there appear to be mild or no respiratory difficulties at birth careful monitoring of oxygen requirements and blood gases allow prompt intervention and treatment if problems arise (This subject is covered in Chapter 4.)

THERMAL ENVIRONMENT

Thermoregulation is one of the most important aspects of the care of preterm babies as they have difficulty in regulating their temperature in response to environmental temperature changes. Temperature can have a significant effect on the intact survival of the baby. Klaus and Fanaroff (1993) found a 50% improvement in survival figures when the baby's temperature was kept between 36°C and 37°C.

Temperature instability

The preterm baby has difficulty maintaining a stable temperature for a number of reasons.

Skin immaturity

One of the main functions of skin is the maintenance of body temperature. Three problems hinder this process in a preterm baby:

- Heat loss through large surface area in relation to mass.
- Poorly developed temperature control from hypothalamus causing poor vascular control.
- Immature skin allowing water loss by diffusion, causing cooling by evaporation.

After 2–3 weeks the preterm infant's skin has matured regardless of the degree of prematurity and is similar to that of a term infant (Cartlidge 1991).

Low fat stores

The baby has little in the way of fat stores and glucose to provide energy. Fat stores are laid down in the last trimester of pregnancy so that babies born before or during the early part of this time are deprived of the benefit.

No shivering response

The motor responses for regulating skin blood flow are immature with a poorly developed shivering mechanism for increasing muscle metabolic rate.

Cold stress

Cold stress slows the circulation in an attempt to conserve heat. This results in reduction of oxygen delivery to vital organs particularly the brain and heart. There is a follow-on effect on the small preterm baby which results in:

- Respiratory distress syndrome, as cold stress delays surfactant production which relies on oxygen, glucose and lung perfusion.
- Hypoglycaemia from using up the glucose stores to keep warm.
- Respiratory acidosis from the metabolism of fat.
- Weight loss as the energy given is being used for warmth instead of growth.
- Increased neonatal mortality.

Heat stress

Heat stress causes the circulation to attempt to cool the body resulting in:

- Dehydration due to increased sweating
- Raised respiratory rate, recurrent apnoea
- Increased metabolic rate
- Increased jaundice
- Increased neonatal mortality

Neutral thermal environment

The provision of a neutral thermal environment is therefore important for the baby's health and growth. It is the ambient temperature suitable for the baby's thermal needs, at which heat requirements are minimal and energy given can be used for growth not maintaining body heat (Sheeran 1996).

It is currently suggested that neutral thermal requirements are met when the baby can maintain body temperature at 36.7°C to 37.3°C (Thomas 1994) when lightly dressed. Some babies' heat regulation mechanisms mature earlier than others so that in practice the incubator is set to its highest setting for admission of a small baby and the heat reduced as the baby's temperature stabilises.

Small babies are usually nursed in enclosed incubators until their thermal requirements are assessed. Babies of 30 weeks and under are routinely nursed in humidity in many units for the first 2 weeks as this prevents the massive heat loss resulting from evaporation from the body surface area. It has been estimated that for every millilitre of water that evaporates from the skin, 2400 KJ (580 kcal) of heat are lost (Marshall 1997) making temperature control difficult. The humidity needs to be in the range of 85–95% to be most effective and can be reduced over a 2-week period according to the baby's tolerance. The use of humidity is associated with the threat of infection from the warm moist atmosphere and the reservoir of water. New devices on the market heat and evaporate water separately then add it to the circulating air in the incubator. This allows greater control of the humidity and is cleaner than the old method of water trays under the mattress.

Managing ongoing thermal needs

Skin temperature needs to be closely monitored as babies can overheat in humidity because perspiration does not evaporate and the baby has no means of cooling. The aim is eventually to reduce the incubator temperature until it approximates room temperature – about 29°C, while keeping the baby's temperature within normal range. This might take days or weeks and depends on the maturing of the baby's heat exchange mechanisms.

When the baby is able to maintain temperature with the incubator temperature at 29°C, transfer to a cot takes place. The baby will be dressed warmly, have a woolly hat to conserve heat (D'Appolito 1994) and covered in warm blankets. If skin temperature is not maintained at over 36.6°C, the baby will be returned to the incubator.

Temperature should be monitored throughout the stay in the neonatal unit. This can be done initially by the servo control mechanism on the incubator and when stable by 4–6 hourly checks with a glass thermometer in the axilla. There is controversy about the length of time needed to obtain an accurate reading but the consensus of opinion is that after 3–5 min the temperature changes will be insignificant (Sheeran 1996). It is necessary to be consistent in the length of time and site for measurement of temperature to obtain a recordable trend for the baby.

Some units take rectal temperatures as part of their admission procedure mainly to obtain a core temperature and to assess the patency of the anus. The risk of cross infection and perforation with this method mean that use of axillary temperatures is safer.

OBSERVATION AND ASSESSMENT

After stabilising and assessing the baby on admission, careful monitoring will detect any irregularities in breathing, heart rate, oxygen requirements, blood pressure or temperature.

If the baby is relatively stable, blood sugar estimation takes place 6–8 hourly with blood for estimating urea and electrolyte status taken daily for the first few days. Preterm babies have immature renal function that can result in phases of fluid and electrolyte imbalances independent of thermal environment or fluid intake in the first few days of life (Lorenz *et al.* 1995). Treatment is not advocated unless this persists, so urine output

should be recorded and urine tested for any electrolyte imbalance that will need correcting. The baby should be passing 3–4 ml per kilogram per hour to be judged as having adequate renal function (Roberton 1993).

To measure the urine output it is easier to weigh nappies before and after use than to stick on bags to collect the urine (Fox 1992). Bowel action will also be recorded. Most infants will have passed meconium in the first 24–48 hours. Failure to do this requires investigation for intestinal obstruction or underlying problem such as cystic fibrosis or Hirschsprung's disease.

DRUG ADMINISTRATION

Therapeutic monitoring

Preterm neonates metabolise drugs more slowly than term babies because of the immaturity of the liver (Patrick 1995). This may cause some drugs to build up toxic levels in the blood and others to be inefficiently absorbed. Many of the drugs given have to be carefully monitored so that optimum therapeutic doses can be given.

Drug monitoring is done by testing the baby's blood for the level of drug and altering the dose if the levels are too high or low. Antibiotics, for example, such as gentamicin and vancomycin, are checked by taking pre- and post-dose blood samples to ascertain the correct dose for the baby. Not every drug is monitored, usually only those with narrow ranges between efficacy and toxicity, such as theophylline and phenobarbitone (Table 3.1). This monitoring must continue for the whole time a baby is on the drug. Neonates keep changing physiologically as they grow (Patrick 1995) and may metabolise drugs at different rates as they mature.

Table 3.1 Therapeutic levels of drugs monitored in the neonatal unit.

Drug	Therapeutic range
Gentamicin	Pre-dose < 2 mg/l Post-dose 5–10 mg/l
Vancomycin	Pre-dose 5–10 mg/l Post-dose 20–30 mg/l
Phenobarbitone	20–40 mg/l
Theophylline	6–12 mg/l
Digoxin	1–2 µg/l

Routinely administered drugs

Some drugs are given prophylactically on admission to mitigate the effects of the complications due to prematurity.

Vitamin K is administered in most units to all new-born babies to prevent haemorrhagic disease of the new-born and intraventricular haemorrhage. In 1992 a link between intramuscular vitamin K and later childhood cancer was reported. Though this was unconfirmed the report caused a review of the current policies. The result of this is that maternity and neonatal units now give an oral dose which is repeated at 28 days to well babies (Barton *et al.* 1995). The preparation available in the United Kingdom is currently unlicensed for intravenous use so sick new-born babies are given one dose of intramuscular vitamin K on admission.

Vitamin E given after admission by intramuscular injection and ethamsylate given intravenously have been shown in controlled trials to decrease the frequency of intraventricular haemorrhage (Fleming *et al.* 1991). Vitamin E stabilises cell membranes and is an antioxidant and ethamsylate reduces capilliary bleeding.

Antibiotics are the most common drugs used in the neonatal unit. Preterm babies have little natural immunity and are susceptible to serious infections from many sources. Antibiotics are given soon after birth to prevent congenital infection, if the mother has had ruptured membranes for more than 24 hours or if the baby has a respiratory problem. Suspected infection is treated immediately with antibiotics after taking blood cultures. The antibiotics can be changed or stopped after 24 hours when the result of the cultures is known. Any baby being given antibiotics should also be prescribed an oral anti-fungicidal drug to prevent systemic *Candida albicans* colonisation.

Routes of adminstration

Drugs can be given to neonates, intravenously, intramuscularly, orally, topically and rectally. Each route will have its advantages and disadvantages. All drugs given must be administered safely in accordance with unit and health authority policies and meet current UKCC standards (UKCC 1992).

Drug safety

Whichever route is chosen for administration:

- Any drug that has a narrow therapeutic range must be monitored.
- Doses must be carefully checked and compatibility with concurrent drugs understood.
- The expiry date of the drug must be checked and the manufacturer's or pharmacy guidelines for use followed.
- The substance to be administered must be clearly specified together with its form (tablet, capsule etc.), with the route and frequency of administration.

- The baby must be properly identified by armband number which should also be on the prescription chart, before receiving the dose.
- The drug chart must clearly identify the baby for whom the medicine is intended.
- The prescription must be clearly written, typed or computer printed with indelible ink and the entry must be dated and signed by the prescribing doctor.
- The prescription chart must be checked to ensure the dose has not already been given (UKCC 1992).

All the factors mentioned above will be carried out by two qualified nurses or in accordance with the Health Authority policy, before each dose is given. After administering the drug the chart must be signed in the correct place. If a drug is to be omitted a note should be made on the chart with the reason for the omission.

Intravenous route

The most efficient method to administer drugs to a sick haemodynamically unstable baby is by intravenous route. During the first few days of life or when the baby is sick, there is decreased blood flow to the extremities, which may alter the absorption rate of intramuscular drugs. There may also be poor enteral absorption because of decreased pancreatic enzymes and impaired bile excretion (Patrick 1995).

Administration

Drugs given intravenously are administered through an intravenous cannula. It is part of the nurse's extended role, after suitable training, to administer intravenous drugs through an already sited cannula.

Before giving the drug the usual safety checks are made. Pressure setting on the infusion pump should be checked for increasing readings which could mean the cannula is becoming blocked, thrombosed or infiltrating the vein. If there is any doubt about the patency of the infusion the drug should not be given.

The entry site of the needle is checked for swelling or redness which may indicate that the needle has slipped out of the vein or that the vein has thrombosed. If this is the case the cannula should be resited in another vein. If the site is satisfactory, the line is flushed with 0.5 ml of normal saline to check patency of the line. If an infusion is running, the drug is given through a three-way tap in the giving set, which can be used to turn the other fluid off before infusing the medication. The dose should be given as near to the baby as possible and followed by a small flush to clear the line. The flush of saline is sometimes omitted if it may give a boost of another drug, such as fentanyl or dopamine already running.

Most drug manufacturers state in their literature the length of time a dose should take to administer. Giving a drug too quickly may have adverse cumulative effects, such as bradycardia. Drugs that take more than a few minutes to administer can be diluted and given with a syringe pump. In many units it is the policy for a doctor to give the first dose of a drug in case of an adverse reaction.

Intramuscular route

The intramuscular route is used as little as possible because of the variable absorption rate and the small muscle mass of the baby. Drugs given this way are those not licensed for intravenous use such as vitamin K and vitamin E.

Injections are usually given in the fattest

part of the upper thigh and must be given with care as damage to underlying bone could result in a painful infection – osteomyelitis. This disease has a long term morbidity and causes painful inflammation of the bone which may only be discovered accidentally on X-ray. Immediate antibiotic therapy and long term follow-up is needed if this occurs.

Oral drugs

Oral drugs are not given to babies who are not on milk feeds to avoid incomplete absorption or gastric irritation. As soon as the baby can tolerate more than half the fluid requirements as milk, drugs can be given orally. Drugs should always be given with feeds so that they do not irritate the gastric lining. Some drugs cause vomiting and may need to be given in another form to suit the baby's digestion or the prescription needs to be changed.

If the drug is palatable babies will often suck it from a teat and most drugs can be mixed with a small amount of milk for this purpose. Breast feeding babies can have their drugs this way. Bottle feeding babies can have their medicines in the milk though if the feed is unfinished it means the complete dose is not taken. Tablets are crushed to a powder before being dissolved in milk or water. Most parents are pleased to learn to give their baby's medicine and gain confidence in giving it.

Rectal drugs

This route is used when the oral or intravenous routes are not accessible. Rectal drugs and suppositories are well tolerated and absorbed by neonates and more drugs are becoming available to use this way. Some antibiotics such as metronidazole are available in this form. Some sedative drugs such as chloral hydrate and paracetamol work more quickly when given by this route.

To give the suppository the nurse should lubricate the end with KY jelly or suitable lubricant and gently insert into the baby's rectum with a gloved finger. Some babies will indignantly protest and the nurse may have to hold the buttocks gently together until the baby has calmed down, to prevent the suppository being expelled.

Topical application

The preterm baby's skin is very thin and any substance used on it is easily absorbed owing to poor barrier properties. Substances such as isopropyl alcohol, e.g. alcohol wipes, should be used sparingly. Skin creams should be used with care especially for babies under photo-therapy. The grease in the cream may cause a burn.

PAIN RELIEF

Human beings of all ages, in hospital, have the right to receive the most effective pain relief that can be safely provided. Before the 1980s there was doubt that neonates felt pain and even as late as 1987 research was being undertaken to find out if babies needed analgesic anaesthesia for surgery (Anand *et al*. 1987). It was common practice to paralyse but not give analgesia up to then. Even now there are still controversial issues that remain a barrier to adequate treatment of pain (Givens-Bell 1994).

It was and may still be a common misconception that neonates, especially preterm babies, do not have the neural physiology to perceive pain. Some authorities justify giving no pain relief by saying that neonates do not remember pain or if they do it has no adverse effect. Reluctance to administer appropriate analgesia also stems from the fear of potentially harmful side-effects. These being respiratory depression, hypotension and withdrawal symptoms.

Indicators of pain

Some of the physiological consequences of pain are sufficiently clear to be useful indicators in neonates of all gestational ages (Van Cleve *et al.* 1995). These symptoms can be evident in quiet still babies who do not appear to be in obvious pain:

- Raised blood pressure
- Increased heart rate
- Sweating
- Pallor
- Dilated pupils

Obvious signs of acute pain include crying, flexing or drawing away from the source of pain, thrashing and/or stiffening the limbs, screwing up the facial muscles in a grimace. These responses can be elicited during painful stimuli such as heel pricks and venepuncture (Sparshott 1991).

Pain management

The neonate cannot verbalise the need for pain relief or express satisfaction at the alleviation of it. Thus units must develop a pain management strategy to make sure all babies get adequate pain relief when they need it. Recent literature highlights the importance of a recognisable tool for assessing pain in babies (Keeble & Twaddle 1995; Sparshot 1996).

Sick babies nursed on ventilators using fast respiratory rates and high pressures are often paralysed so that there is good lung compliance. The paralysis makes the baby appear relaxed and unresponsive but the paralysis affects only the muscles and has no analgesic effect leaving the baby frightened and in pain. This is inhumane and it should be unit policy that paralysed babies are routinely given pain relief.

Babies undergoing major procedures such as peritoneal dialysis or chest drain insertion, may be too ill or shocked to show obvious signs of pain. Routine pain relief should be a policy for these babies too. Even if not ventilated, babies should be given pain relief after surgery for the first few days for physiological and ethical reasons.

Babies undergoing painful procedures or with irritability caused by chronic painful stimuli are helped by the use of pain relieving drugs (Pokela 1994). These can be given after comforting measures such as cuddling, positioning and non-nutritive sucking have failed and the baby remains distressed and agitated.

Opioid drugs

Systemic opioid drugs, given intravenously, provide the most effective pain relief during the acute stages of the baby's illness or after surgery. Their use may cause apnoea and respiratory depression in unventilated babies so careful observation and access to full resuscitation facilities are necessary.

Care has to be taken with the use and management of opiate drugs such as fentanyl or morphine. They provide excellent pain relief in ventilated babies but weaning can be a problem, if they have been needed for many days. The baby can be left with distressing withdrawal symptoms of hyperactivity, irritability and altered sleep patterns (Franck & Vilardi 1995). As a result more oxygen and increased ventilatory support may be needed as continual agitation disturbs respiratory efforts. These drugs are most successfully used with a planned system of withdrawal. Gradually reducing the infusion over a number of days is often sufficient. If the baby starts showing signs of withdrawal, another drug, such as midazolam, can be substituted which is not so addictive and has a sedative rather than a pain relieving effect.

Midazolam is a relatively new drug, a short acting benzodiazepine which acts as a central nervous system depressant causing sedation. It is not an analgesic but is increasingly used in neonatal units to wean babies from opioid drugs. This drug can cause respiratory arrest and must be used with care in unventilated babies. It also has addictive properties and if used for more than 7 days should be reduced slowly (Noerr 1995). As it has a shorter half-life in the body it is easier to wean the baby off this drug. While the dose is being reduced oral or rectal drugs such as paracetamol or chloral hydrate can be given to relieve pain or agitation.

Sedatives and analgesics

Paracetamol can be used orally or in suppository form. It must be used only as prescribed, as overdosage causes liver damage. Chloral hydrate is a sedative drug that can be given in conjunction with paracetamol to calm a baby who is in pain. This is available in oral or suppository form.

Oral and rectal pain relieving drugs can be given to babies who have had minor surgery or are being weaned from intravenous pain relief. If a painful procedure such as lumbar puncture or ventricular tap is to be done a dose of paracetamol given half an hour before is efficacious.

When first prescribed for weaning or postoperative pain relief, regular rather than 'as needed' prescriptions should be given (Andrews & Wills 1992). As the baby improves the time between doses can be lengthened with the aim of enabling the baby to be relaxed but responsive (Andrews & Wills 1992).

Non-pharmaceutical methods of pain relief

Babies who are a few days post-surgery or are irritable because of chronic painful stimuli may need pain relief, but nursing measures can often help. This is often where pain relief can be misused (Givens-Bell 1994). No baby should be left to cry or be given pain relief just for quiet. If the situation is not clear, comforting measures should be tried first. Repositioning, or swaddling may help, or sucking on a dummy. Sparshott (1989) found that cupping a baby's head with the hand, soothed and relaxed. D'Appolito (1991) discovered that putting babies' fingers to their mouths helped them find comfort.

A baby in the neonatal unit should never be left to cry whether in pain or discomfort. Effective pain relief helps the baby to behave in a normal manner and promotes normal neurological behaviour in response to having needs met.

SKIN INTEGRITY

The immature skin of the preterm infant causes problems with thermoregulation and absorption which will be further exacerbated by skin trauma (Cartlidge 1991). During the second trimester of pregnancy, the epidermis consists of peridermal cells providing a weak barrier. By 24 weeks gestation a thin poorly functioning stratum corneum has developed and it is not until 34 weeks gestation that the stratum corneum is well developed.

Thermoregulation

The neonate loses water through the skin by a process of diffusion: as water is lost through the skin by diffusion, evaporative heat loss occurs. When the water turns into a vapour, heat is taken with it causing the baby to become hypothermic. Nursing babies in humidity for 2–3 weeks helps reduce this water loss and stabilise body temperature (Marshall 1997). Skin temperature needs to be closely monitored as the babies can actually overheat in high humidity as sweat cannot evaporate.

Absorption

Preterm infants are at risk of absorbing toxic substances through their skin because of its poor barrier properties. Substances such as isopropyl alcohol, e.g. alcohol wipes, should be not be used. Aqueous preparations should be used for preparing the skin for sterile procedures.

The absorption properties of the skin can be used to the neonate's advantage. Carbon dioxide can be excreted through the skin in the first few weeks of life (Cartlidge 1991) and oxygen can be absorbed. By nursing the very immature ventilated infant in ambient oxygen up to 90%, arterial oxygen tension can be increased (Cartlidge & Rutter 1988). These factors may reduce the need for high levels of ventilation and high inspired oxygen levels.

Causes of skin trauma

The preterm skin is extremely vulnerable to trauma such as infections and ulcers caused by pressure and scarring. Neonatal intensive care has the potential to cause permanent damage to the skin. Preventative measures must be a priority. The actions carried out by neonatal staff can be classified into:

- Non-invasive, such as monitoring, electrodes and urine collecting bags.
- Invasive, such as chest drain insertion, heel prick or cannulation which penetrate the skin.

Non-invasive actions

Despite being referred to as non-invasive, surface monitoring devices such as transcutaneous O_2, CO_2 monitors, saturation monitors and ECG monitors have to be fixed to the skin with adhesive electrodes. When removed, the stratum corneum is stripped, weakening the epidermal barrier. This results in a higher skin water loss, increased permeability to potentially toxic drugs and chemicals, susceptibility to infection and scarring from damage to the epidermal junction (Cartlidge & Rutter 1990). The greatest care must be used in the use and removal of adhesive electrodes. Some probes that require a change of site every 3–4 hours may have the adhesive ring left in place so that the probe can be alternated between sites.

Urine specimens for culture and sensitivity must be sterile. This necessitates the use of an adhesive bag for collection. To collect sterile samples, the adhesive area should be cut to the smallest functional expanse required to stick and removed very carefully to minimise trauma. Before applying the bag the area should be cleaned with water and dried thoroughly. This will reduce the risk of contamination and prevent having to repeat the procedure. The specimen should be decanted into a sterile bottle as soon as possible after voiding (Roberton 1993). For boys, fingers can be cut from sterile gloves and placed over the penis (Sparshott 1991). Other urine specimens for urea, electrolytes and osmolality do not need to be sterile so clean cotton wool balls may be placed in the nappy and squeezed out later when wet.

Invasive procedures

Invasive procedures involve penetration of the skin surface. They include heel pricks, siting intravenous cannulae, insertion of chest drains and lumbar punctures. The poor integrity of a preterm infant's skin allows scarring from these procedures many of which will be visible in later childhood and can result in permanent deformity (Bernbaum & Hoffman-Williamson 1991).

Chest drains

Insertion of a chest drain is a commonly used invasive practice to resolve a pneumothorax in a preterm infant. This has great potential for causing disfiguring scarring depending on site of entry and choice of wound closure. Purse string sutures pucker the skin and can cause ugly scars, despite this they are often recommended in neonatal books. Wound edges can be closed by simple suturing or adhesive strips (Steristrips), as an airtight seal is not necessary (Cartlidge & Rutter 1990).

Waterproof strapping should not be used to fix the drain in position as on removal the skin is stripped. Tegaderm or Opsite causes less scarring. Chest drains should be placed with great caution in girls to prevent problems with future breast development (Cartlidge 1991). This is an area where nurses can act as the patient's advocate reminding doctors to take care during such procedures.

Heel stabs

Heel stabs are frequently used to obtain blood for blood gases, glucose levels, drug levels and other routine tests. Heel stabs can cause

osteomyelitis of the os calcis, tissue atrophy and painful dermoid cysts if performed incorrectly and it is possible that the child will have problems with shoe fitting and walking later (Bernbaum & Hoffman-Williamson 1991). The area that should be used is shown in the diagram (Fig. 3.1). This is the area where bone is unlikely to be damaged.

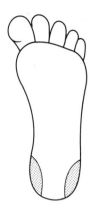

Fig. 3.1 Heel stab should be performed on the plantar surface of the heel in the shaded area of the diagram.

Intravenous cannula

The success of siting an intravenous cannula depends upon skill and ideally should be done by experienced doctors or nurse practitioners. Repeated resitings of cannulae leave the baby with scars which appear as small white pinpricks when growing (Bernbaum & Hoffman-Williamson 1991). Scalp veins may be used but the forehead should be avoided as extravasation may cause facial scars. The scalp vein cannula needs to be securely fixed but still visible. A plastic pot (gallipot) can be placed over the cannula with two pieces cut out to allow for the entry site and the T-connectors, and then taped down.

Extravasation occurs when fluid leaks out of the cannula into the surrounding tissue. It occurs when the cannula becomes displaced from the vein and is seen at first as a red swelling over the area. If there is no treatment this can change in a few hours to a black blister which will later slough leaving a deep scar. Extravasation injuries sometimes damage a full thickness of the skin, causing scarring and loss of function (Cartlidge & Rutter 1990). The burn is worse when associated with fluid containing calcium and amino acids.

Rowe *et al.* (1987) advocated the use of Intrasitegel to help reduce contractures caused when the wound heals. Intrasite gel provides a moist environment which promotes the healing of the injury with the least scarring. Intrasite gel is liberally applied to the area affected immediately after the extravasation, the affected part enclosed in a sterile plastic bag and secured with tape. The wound is easily observed and can be left intact for 2–3 days. If infection occurs then daily dressings are performed. The wound is irrigated with saline to clean it when being re-dressed but should not be dried to prevent damage to the new forming epithelium. Treatment needs to be prompt to prevent further damage occurring. Untreated wounds can result in permanent damage and disfigurement and contracture of the underlying joint may occur (Bernbaum & Hoffman-Williamson 1991).

Extravasation is best prevented by close observation of the infusion site and the use of pressure sensitive infusion pumps. The infusion should be discontinued when pressure rises or there is any redness or swelling around the site.

Good immobilisation of the cannula helps prevent such accidents, foam covered plastic splints can be bent to fit arm or leg. They should be carefully placed and well padded to prevent rubbing of the skin and pressure on bony prominences. Splints can be held in place by using double-sided adhesive tape, or tape padded with cotton wool where it crosses the skin to prevent stripping of the skin on

removal. A pectin based barrier (Stomahesive or Coloplast) can be placed between the skin and the tape to protect the skin if necessary (Sparshott 1991). The site of the needle must always be clear for observation.

General hygiene of the skin

In the very preterm or sick infant, minimal hygiene procedures are performed until temperature control is established and handling can be tolerated. Even then cleaning and position changes should only take place 6–8 hourly until the baby is strong enough to tolerate them without adverse reactions. Parents should be allowed to assist with nappy changes and mouth care as they feel able and must be supported and encouraged by the baby's nurse. The small baby can be 'freshened up' by gently sponging face and body with warm water and cotton wool swabs. The addition of 'baby bubble bath' is safe. Clothes or bedding should only be changed when soiled or damp to ensure minimal handling of the baby. Lips can be kept moist by cleaning with cotton buds dipped into sterile water.

Until fairly recently it was common practice to use talcum powder in routine care. Research has highlighted the dangers of inhalation and respiratory problems with talcum powder (Pairaudeau *et al.* 1991). There have been 30 cases of symptomatic talcum powder inhalation reported including eight deaths. The main reason for powder use was to keep the nappy area dry and to make the baby smell nice. Considering the dangers associated with the talcum powder use, health workers should discourage its use.

Umbilical cord care

This has been the subject of much research in recent times especially into infection and separation rates. It has been shown that the best cord care is to allow a natural drying and separation to occur (Salariya & Kowbus 1988; Bain 1993). If there are signs of infection a swab will be sent for culture. The umbilical cord clamp will be removed when the cord is dry, stiff and unlikely to bleed.

POSITIONING

Preterm babies are excessively hypotonic. They have not experienced the natural flexion and immobility that occurs during the last weeks of intra-uterine life when adaption to the restricted space of the uterus occurs. Muscle tone is also lacking as this is thought to develop from 36 weeks gestation (Downs *et al.* 1991). This means preterm babies have little power to move themselves once put in any position and are at risk of skeletal and joint deformities which could affect their future development (Fig. 3.2). It is important, therefore, that the positioning of the baby is

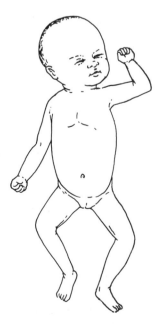

Fig. 3.2 Preterm baby in resting position showing shoulder retraction and frog-leg position.

considered during this vulnerable stage to ensure present and future welfare. Mal-positioning of babies causes problems with neuromuscular development that result in physical, psychological and social implications for the baby and family. These problems can be reduced with minimal cost and nursing time by frequent position changes that support the baby while allowing movement and natural flexion.

It is important that the baby is moved into different positions at least every nappy change time to prevent positional disorders of joints and limbs. All positions have good and bad points so must be used in rotation to maximise the benefits and minimise the disadvantages.

The prone position

The chest wall in a preterm baby is highly compliant offering little or no resistance against expansion on inspiration and poor support on expiration to oppose lung collapse or atelectasis. The prone position helps by stabilising the rib cage and so improving lung function (Kurlak *et al.* 1994). Less oxygen is needed by ventilated and unventilated babies in this position. More time is spent asleep and comfortable this way, so less of the baby's valuable energy is wasted.

There are disadvantages of nursing the baby in this position. There may be obstruction of the airway as the head is turned to one side and segmental lung collapse may occur if a small baby is nursed for several weeks in this position. Observation of the chest wall movement is difficult and there can be delay in recognising abdominal distension. If the baby has an umbilical catheter the site is not visible and bleeding could pass unnoticed. The prone position is thought to be a causative factor in cot death.

In a persistent prone position, the head

becomes compressed at the sides, there is flattening of the thorax and pelvis, the legs are abducted and the shoulders are retracted. A flattened 'frog' position results. As the baby grows this abduction of the shoulders and legs will cause problems with walking and eye, hand, mouth co-ordination (Turill 1992) which will delay future development.

The problems with the prone position can be counteracted to maximise benefits. When placing the baby prone, the arms should be close to the body with the hands symmetrically close up to the mouth. This provides hand to mouth orientation and can have a soothing effect. Flexion of the legs can be encouraged with the knees brought up to the chest, raising the hips slightly. This position can be maintained by using a rolled up sheet at the feet for the baby to press against (Turill 1992) (Fig. 3.3).

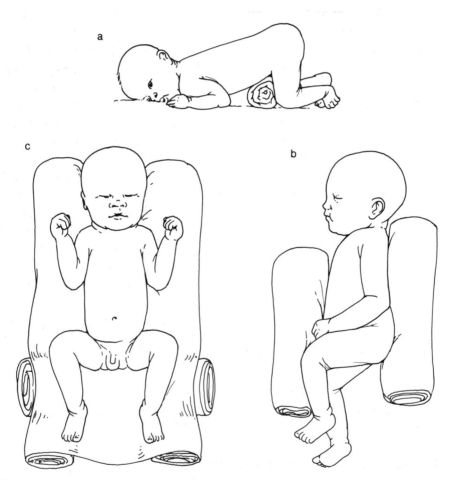

Fig. 3.3 Diagram showing prone, side and supine positioning.
(a) Prone position with roll under hips, and hands brought to mouth.
(b) Side position with roll behind back and head. Another roll in front of the baby with the upper leg over the roll.
(c) Supine position with rolls on either side and under the knees. This provides boundaries and promotes flexion.

The supine position

The supine position allows carers easy access to and observation of the baby. It is necessary for certain procedures such as insertion of intravenous lines. This position does not promote flexion and may be stressful to the baby. There is an increased risk of hyperextension of the baby's unsupported neck, head and shoulder and arching behaviour often seen in chronically ill babies is encouraged. The startle response is more frequent and may occur with exposure to light and noise causing agitation and disturbed sleep.

To minimise the disadvantages if the baby needs to lie in the supine position, the body should be maintained in a state of flexion. The head, feet and body can be supported in the midline using soft blanket rolls positioned close to the baby. Small rolls can be placed under the knees to support flexion of the legs. A roll under the occiput supports the baby's airway and allows slight forward flexion of the head.

Lateral position

Babies can be nursed comfortably on their sides. They have free movement of legs and arms in this position and can achieve a naturally flexed fetal position. The baby may not tolerate this position if sick or unstable and access is not easy for the carers.

The baby can be secured with a blanket pulled securely over the pelvis and tucked in either side of the mattress. This position helps counteract the splinting of the hips in abduction that the use of nappies causes. A rolled blanket can be used for back support (Fig. 3.3). A soft toy between the baby's arms will help maintain flexion and provide a stimulus to flex forwards.

Ideal positioning

Babies very quickly get used to one position and are not happy in any other, so changes should start as soon as possible after the baby is born (Turill 1992). Good positioning should support the baby's limbs comfortably in a normal position close to the body. There should be a change of position 6 hourly to ensure that the baby does not get the problems associated with any particular position.

All preterm babies are at risk from positional and tonal disorders. The effects may be further reduced by the use of sheepskins, quilted mattresses or beanbags. These support the weight of the body and in the case of sheepskins provide tactile stimulation promoting flexion. The use of water beds and air mattresses help reduce craniofacial deformation.

An American study tried swaddling well preterm babies in a flexed position and compared the results with standard positioning. It was found that this confining position simulated the position of the baby in the uterus and promoted hypertonicity. Other benefits included increased self-quieting behaviour and more eye–hand–mouth control. The study concluded that there were important benefits in this type of swaddling that could be used for advantage of the baby (Short *et al.* 1996).

PARENTAL INVOLVEMENT

Parents are encouraged to help with their baby's care from the first day. Nappy changes and mouth hygiene can be done on even the sickest babies with the nurse's support and help. The baby will recognise their voices from intrauterine life and will be comforted by their familiar sound. Parents can bring in a recording of their voices which can be played when they are away from the unit. Small soft toys can be put in the incubator and musical toys brought in to soothe the baby. Siblings can make drawings to put on the cot. Any measures which help the parents familiarise themselves with their baby, help soften the austerity of the unit for them.

As soon as the baby is reasonably stable parents can give the baby their first cuddle. Most parents are nervous of caring for the baby and need a great deal of support and encouragement, which they will continue to need throughout the baby's stay (Farrell & Frost 1992). Medical and nursing staff will frequently discuss the baby's progress and treatments and maintain a supportive informative attitude with the family.

COMPLICATIONS THAT ARISE FROM PREMATURITY

The nursing care of a small baby will take into account the complications that can arise from prematurity and the treatment needed to keep the baby alive. It is important that as well as helping small babies survive, their quality of life is maximised. The main complications of prematurity are:

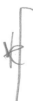

- Bronchopulmonary dysplasia
- Intraventricular haemorrhage
- Retinopathy of prematurity
- Jaundice (see Chapter 12)
- Necrotising enterocolitis (see Chapter 4)
- Behavioural problems

Bronchopulmonary dysplasia

Bronchopulmonary dysplasia (BPD) is the most common complication of respiratory distress syndrome. It occurs in approximately

20% of infants who have required assisted ventilation (McClure *et al*. 1988). It is discussed in Chapter 4.

Periventricular/intraventricular haemorrhage

The increased survival rate of very low birth weight babies due to improvements in technology has resulted in a rise in the number who suffer from intercranial haemorrhage. The disease is seen almost exclusively in preterm babies with up to 50% of very low birth weight babies affected. The handicaps caused by the haemorrhage range from failure to do well at school to severe spastic cerebral palsy (Emery 1996).

Aetiology

The germinal matrix of the brain is a primitive, fragile and highly vascular layer which is thought to be most active in brain development during 24–32 weeks gestation. Its function is diminishing by 34 weeks and it is redundant by term, the cerebral blood flow being then directed mainly to the cerebral cortex (Emery 1996). Thus periventricular haemorrhage is rare in babies over 32 weeks gestation.

Periventricular haemorrhage occurs in the rich vascular network (germinal layer) lying on the floor of the lateral ventricles of the brain and can spread through all the ventricles. In the most badly affected babies, the haemorrhage eventually reaches the brain tissue (Fig. 3.4). Haemorrhage appears to be caused by fluctuations in cerebral and systemic blood flow which damage the fragile blood vessels in the germinal layer.

Decreased cerebral blood flow

The germinal layer needs adequate oxygen to

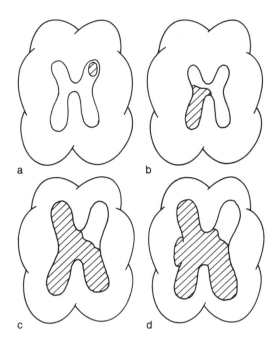

Fig. 3.4 Grades of cerebral haemorrhage. (Adapted from Merenstein and Gardner, (1993).)
(a) Grade 1 Subependymal haemorrhage only.
(b) Grade 2 IVH without ventricular dilatation.
(c) Grade 3 IVH with ventricular dilatation.
(d) Grade 4 IVH with bleeding into the brain.

function. When the baby is hypoxic cerebral blood flow is decreased and ischaemia of the brain tissue can result. Cerebral hypoxia occurs when the baby suffers circulatory depression and hypotension caused by major illness or by such events as blocked airway/endotracheal tube, suctioning or pneumothorax.

Increased cerebral blood flow

Abrupt increases in systemic arterial blood pressure complicated by the effects of hypoxia and hypercapnia, dilate the cerebral blood vessels allowing a large blood flow to the periventricular region. The fragile highly vascular and fragile vessels then rupture causing haemorrhage (Dietch 1993). A rapid rise in fluid volume given intravenously to the baby causes over-distention of the cerebral blood vessels which may result in rupture (Emery 1996).

Fluctuations in systemic pressure

Increased venous pressure can be a result of positive pressure ventilation when the baby attempts to breathe against the ventilator or as a result of cardiac failure. Both these factors can impede cerebral venous return causing stasis and congestion leading to rupture of fragile vessels.

Pressure on the head may be caused by long labour, breech or instrumental delivery which could distort the soft cranial bones of the preterm baby. These factors may obstruct cerebral venous blood flow with a subsequent increase in cerebral venous pressure (Emery 1996). Skull compression from postnatal events such as holding the head for intubation and scalp vein cannulation may obstruct cerebral flow. Tight phototherapy caps, encircling phototherapy masks, and unsupported supine positioning are also implicated (Dietch 1993).

The severity of the haemorrhage

Periventricular haemorrhage can be graded into four categories according to severity:

- Grade 1. This is a haemorrhage into the germinal layer bed only.
- Grade 2. Blood has ruptured into the ventricular system starting with the lateral ventricles.
- Grade 3. The haemorrhage has filled the ventricles causing them to dilate.
- Grade 4. The blood from the haemorrhage has dilated the ventricles and is extending into the white matter of the cerebrum.

Clinical features

Though there is a possibility that some damage may occur *in utero* (Murphy *et al.* 1997). The greatest risk for intraventricular haemorrhage occurs during the first 72 hours of life when the germinal matrix is at its most fragile. There may be another bleed, extending the original haemorrhage during the first week to 10 days of life. The clinical features may vary from a sudden collapse with obvious neurological signs, to a slower, more subtle presentation of symptoms.

A sudden catastrophic bleed occurs with neurological deterioration developing within minutes or hours. The baby may appear limp and unresponsive, apnoeic, have respiratory disturbances or develop fits. The anterior fontanelle will be bulging and there will be systemic hypotension, bradycardia and temperature instability. Metabolic acidosis, glucose abnormalities and fluid retention often accompany the event. The outcome for this type of haemorrhage is likely to be poor.

The more subtle presentation is characterised by a change in alertness, decrease in spontaneous movements and hypotonia. The outcome is usually more favourable depending on the severity of the haemorrhage.

A clinically silent haemorrhage may occur with the infant showing no obvious deterioration. This type may only show up on a routine scan. Care must be taken not to expose the baby to any further factors that might extend this bleed in the next week to 10 days.

Prophylaxis

A significant reduction in the incidence and severity of periventricular haemorrhage is obtained if the mother has had at least 24 hours of steroid treatment (Hediger *et al.* 1995). Steroid treatment is given to mature the lungs of the baby and appears to help mature other organs including the germinal matrix.

Vitamin E given on admission to the neonatal unit by intramuscular injection and ethamsylate given intravenously have been shown in controlled trials to decrease the frequency of intraventricular haemorrhage (Fleming *et al.* 1991).

Awareness of risk factors during delivery, resuscitation and stabilisation in the delivery room and the neonatal unit, is of critical importance in the prevention of periventricular and intraventricular haemorrhage. Particular factors to be observed are:

- Efficient resuscitation at birth to prevent hypoxia.
- Patent airway must be maintained on ventilated babies.
- Suctioning the endotracheal tube can raise the blood pressure and decrease the oxygen saturation so the need for it must be carefully assessed.
- Pneumothorax and air leaks in a ventilated baby cause hypoxia and stress and need to be recognised and treated promptly.
- Blood gases should be maintained within normal limits by ventilatory management.
- Blood pressure must be monitored and hypotension quickly corrected with colloid and/or inotropes.
- Sick ventilated babies should be paralysed and given pain relief to stop them fighting the ventilator and becoming hypoxic with fluctuations in blood pressure.
- Temperature should be maintained within normal limits to prevent fluctuations in blood flow.
- Sudden changes in the baby's condition should be avoided and minimal handling is necessary.
- Over hydration should be avoided to prevent over distention of the blood vessels.

Diagnosis

Periventricular haemorrhage can now be diagnosed on ultrasound scan. In some units all small babies at risk have routine head scans throughout their stay on the unit. The extent of the damage and the healing process can then be observed.

Acute management

The immediate concern is for maintenance of cerebral perfusion and to prevent fluctuations in cerebral blood flow. An adequate blood pressure needs to be maintained while the intercranial pressure is kept from rising too high. Blood volume expanders such as fresh frozen plasma, must be given with care to prevent a sudden rise in blood pressure which may change a moderate bleed into a severe one. Prompt evaluation and treatment of seizures and pneumothoraces help to prevent extension of the existing haemorrhage.

Babies with sudden catastrophic intraventricular haemorrhage must be evaluated clinically and diagnostically by ultrasound scan. Ethical issues about continuing treatment should be considered when a poor prognosis is made (Doyal & Wilsher 1994). The severity of the bleed may cause profound pathophysiological changes from which the baby, even if responding initially to resuscitation, will not recover. In these cases intensive care should not be continued (Roberton 1993).

Babies with mild symptoms or whose bleed is only discovered on scan need no treatment or intervention in the acute stage.

Longer term management

Post-haemorrhagic hydrocephalus
Babies who survive a severe bleed are likely to develop ventricular dilatation which can be seen on ultrasound scan. This can lead to post-haemorrhagic hydrocephalus where the cerebrospinal fluid (CSF) cannot drain freely because of damage from the original haemorrhage. If this is not associated with abnormal head growth no treatment is required but careful head circumference and weight charts need to be kept. If the head growth exceeds body growth then treatment will begin to prevent head growth and further damage to the brain from the pressure of the fluid. Treatment will consist initially of lumbar punctures or ventricular taps to drain CSF to control seizures or rapid head growth.

Drug treatment with acetazolamide can temporarily reduce CSF production but is of little long term benefit (Emery 1996).

When the protein in the CSF reaches a suitably low level, a ventriculo-peritoneal shunt may be inserted for long term drainage. If the protein level is high the shunt will block.

Periventricular leukomalacia
This occurs when the haemorrhage has been large enough to encroach on the white matter of the brain. As the blood is absorbed, cysts which can be seen on scan form in the brain matter. These cysts appear from 2 to 8 weeks after the original haemorrhage. Resolution is highly variable and some will never resolve causing areas of brain damage (Bernbaum & Hoffman-Williamson 1991).

Outcome

Babies with grade I or II haemorrhages usually have no problems from the haemorrhage. Babies with grade III or IV often have long term morbidity with abnormalities in neuromotor and cognitive function. It is impossible to predict how a particular child will be affected. Figures show that about 50% of babies with a grade III or IV haemorrhage will go on to develop cerebral palsy and/or learning difficulties. The type and severity will depend on the severity of the haemorrhages and the resulting degree of hydrocephalus or periventricular leukomalacia (Bernbaum & Hoffman-Williamson 1991). Long term follow-up in the community is essential for all babies with unresolved cystic changes and hydrocephalus.

Parents

Parents need to know if their baby has had any kind of intraventricular bleed and what the outcome is likely to be. For most parents of sick babies the worry of having a handicapped child is paramount and they are anxious about being able to cope.

It is possible to paint a positive picture for parents as a mild haemorrhage often resolves with no sequelae. Even if the baby has a fairly severe haemorrhage it is not clear at the time what the damage will be. A 'wait and see' policy is often the only prognosis that can be made to the parents. Ultrasound scanning is an essential tool in observing the area affected and parents will eagerly await the results.

Retinopathy of prematurity

Retinopathy of prematurity (ROP) is the commonest cause of acquired blindness in the neonatal period. Babies most commonly affected are below 28 weeks and it is rare after 32 weeks gestation (Fleming *et al.* 1991). As the gestational age and birth weight falls, the incidence increases and it is now becoming common for babies surviving below 28 weeks to have some degree of ROP (Roberton 1993).

The exact cause is not known but it is thought to be a multifactorial disorder resulting from the treatment given and the course of the baby's illness. Researchers suspect that

prematurity with low birth weight, blood transfusions, intraventricular haemorrhage, patent ductus arteriosus, hypoxia, apnoeic episodes, infection and bronchopulmonary dysplasia are among the contributing factors (Hunsucker *et al.* 1995). These high risk babies who will have been given oxygen during their treatment are most at risk of developing ROP.

Aetiology

Retinal growth and vascularisation are not complete until after term, so in the premature infant these developments are still in progress. High levels of oxygen in the blood cause the developing vasculature of the retina to have a rapid irregular bout of growth. On returning to normal oxygen tensions, the vessels continue to proliferate intensely with new capillary formation which may cause retinal detachment and blindness. The resulting damage to the peripheral retina may become irreversible. However, as vascularisation continues until the 44th week of gestational age, acute cases often resolve spontaneously (Hunsucker *et al.* 1995).

Prevention

The most likely cause of ROP is thought to be concerned with the administration of oxygen. Oxygen is a life saving therapy and as such is essential in the treatment of sick preterm babies. There is no known safe level to prevent ROP (Greenough 1994) but the incidence of the disease can be minimised by constant vigilance and careful monitoring of oxygen. It must be remembered that babies are at risk until they are over 34 weeks gestation and care must be taken with oxygen administration until that time. It often happens that a baby may need oxygen for many weeks if there is chronic lung disease but on reaching the 34 week gestational age the risk for retinopathy is greatly reduced.

Pulse oximetry

The development of pulse oximetry for babies who are receiving oxygen makes accurate monitoring possible. The machine provides a continuous display of the percentage of oxygen saturation in the tissues (Greenough 1994). The saturation probe consists of a light emitter and a light sensor. The probe should be fitted on a hand or foot with sensor and emitter opposite each other. In the very small baby it can be used on wrist or ankle. The probe site should be changed at least 6 hourly to prevent pressure areas and skin infections under the strapping.

As the pulse oximeter calculates arterial blood oxygen levels during peak arterial pulses, it can give false readings when the baby moves or the sensor becomes partly detached from the skin. Hypothermia and anaemia can also give false low readings as hands and feet are likely to be poorly perfused. Oxygen saturation readings should be kept as near to 95% as possible as this level appears to approximate the needs of healthy babies who have been monitored in air (Greenough 1994).

Transcutaneous monitoring

Another method of oxygen measurement is by transcutaneous probe which uses a heated electrode to measure oxygen tension across the skin. The disadvantage of this method is that it has to be stuck on to the baby's chest or abdomen and leaves small burn marks even when changed 4 hourly. The advantage is that some probes incorporate a carbon dioxide sensor which is helpful in gauging the respiratory status of a very sick baby.

Diagnosis

Units should have a screening policy to diagnose and treat babies at risk of retinopathy of prematurity with the aim of preventing irreversible damage. The most vulnerable babies are those born before 32 weeks who have been given oxygen. They need to be examined by an ophthalmologist at 1 month old and should have repeat examinations every 2 weeks or so while they need oxygen therapy. There are no figures for the length of time the oxygen takes to cause damage (Roberton 1993).

There are five stages of retinopathy of

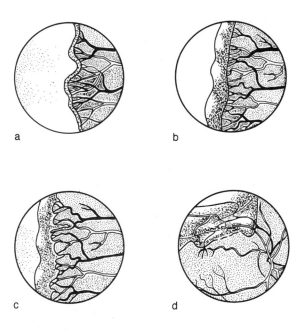

Fig. 3.5 Showing the stages of retinopathy. (Adapted from Bernbaum and Hoffman-Williamson (1991).)
(a) Stage 1 Demarcation line between vascularised and avascularised retina.
(b) Stage 2 Ridge at the edge of the avascularised retina.
(c) Stage 3 Ridge with extraretinal proliferation.
(d) Stage 4 and 5 Peripheral and total retinal detachment. Total detachment is shown.

prematurity (Fig. 3.5) which can be seen on ophthalmic examination:

(1) A demarcation line between vascularised and avascularised retina.
(2) A ridge at the edge of the avascularised retina.
(3) A ridge with extraretinal proliferation.
(4) Subtotal retinal detachment.
(5) Total retinal detachment.

Treatment

For most babies stages 1 and 2 regress spontaneously. Once stage 3 has been reached the disease continues to proliferate and treatment is needed if blindness is to be prevented.

There are two methods of treatment. The first to be tried with any success was cryotherapy. This operation is carried out under general anaesthetic. The retina is transclerally frozen with a probe cooled by nitrous oxide. The probe is applied through the sclera to destroy the avascular retina in front of the ridge (Gracey *et al.* 1991). The probe has to be repeatedly withdrawn and reinserted to prevent compromise of blood supply. This treatment effectively prevents further proliferation. Complications of this treatment include retinal scarring, detachment of the retina and damage to the peripheral vision.

Since the early 1990s laser therapy has been used. This treatment causes less trauma to the eye and is more accurate. It involves the use of a laser beam, which is a highly focused powerful red light, to perform photocoagulation of the avascular periphery of the retina. Photocoagulation means that the proliferation of cells along the retinal ridge is condensed. It allows deeper penetration into the tissues and is more controllable. This type of surgery is less painful for the baby as there is less tissue penetration and it does not require a general anaesthetic.

Complications

All babies who have any of the stages of retinopathy of prematurity are at risk of developing vision problems. These encompass some impairment of vision and include myopia (nearsightedness), amblyopia (reduction or dimness in the amount of vision), strabismus, glaucoma, cataract formation and possible detachment of retina at a later date (Gracey *et al.* 1991). Treatment with laser surgery appears to have good follow-up results so far, with most babies retaining normal vision (Hunsucker *et al.* 1995). These babies will be followed up in the community as there is some concern about the development of cataracts (Palmer 1996).

Parents

The diagnosis of retinopathy comes at a time when the baby is making progress and seems well. The parents are naturally anxious at the thought that their child will be visually impaired and possibly blind. The operation, if cryotherapy, needs an anaesthetic and their baby may have to return to the intensive care nursery once more. They may feel angry that their baby has to undergo this treatment after the suffering of the primary illness and need to express this anger by talking about their feelings. Counselling can be offered at this stage or there may be a family support sister on the unit who will help. There are a number of societies which help visually impaired children and their families and the parents should be given this information so that they can make contact when they feel ready (see Appendix 1).

BEHAVIOURAL PROBLEMS

Babies treated in the neonatal unit have often undergone lengthy and painful treatment. They have been deprived for the most part of the loving nurturing of their parents and have been subjected to an environment that does not enhance normal behavioural responses. It is small wonder that they and their family need help to return to a normal way of life.

The environment

The environment in neonatal units is noisy, bright and intrusive. Actions necessary to promote the health of the baby are often painful and prolonged. The incubator the baby lies in is noisy and magnifies sound from the unit (Weibley 1989). The baby's rest is interrupted frequently and often uncomfortably during a vulnerable time. In a vain attempt to cope with this environment the baby's responses become disorganised (D'Appolito 1991) when handled. There may be lethargy, bradycardia or cyanosis, alternatively there may be overactivity and irritability with difficulty in settling.

These behavioural mechanisms are not helpful to the baby and could lead to further intervention such as more oxygen if the baby becomes cyanosed, or sedative drugs if comfort measures such as dummies and position changes fail to prevent the baby getting exhausted. Later, feeding becomes difficult as the baby struggles to cope with sucking, swallowing and being handled. If this behaviour continues as the baby grows it can disrupt good interactions with parents.

Systems of care

Parents have been found to be unwilling to cuddle, play and talk with a baby who reacts badly or not at all, and this tends to delay development. Nurses are in an ideal position to provide a psychologically nurturing environment to improve the baby's responses. This can be done by using a system that takes into account the effects of environment and medical intervention on the baby's behaviour (Sparshott 1991; Becker *et al.* 1993). These programmes of care are gaining success in neonatal units and are increasingly being used to help the babies normalise their reactions. American nurses worked out a system called the Neonatal Individualised Developmental Care and Assessment Programme (NIDCAP). This is a system of care widely used in America. Each baby is assessed and care is given to meet psychological needs. The assessment includes such issues as:

- Environment and noise
- Bedspace and bedding
- Handling techniques
- Positioning
- Feeding
- Chronic disease management
- Family support
- Education of parents

This system has gained wide approval in America but is not greatly used, as yet, in Britain. It is expensive to set up and use as the carers need special training in assessment skills.

Many of the areas covered by the NIDCAP are being addressed by neonatal units and there has been an improvement in the previously medically orientated care these babies had been given (Padden 1996). Fewer babies and their families are now psychologically damaged by the care given. This results in more natural relationships and easier acceptance of the small baby into the family.

TOUCH

Minimal handling

A baby is likely to get handled a great deal initially, as investigations and procedures are carried out. For this reason a policy that limits unnecessary handling should be undertaken wherever possible. The baby should be allowed periods of uninterrupted sleep in a darkened room. Hygiene needs only require to be carried out 6–8 hourly on sick babies. Ideally the baby should be attended to when awake and afterwards helped smoothly back to sleep by comfortable positioning in a nest of sheets to create a feeling of security.

When parents visit it is difficult for them to understand the importance of not disturbing the baby. Careful explanations help them to see this as part of the baby's care and treatment. The majority of parents will soon learn their baby's needs and will learn when to touch and what form of stroking is best tolerated.

Comforting touch

The skin is a medium through which the baby experiences contact with other people. It is through the skin that experiences both pleasant and painful will be felt. Preterm or very ill babies are usually deprived of the pleasant touch because of their condition. Instead they are subjected to painful invasive procedures and limitation of movements.

Some form of good skin contact is essential to balance these experiences. Some units use massage on their sick babies. According to Hartelius *et al.* (1992) preterm infants found it difficult to tolerate massage but responded positively to containment techniques which do not require any response or stimulate

reflexes. Their blood oxygen level increased and a quiet alert state resulted. If the baby is too unstable for even gentle stimulation the parents or nurse can use the technique of containment to help the baby get used to human contact. This involves placing the hand very gently on the baby's head and the other over the trunk thus 'containing' the body.

One study looked at the technique of stroking and passive limb movement (Russell 1993). This resulted in 47% greater weight gain than the control group and babies went home on average 6 days earlier.

Kangaroo care

Kangaroo care is a form of skin contact where the baby, dressed only in a nappy, is placed upright between the mother's breasts. This kind of care is not carried out in every hospital but studies have shown that babies had fewer apnoeic attacks and lower oxygen needs while being nursed in this way. It has also been shown to promote parental attachment even in parents who were at high risk of attachment impairment (D'Affonso *et al.* 1993).

Research done in America (Ludington-Hoe *et al.* 1994) shows that babies' behavioural and thermal states were improved during kangaroo care. The babies were calmer and did not react to environmental disruptions. Hats were not needed for warmth as the mothers' body temperature was sufficient.

Kangaroo care is useful for stable relatively healthy long stay infants being nursed in open incubators or cots. It is not advised for ventilated babies, those on low flow oxygen, or with significant apnoeas or bradycardias who need careful observation. If the baby has an umbilical artery catheter *in situ* or an unstable metabolism then this kind of care is not recommended (Ludington-Hoe *et al.* 1994).

Parental feelings

The small preterm baby has the same basic needs for nurturing and care as all human beings but the size and illness of the baby, and the staff, machinery and technology in the unit blunt the normal reactions of parents or paralyse them with fear and anxiety. They often need assistance to see the baby as their baby (Orford 1996). Parents need to feel involved from the beginning of their baby's stay in the neonatal unit and be given information about the condition, treatment and prognosis at all stages. They need to understand the baby's basic needs for food, warmth and love and how they can help to supply these. The response of the baby to their caring handling will help them gain skills in parenting while having the nurses close at hand for support (Graham 1995).

REFERENCES

Anand KJS, Sippell WG, Aynsley-Green A. (1987) A randomised trial of Fentanyl anaesthesia. *Lancet*, i, 243–248.

Andrews K, Wills B. (1992) A systematic approach can reduce the side-effects: a protocol for pain relief in neonates. *Professional Nurse* 8 (8), 528–529.

Bain J. (1993) Umbilical care in pre-term babies. *Neonatal Nurses Year Book*. CMA Medical Data, Cambridge.

Barton JS, Tripp JH, McNinch AW. (1995) Neonatal vitamin K prophylaxis in the British Isles: current practice and trends. *British Medical Journal*, 310 (6980), 632–633.

Becker PT, Grunwald PC, Moorman J. (1993) Effects of developmental care on behavioural organisation in very low birth weight infants. *Nursing Research*, 42 (4), 214–220.

Bernbaum JC, Hoffman-Williamson M. (1991) *Primary Care of the Pre-term Infant*. Mosby Year Book, St Louis.

Cartlidge PHT. (1991) Newborn skin. *Current Paediatrics*, 1, 153–154.

Cartlidge PHT, Rutter N. (1988) Percutaneous oxygen delivery to the pre-term infant. *Lancet*, i, 315–317.

Cartlidge PHT, Rutter N. (1990) The scars of newborn intensive care. *Early Human Development*, 21, 1–10.

D'Affonso D, Bosque E, Wahlberg V, Brady J. (1993) Reconciliation and healing for mothers through skin to skin contact. *Neonatal Network*, 12 (3), 25–32.

D'Appolito K. (1991) What is an organised infant. *Neonatal Network*, 10 (1), 23–29.

D'Appolito K. (1994) Hats used to maintain body temperature. *Neonatal Network*, 13 (5), 93–94.

Dietch JS. (1993) Periventricular intraventricular haemorrhage in the very low birthweight infant. *Neonatal Network*, 12 (1), 7–19.

Downs JA, Edwards AD, McKormick DC, Roth SC, Stewart AL. (1991) Effective intervention on development of hip posture in very pre-term babies. *Archives of Disease in Childhood*, 66 (7), 797–801.

Doyal L, Wilsher D. (1994) Towards guidelines for withholding and withdrawal of life prolonging treatment in neonatal medicine. *Archives of Disease in Childhood, Fetal and Neonatal Edition*, 70, 66–70.

Emery M. (1996) Periventricular/ventricular haemorrhage in the pre-term infant. *Journal of Neonatal Nursing*, 2 (1), 16–18.

Farrell MF, Frost C. (1992) The most important needs of parents of critically ill children. *Intensive and Critical Care Nursing*, 8, 130–139.

Fleming PJ, Speidel BD, Marlow N, Dunn PM. (1991) *A Neonatal Vade Mecum*, Second Edition. Edward Arnold, London.

Fox MD. (1992) Measurement of urine. *Neonatal Network*, 12 (2), 11–18.

Franck L, Vilardi J. (1995) Assessment and management of opioid withdrawal in ill neonates. *Neonatal Network*, 14 (2), 39–48.

Givens-Bell S. (1994) The national pain management guidelines. Implications for neonatal care. *Neonatal Network*, 13 (3), 9–17.

Gracey K, McLaughlin KL, Smiley JM. (1991) Caring for the infant with retinopathy of prematurity undergoing cryotherapy. *Neonatal Network*, **9** (7), 7–11.

Graham S. (1995) Psychological need of families with babies in the neonatal unit. *Journal of Neonatal Nursing*, **1** (5), 15–18.

Greenough A. (1994) Pulse oximetry. *Current Paediatrics*, **4**, 196–199.

Hartelius I, Rasmussen L, Odelise OS. (1992) How little you are. *Neonatal Network*, **11** (8), 33–37.

Hediger ML, Scholl TO, Schall JI. (1995) Fetal growth and the etiology of pre-term delivery. *Obstetrics and Gynaecology*, **85** (2), 175–182.

Hunsucker K, King C, Stamm S, Cisneros N. (1995) Laser treatment for retinopathy of prematurity. *Neonatal Network*, **14** (4), 21–25.

Keeble S, Twaddle R. (1995) Assessing neonatal pain. *Nursing Standard*, **10** (1), 16–18.

Klaus MH, Fanaroff AA. (1993) *Care of the High Risk Neonate*, Fourth Edition. WB Saunders, Philadelphia.

Kurlack LO, Ruggins NR, Stephenson TJ. (1994) Effect of nursing position on incidence type and duration of clinically significant apnoea in pre-term infants. *Archives of Disease in Childhood, Fetal and Neonatal Edition*, **71** (1), 16–19.

Lorenz JM, Kleinman LI, Ahmed G, Markarian K. (1995) Phases of fluid and electrolyte homeostasis in the extremely low birthweight infant. *Pediatrics*, **96** (3), 484–489.

Ludington-Hoe SM, Thompson C, Swinth J, Hadeed AJ, Anderson GC. (1994) Kangaroo care – research results. *Neonatal Network*, **13** (1), 19–27.

McClure G, Halliday H, Thompson W. (1988) *Perinatal Medicine*. Baillière Tindall, London.

Marshall A. (1997) Humidifying the environment for the premature neonate. *Journal of Neonatal Nursing*, **3** (1), 31–36.

Merenstein GB, Gardner SL (1993) *Handbook of Neonatal Intensive Care* 3rd edn, Mosby Year Book, St. Louis.

Murphy DJ, Hope PL, Johnson A. (1997) Neonatal risk factors for cerebral palsy in very preterm babies. *British Medical Journal*, **314**, 404–408.

Noerr B. (1995) Midazolam. *Neonatal Network*, **14** (1), 65–67.

Orford T. (1996) Crisis and crisis intervention: psychological support for parents whose children require neonatal intensive care. *Journal of Neonatal Nursing*, **2** (1), 11–13.

Padden T. (1996) Developmental issues in neonatal nursing. In: *Neonatal Nurses Year Book 1996*. pp. 2-47–2-52. CMA Medical Data, Cambridge.

Pairaudeau PW, Wilson RG, Hall MA, Milne M. (1991) Inhalation of baby powder; an unappreciated hazard. *British Medical Journal*, **302**, 1200–1201.

Palmer E. (1996) The continuing threat of retinopathy of prematurity. *American Journal of Ophthalmology*, **122**, 420–423.

Patrick CH. (1995) Therapeutic drug monitoring in neonates. *Neonatal Network*, **14** (2), 21–26.

Pokela M (1994) Pain relief can reduce hypoxaemia in distressed neonates during routine treatment procedures. *Pediatrics*, **93** (3), 379–383.

Polak JD. (1992) Surfactant replacement: An old idea breathes new life into neonatology. *Neonatal Network*, **11** (4), 1–6.

Roberton NCR. (1993) *A Manual of Neonatal Care*, 3rd edn. Edward Arnold, London.

Rowe T, Keats J, Morgan J. (1987) A new approach to the management of extravasation injury in neonates. *Pharmaceutical Journal*, Nov 14th.

Russell J. (1993) Touch and infant massage. *Paediatric Nursing*, **5** (3), 8–11.

Salariya EM, Kowbus NM. (1988) Variable umbilical cord care. *Midwifery*, **4**, 70–76.

Schwartz RM, Luby AM, Scanlon JW, Kellogg RJ. (1994) Effect of surfactant on morbidity, mortality and resource use in newborn infants weighing 500–1,500g. *New England Journal of Medicine*, **330** (21), 1476–1480.

Sheeran M (1996) Thermoregulation in neonates. *Journal of Neonatal Nursing*, **2** (4), 6–9.

Short MA, Brooks-Brunn JA, Reeves DS *et al.* (1996) The effects of swaddling versus standard positioning on neuromuscular development of very low birth weight infants. *Neonatal Network*, **15** (4), 25–31.

Sparshott M. (1989) Pain and the special care baby unit. *Nursing Times*, **85** (41), 61–64.

Sparshott M. (1991) Maintaining skin integrity. *Paediatric Nursing,* **3** (2), 12–13.

Sparshott MM. (1996) The development of a clinical distress scale for ventilated newborn infants. *Journal of Neonatal Nursing,* **2** (2), 5–10.

Thomas K. (1994) Thermoregulation in neonates. *Neonatal Network,* **13** (2), 15–22.

Turrill S. (1992) Supported positioning in intensive care. *Paediatric Nursing,* **4** (4), 24–27.

United Kingdom Central Council for Nursing, Midwifery and Health Visiting. (1992) *Standards for the Administrations of Medicines.* UKCC, 23 Portland Place, London.

Van Cleve L, Johnson L, Andrews S, Hawkins S, Newbold J. (1995) Pain responses of hospitalised neonates to venipuncture. *Neonatal Network,* **14** (6), 31–36.

Weibley T. (1989) Inside the incubator. *American Journal of Maternal Child Nursing,* **14** (2), 96–100.

4 | Nursing Management of Babies with Respiratory Problems

LEARNING OUTCOMES

When this chapter has been read and understood the reader should be able to:

O Describe development of the lungs and the changes at birth.
O List factors that influence surfactant production.
O Discuss the care of a ventilated baby.
O Discuss new ways currently used to ventilate babies.
O Identify common respiratory diseases in the neonatal unit.
O Describe the management of bronchopulmonary dysplasia.

LUNG FUNCTION IN THE NEW-BORN

Respiratory difficulties present the most common problems in the neonatal unit and are a significant factor in the morbidity and mortality of the neonatal population. Despite recent advances they continue to be a major problem to the preterm and full term sick baby.

Embryological maturation of the lungs

In order to understand why respiratory problems develop it is necessary to look at the development and maturation of the lungs in late fetal life.

Canicular stage

This stage occurs between 17 and 24 weeks gestation and involves the development of the respiratory bronchioles and alveolar ducts; enlargement of the lumina of the bronchi and terminal bronchioles and vascularisation of lung tissue (Fig. 4.1). A baby born at the end of this stage usually has no natural surfactant and survival rate is low even with treatment.

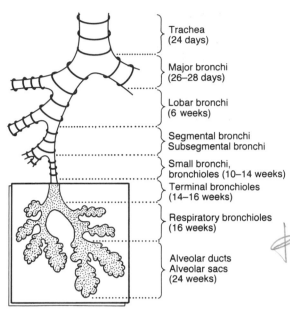

Trachea
(24 days)

Major bronchi
(26–28 days)

Lobar bronchi
(6 weeks)

Segmental bronchi
Subsegmental bronchi

Small bronchi,
bronchioles (10–14 weeks)
Terminal bronchioles
(14–16 weeks)

Respiratory bronchioles
(16 weeks)

Alveolar ducts
Alveolar sacs
(24 weeks)

Fig. 4.1 Respiratory tract with approximate gestational ages of formation. (Adapted from Korones and Lancaster (1986).)

Saccular stage

This stage occurs between 24 and 38 weeks gestation. The alveolar ducts give rise to terminal sacs which are initially lined with cuboidal epithelium. This changes to squamous epithelium at around the 26th week. Surfactant production commences slowly in the alveolar epithelium. There is a surge of production between weeks 30 and 34. If a fetus is born prematurely at this stage, its lungs are usually sufficiently developed for survival.

Alveolar stage

This stage takes place from 36 weeks gestation. New alveoli are formed as the lungs grow. This process continues up to about the age of 8 years, after which time the alveoli grow in size but do not increase in number (Beck *et al.* 1985).

Mechanics of respiration in a newborn baby

A newborn baby and especially a premature infant, has a highly compliant chest wall. Little or no resistance is offered against expansion on inspiration and there is insufficient support on expiration to oppose lung collapse or atelectasis. In full term neonates, the major force contributing to elastic recoil of the lungs is surface tension at the air–liquid boundaries in the distal bronchioles and alveoli. This surface tension is provided by surfactant.

In the healthy full term baby, who has had a normal delivery, there is no problem with surfactant production and the baby progresses well. In a preterm baby or a baby with fetal distress from pregnancy, labour or delivery, surfactant production is absent, delayed or halted by the illness. Then the lack of surface tension combined with the compliant chest wall means that lungs fail to retain air in some alveoli, and gas is trapped in others. Failure to retain air leads to alveolar collapse which leads to more gas trapping. Thus each breath requires great effort to obtain sufficient oxygen. The infant tires easily and needs assisted ventilation in order to survive.

The first breath

During intrauterine life gaseous exchange occurs transplacentally between the fetal and maternal blood. Postnatally, exchange occurs across the alveolar membrane from a gaseous to a liquid medium. There are a number of physical stimuli that play a role in respiratory initiation. As the infant is propelled down the birth canal a negative intrathoracic pressure is exerted so that on delivery air is sucked into the lungs causing the infant to breathe. Asphyxial changes resulting from cord clamping help stimulate the onset of respiration.

The aortic and carotid bodies are sensitive to the reduction in the partial pressure of oxygen and pH levels, and so stimulate the respiratory centre in the medulla oblongata to initiate the first breath (Roberton 1993a). Pressure in the alveoli would lead to widespread alveolar collapse if surfactant were not present to reduce surface tension. Initial inflation of the lungs mediates the release of vasodilators which together with the rising PaO_2 and falling $PaCO_2$ establish pulmonary perfusion with the onset of respiration (Roberton 1993a).

Surfactant

Most respiratory problems of the new-born whether preterm or full term are affected by the amount of surfactant produced in the lungs. Surfactants line the lungs of all animals to maintain a constant alveolar pressure and lower surface tension.

Surfactant is made in the granular pneumocytes of the alveolar epithelium. It is a complex mixture of lipids and protein and occupies approximately 5% of the alveolar surface. The expansion of the lungs at birth helps release surfactant and once released it is recycled unless exposed to adverse conditions.

Factors affecting surfactant production

Prematurity

This is a major factor, as active surfactant production does not occur till the third trimester. The administration of steroids to the mother at least 24 hours before delivery lessens the severity of respiratory distress by encouraging the production of surfactant (Crowley *et al.* 1990).

Perinatal asphyxia

Perinatal asphyxia predisposes to surfactant deficiency as hypoxia and acidaemia caused by the asphyxia, slow down surfactant synthesis. In addition asphyxia damages the pulmonary blood vessels allowing proteins from the blood to seep out into the alveoli thus inhibiting surfactant activities.

Maternal diabetes

Surfactant production has been shown to be delayed in diabetes (Roberton 1993b). There is also the possibility of the mother having to have a Caesarian section owing to the size of the baby.

Caesarian section

If a Caesarian section is carried out in women with preterm babies, surfactant production may not be complete. Often a Caesarian section will be carried out for fetal distress so the baby may be hypoxic with the resultant reduction in surfactant production. In addition the mechanical squeezing of the baby's chest, which clears lung fluids during descent through the birth canal is denied, resulting in retention of lung fluid and inhibition of surfactant activities. Babies are also denied the beta-adrenergic mediated release and reduction in fetal lung liquid which occurs 24–48 hours before spontaneous labour.

Second twin

There is faster surfactant maturation in the first twin presenting possibly because of the stress of labour (Roberton 1993b).

Factors thought to increase surfactant production

Drug abuse

Acceleration in surfactant production is seen in infants of mothers addicted to heroin or cocaine. The reason for this is not clear but it is thought to be because such drugs influence surfactant production (Roberton 1993b).

Maternal factors

Hypertension, maternal infection and rupture of membranes longer than 48 hours can cause the baby to have increased surfactant production. This is thought to be the result of the stress caused to the baby which gives a natural surge of surfactant production (Merenstein & Gardener 1993).

MANAGEMENT OF A BABY WITH A RESPIRATORY DISEASE

Delivery

A paediatrician/neonatal nurse practitioner and a neonatal nurse should attend all preterm births or any delivery where there is a known problem with the baby. Resuscitation equipment such as endotracheal tubes, laryngoscope, bag and mask, oxygen and suction should be checked and ready before the delivery. A warm portable incubator with ventilation facilities should be plugged in near the delivery room. When the baby is born the establishment of respiration is paramount and prevention of cold stress, which slows surfactant production, is also vital.

Resuscitation

Prompt efficient resuscitation in the labour ward will reduce the severity of respiratory distress. If the baby does not start breathing spontaneously after oral and nasopharyngeal suction, a bag and mask should be used. The baby should be placed supine with neck extended (Fig. 4.2). The mask must fit snugly over the baby's nose and mouth so that air can be forced into the lungs. The bag must be connected to oxygen and should be compressed at a rate of 60 per minute with just enough pressure to inflate the chest. Too vigorous a bagging will give the baby a pneumothorax from over-inflation of inelastic alveoli. Care needs to be taken with babies who have secondary apnoea possibly from diaphragmatic hernia as bagging inflates the gut causing even more respiratory problems. Babies with suspected diaphragmatic hernia should be intubated and ventilated immediately.

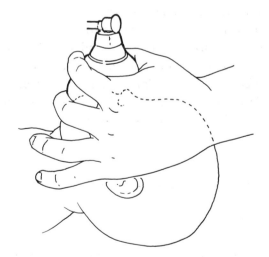

Fig. 4.2 Position for bag and mask ventilation.

If bagging does not stimulate breathing after 2–3 min, an endotracheal tube must be passed and manually bagged to provide more efficient oxygenation of the lungs. Once the baby is well oxygenated, breathing may commence spontaneously and the tube can be withdrawn. If this is not the case, bagging or ventilation will continue and the baby will be taken to the neonatal unit in a warmed incubator for treatment.

It is vital that during resuscitation the baby is kept warm and dry. Cold stress worsens all respiratory problems by slowing surfactant production. Cold also causes physiological problems such as hypoglycaemia because of physiological compensatory mechanisms. The baby uses energy to try and maintain temperature, using stores of glucose and causing anaerobic glycolysis, a process which can also be caused by hypoxia. A by-product of this action is lactic acid which causes metabolic acidosis. Further compensatory mechanisms turn this into a respiratory acidosis. This then can cause diminished pulmonary perfusion leading to alveolar damage and the impaired production of surfactant.

Admission

All babies admitted to the neonatal intensive care unit will have cardiopulmonary and oxygen saturation monitoring to observe and assess the need for treatment and intervention. The prevention of hypoxia, cold stress and hypoglycaemia, keeping vital signs stable and normal and minimal handling ensure the best outcome for the baby.

Headbox oxygen therapy

If continuous, ambient oxygen is needed to keep the baby's saturations around 95%, warmed humidified oxygen in a head box should be given. A steady flow of oxygen can then be maintained even when the incubator doors have to be opened.

The oxygen requirements and baby's saturations, must be monitored and recorded. Blood gases should be measured regularly to assess respiratory status particularly if oxygen requirements increase. This could mean that the baby needs more help with breathing.

Continuous positive airways pressure (CPAP)

This is a mechanical device used to prevent the alveoli collapsing during expiration thus easing the inspiratory effort for the baby. It increases intrapulmonary pressure and blows open collapsed alveoli to improve oxygenation. The alveoli are splinted open with applied pressures of up to $10\,cmH_2O$ and humidified oxygen can be given if necessary. CPAP can be given by nasal prong or less commonly through the endotracheal tube (ETT). Most ventilators have a CPAP mode using the same tubing as the ventilation circuit.

Indications for use

CPAP is useful during the first few hours after birth for babies under 1500 g (3 lb 5 oz) with mild respiratory problems indicated by a rising $PaCO_2$ and ambient oxygen needs of 30–40%. It can be used for larger babies with mild respiratory problems who need up to 60% in the first few days after birth. CPAP may prevent a more serious progression of respiratory distress syndrome, as the splinting effect helps to preserve alveolar surfactant.

Babies who are being weaned off ventilation may be given CPAP by the ETT for an hour or two. If this is satisfactory, extubation can take place and a nasal prong used. CPAP can be used to assist babies who are having recurrent apnoea with or without RDS (Roberton 1993b). It can be used continuously or intermittently for babies with chronic lung disease until they are able to cope fully on their own.

Methods of administration

CPAP can be given by a single prong inserted into the nose and into the nasopharynx, or by short 'piggy' prongs which fit just inside the nostrils. The single prong can be cut from the smallest size endotracheal tube, measured 3 cm shorter than that which the baby would need for intubation. The holder is put on and the prong lubricated with a small amount of antimicrobial Naseptin cream. It is then inserted gently into the nostril, secured in the unit's usual way and attached to the ventilator tubing. Short double 'piggy' prongs are more comfortable but difficult to keep in place if the baby is active.

The gas flow rate is set to give a pressure of 5–6 cmH$_2$O and oxygen given to keep the baby's saturations around 95%. Blood gases should be checked an hour after commencement and then 6–8 hourly unless there is any deterioration in condition or rise in oxygen requirements before that time.

Complications

CPAP may cause distension of the stomach from the gas flow so the nasogastric tube should be aspirated frequently. If the CPAP is being used after the acute stage of RDS, for chronic lung disease or recurrent apnoea, tube feeding is usually well tolerated.

Pneumothorax may occur with the use of CPAP and a sudden deterioration in oxygen saturation levels may mean that this has occurred. The chest can be transilluminated and a butterfly needle inserted in the appropriate part of the chest with the end to be in water to allow the air to escape temporarily. Chest X-ray will reveal the pneumothorax and

an indwelling chest drain may be necessary. CPAP may need to be stopped and ventilation started.

Flow drivers

A flow driver is a specially designed machine that acts in a similar manner to CPAP. It is characterised by a mechanism that causes the direction of the gas flow to change with the baby's breathing while maintaining a constant pressure to the lungs (Blease 1997). This minimises the work of breathing for the baby and is used to treat mild RDS and chronic lung disease.

All machines have a gas flow meter for the air/oxygen pressure, a humidifier and a set of tubing which includes soft, plastic, short, nasal prongs with Velcro attachments for securing to the baby's hat. The prongs are well tolerated and comfortable, especially for small babies with chronic lung disease who may need this treatment for weeks.

Flow drivers are gaining popularity in neonatal units and do not cause the abdominal distension that conventional CPAP does. There is however some worry about nasal deformities and necrosis caused by the designs on the market at the time of writing. Babies who are being treated with these devices should be examined frequently for signs of reddening, snubbing or flaring of nostrils (Robertson *et al.* 1996). Flow drivers should ideally not be used in units where there are no facilities for resuscitation and ventilation in case of pneumothorax or worsening respiratory distress requiring full ventilatory support.

Nursing a baby on CPAP or flow driver

Oxygen and pressure should be monitored and recorded hourly, the humidifier should be turned on and kept topped up, if it does not refill automatically, to ensure a continuous supply of warmed, humidified gas.

The prong or 'piggy' prongs can be removed briefly if there is a need to suction the nostrils. This should be carried out with care, using a small bore catheter to prevent trauma and bleeding of the nasal cavities. Oral suction can be carried out with the prongs in place. The baby can otherwise be tube fed, nursed and positioned as usual. Normal handling is easy so that cuddling and even bathing (if the baby tolerates it) can be done.

Weaning off CPAP

As the blood gases (Table 4.2) improve, the pressure is reduced. When the gases are good and the baby is in air the prong/prongs can be removed and head box or low flow oxygen used if necessary.

If the baby develops apnoea and brady-cardia after discontinuing CPAP, caffeine or aminophylline can be started to stimulate the respiratory centre. A record should be kept of apnoeic and bradycardic episodes as the baby may need a further period on CPAP or an increase in the dose of aminophylline. Ther-apeutic levels of aminophylline should be checked at least weekly.

Babies with chronic lung disease may have been ventilated for a long time and then progressed to CPAP. These babies may need to be weaned off CPAP by learning to cope a few hours at a time in low flow oxygen. They will be returned to CPAP after a set time or if oxygen needs and respiratory rate rise. Gradually tolerance increases until they can cope without it. It may take many weeks before a baby can cope completely.

Conventional mechanical ventilation

Indications for mechanical ventilation

- Poor respiratory effort at birth or elective intubation of a baby under 800 g (1 lb 12 oz).
- A baby on CPAP needing more than 60% oxygen to maintain a partial pressure of oxygen (PaO_2) above 60 mmHg (7.8 kPa).
- Any baby whose gases show a significant rise in $PaCO_2$ and drop in pH, indicating poor exchange of gases in the lungs.
- Sudden deterioration with apnoea or irre-gular gasping respirations.

Intubation

An endotracheal tube can be passed orally or nasally. The result is the same, that of giving access to the lower airways for oxygenation and suction. Both nasal and oral methods have their advantages and disadvantages.

Nasal intubation

It is more difficult to intubate this way as the vocal cords cannot be seen so easily. The tube is easier to secure with strapping on the baby's face but makes this an unpopular method with parents. Stripping of the skin occurs when the strapping is removed and pressure necrosis to the anterior nares sometimes cau-ses severe deformity requiring plastic surgery later (Crawford & Morris 1994).

Oral intubation

It is easier to intubate a baby orally as the mouth can be held wide open and the vocal cords visualised making this a safer and less traumatic method to use. Oral tubes used for long term ventilation may be responsible for distortion of the roof of the mouth in the form of a groove along the track of the tube, which may cause feeding and speech problems later

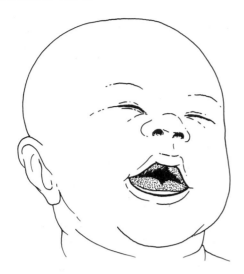

Fig. 4.3 Palatal groove from oral intubation.

(Crawford & Morris 1994) (Fig. 4.3). Some units use an orthodontic plate of plastic specially made for each baby in an effort to prevent this happening. As this groove only occurs in small preterm babies, it may be caused by moulding of the bones and not by the endotracheal tube.

Oral intubation may make the tube less secure and can cause tracheal abrasion owing to the amount of movement the tube can make. Problems occur later when areas of the trachea loose their elasticity and collapse. This is known as tracheomalacia, and can cause serious upper airway problems which may necessitate the formation of a tracheostomy until the damage repairs itself.

Conventional ventilator settings

The aim of ventilation is to maintain adequate exchange of gases in the lungs with minimum pressures and oxygen. Initial settings (Table 4.1) will be altered to suit the baby. Subsequent changes are made on assessment of blood gases and settings adjusted accordingly. Management of peak inspiratory pressure, peak end expiratory pressure, inspiratory and expiratory time ratio, breaths a minute or rate, and oxygen levels are needed during ventilatory treatment.

Peak inspiratory pressure (PIP)
This is the pressure needed to inflate the lungs. If the gases show hypercarbia and hypoxia the PIP may be increased to 'blow off' the carbon dioxide (CO_2) by further inflating the lungs. The aim is to use the lowest pressure that works and to get the pressures down as soon as possible to prevent lung damage. The normal PIP range is 18–30 cmH$_2$O but can go from 15 to 40+ cmH$_2$O. High pressures cause barotrauma (lung damage from the ventilator) increasing the risk of pneumothorax and bronchopulmonary dysplasia (BPD).

Positive end expiratory pressure (PEEP)
This is the volume to which the ventilator returns after it has delivered a breath. In babies with RDS it is normally kept at 5–6 cmH$_2$O and prevents a complete exhalation which could lead to collapse of the alveoli.

Inspiratory and expiratory ratio (I:E ratio)
This is the length of time each breath takes on the ventilator, normally a ratio of 1:1 is used so that the inspiratory breath is the same as the expiratory one. Increases or decreases of this ratio do not improve the overall efficiency of ventilation as well as an increase in the PEEP or PIP.

Rate
The usual rate is 30–40 breaths a minute which may be increased to 60–120. Higher rates combined with lower pressures appear to reduce the incidence of pulmonary interstitial oedema and pneumothorax (Fleming *et al.* 1991).

Oxygen

High levels of inspired oxygen cause atelectasis (collapse of some of the alveoli), by decreasing ciliary activity in the airways which then causes an increase in capillary leakage. The aim is to improve oxygenation of the lungs by altering ventilator settings. High inspired oxygen levels are also implicated in retinopathy of prematurity.

Table 4.1 Typical settings for conventional ventilation.

Oxygen	40–50%
Inspiratory time	0.8–0.6 seconds
Expiratory time	0.8–0.6 seconds
I:E ratio	1:1
Rate	37–50/minute
Inspiratory pressure (PIP)	18–20 cmH$_2$O
Expiratory pressure (PEEP)	4 cmH$_2$O
Gas flow	8 litres/minutes

Making changes in the ventilator settings

Initial settings for the ventilator for an admission of a new-born baby are seen in Table 4.1. These will be adjusted to meet the needs of the baby after taking blood gas readings.

Settings should only be changed in response to blood gas readings. Exceptions to this rule are emergency alterations made in rate and pressure during sudden collapse or deterioration. Inspired oxygen percentage may also be increased or decreased according to the baby's immediate needs during suction, handling or crying.

Alterations in rate or pressure should be followed by blood gas assessment in one hour or less if the baby is still in obvious difficulty. Ideally a ventilated baby should have an arterial umbilical catheter or peripheral arterial line inserted for the accurate measurement of blood gases. The baby does not then have to suffer frequent heel stabbing for capillary samples, which can be unreliable in cases of hypotension, poor peripheral perfusion and cold stress.

Blood gases

Blood taken for gases reveals the state of exchange of oxygen and carbon dioxide gases in the lungs. Blood is taken from capillary samples, usually from the heel, or from arterial blood from a peripheral or umbilical line. At least 4-hourly checks are needed during the acute stage of the illness, so that ventilatory changes can be made to improve gases or wean down the ventilation. Results are compared with the normal readings expected (Table 4.2).

If the pH falls below 7.25, a metabolic acidosis results, which halts the production of surfactant. It can be corrected by an infusion of colloid, fresh frozen plasma or human albumin or more rarely by the use of sodium bicarbonate infusion.

If the gases show low PaO$_2$, the inspired oxygen should be raised. If this does not help, the PEEP and/or the rate can be raised.

If the PaCO$_2$ is high then there are three actions which could help:

- If it is very high the baby may need hand bagging to reduce the level.
- The ventilator rate can be increased to blow it off.
- The peak inspiratory pressure may be raised.

If the PaCO$_2$ is low, under 4.5 kPa, the baby may be over ventilated and needs lower rates and pressures.

Table 4.2 Normal blood gases.

pH	7.35–7.45
PaO^2	50–70 mmHg, 6–10 kPa
$PaCO_2$	35–45 mmHg, 4.5–6.5 kPa
Bicarbonate	18–25 µmol/l

Management

The aim is to improve lung function and get the baby weaned on to low settings as soon as possible to lessen the risk of lung damage and repeated chest infections.

NURSING A BABY ON CONVENTIONAL VENTILATION

All babies on ventilatory support are initially acutely ill and as such require expert nursing by experienced staff to maximise their potential. Good nursing care at this stage reduces mortality and morbidity by initiating prompt intervention when problems occur. Vigilance is essential and no ventilated baby should be left unattended. If the tube blocks or the baby deteriorates it must be seen and acted on immediately.

Ventilated babies are nursed in an incubator or in a cot with an overhead heater. They must be nursed in a neutral thermal environment which is the temperature at which least oxygen and energy are needed. To assess ideal temperature, neonatal incubators have a servo-control mode which will keep the baby's temperature around 37°C.

Minimal handling is essential as any disturbance may increase or decrease vital signs, oxygen and temperature levels. Vital signs, ventilator settings and fluid balance should be recorded hourly. Nursing a baby on a ventilator will encompass:

- Intubating the baby
- Observations to check deterioration on the ventilator
- Care of the endotracheal tube
- Blood pressure monitoring
- Nutrition
- Drugs
- Positioning and comfort
- Care of a paralysed baby
- Supporting parents
- Weaning off ventilation
- Extubation of the baby

Intubation

The baby may have been intubated on the labour ward and will be admitted with an endotracheal tube already in place. Others will need an endotracheal tube inserted on the unit. A trolley containing the basic items for emergency intubation and resuscitation should always be ready for use in neonatal units.

When the decision is taken to intubate a baby the equipment will include:

- The correct size tube and holder (Table 4.3). An introducer if used.
- A laryngoscope with bright bulb and a suitable size blade.
- A scalpel to cut the tube to the correct size.
- Tapes to secure.
- A hat if used to attach the tube holder.

Suction will be on and working with a clean suction catheter attached. The baby's stomach is emptied of air that might have accumulated from a previous hand bagging. If milk feeds have been given, the stomach should be aspirated to prevent vomiting during intubation. When ready the baby will be placed on

Table 4.3 Endotracheal tube (ETT) sizes.	
Baby's weight	**ETT size**
< 1000 g	2.5 mm
1000–2000 g	3.0 mm
2000–3000 g	3.0 or 3.5 mm
> 3000 g	3.5 mm

the back with the neck extended while the tube is inserted by a paediatrician or neonatal nurse practitioner.

After insertion, a stethoscope auscultation of both sides of the chest, while the baby is hand bagged, will ascertain the position of the tube. When the tube position is correct and the baby's saturations improved, the tube is secured in the normal way. Some units use holders which can be threaded with tapes and attached to a hat, others use strapping to secure the tubes (Fig. 4.4).

A chest X-ray should be taken to ascertain the length and position of the tube. Tube changes should only take place if there is a deterioration in the baby's condition or if the tube is obviously blocked with secretions. Intubation is a very traumatic event for the baby. If the tube is too short, it is in danger of slipping out of the lungs into the oesophagus. It may not always be necessary to re-intubate unless the baby is not being efficiently ventilated. A note should be made to cut the next tube to a longer length. If the tube is too long it could slip down into one of the bronchi. This will then cause over-inflation of the lung on that side. Small, firm, cotton wool wads or dental rolls will raise the tube into the correct position. The next tube passed should then be cut shorter.

Deterioration on the ventilator

Nursing observation of vital signs is an intrinsic part of the care. Sudden deteriora-

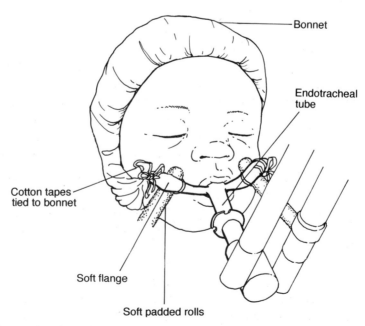

Fig. 4.4 Fixing of an oral endotracheal tube.

tions may be obvious but small changes may occur that may lead to major problems if not dealt with promptly.

Sudden deterioration on the ventilator with a fall in PaO_2 and rise in $PaCO_2$ may be caused by displaced or blocked endotracheal tube or pneumothorax. Slower deterioration accompanied by a slow fall in PaO_2 and rise in $PaCO_2$ may also be caused by the above factors or by the baby breathing against the ventilator. Other likely causes include intraventricular haemorrhage, patent ductus arteriosus, infection, hypotension, anaemia, metabolic imbalance, over-handling. These causes can be checked on and eliminated or corrected.

Blocked airway

When the airway is blocked or the tube is out of position there will be a sudden drop in oxygen saturations possibly accompanied by bradycardia, there may be no movement of the chest wall. Emergency treatment will involve detaching the endotracheal tube from the ventilator tubing and using a manual ventilation bag with oxygen to ventilate the endotracheal tube.

The baby's stomach should be emptied to prevent vomiting and aspiration. The chest should be auscultated for air entry. If the endotracheal tube is in the stomach, it should be removed forthwith and the baby reintubated. If the tube has slipped into either left or right bronchus, the problem may be relieved by lifting the tube with small cotton wool pads or dental rolls.

Hand bagging

It is important to use the correct size resuscitation bag. A small bag should be used for tiny babies to prevent lung damage from too much pressure. It is easy to cause a pneumothorax by over vigorous use. A larger baby will need a bigger bag to ensure adequate pressure. Ideally each ventilated baby should be provided with a bag. If this is not possible, at least two different sized bags properly connected to oxygen for emergency use should be available on a nearby resuscitation trolley. Bagging should commence with a rate similar to that of the ventilator and increased if this does not bring the oxygen saturation levels up quickly.

The endotracheal tube can be irrigated with saline in an attempt to clear it. This may be needed more than once if there are a lot of thick secretions. The hand bagging should continue in between each suctioning so that the baby does not get hypoxic. If the tube does not clear the baby will need re-intubating.

Care of the endotracheal tube

Maintaining patency of the airway is paramount in preventing hypoxia and enabling efficient ventilation to take place.

Endotracheal tube suction

The purpose of suctioning the endotracheal tube is to remove airway secretions in order to prevent obstruction, lung damage and decreased lung compliance. This should improve oxygenation and ventilation. Suction is an important part of the care of the baby on the ventilator. However, suction has the potential to cause hypoxia, lung damage, periventricular haemorrhage and infection so should be done with care and knowledge.

Frequency
Suctioning the endotracheal tube should not be carried out routinely as it is a traumatic event for the baby, causing bradycardia, drop in oxygen levels and often a long recovery

time afterwards. The need for suction should be assessed on increasing oxygen needs, alterations in heart or respiratory rates, if there are visible secretions in the endotracheal tube, or if the gases show rising $PaCO_2$ levels which could mean that the tube is blocked.

Oxygen saturation

When suctioning a baby the endotracheal tube is detached from the ventilator so that no oxygen is being delivered to the airway. The airway is then blocked by the catheter used and suctioning removes the oxygen that is there, causing hypoxia. Hodge (1991) found that pre-oxygenation of 10–20% above the maintenance oxygen level for about 1 min before suction and continued afterwards till the baby had regained pre-suctioning heart rate and saturations, stopped hypoxia during suction. The problem with increasing the oxygen is the risk of retinopathy of prematurity for the preterm baby. A careful watch must be kept on the saturations and the oxygen level turned down as soon as possible.

Depth of suction

Deep endotracheal suction, which passes the end of the tube, can cause mucosal damage and bradycardia from vagal nerve stimulation. Ideally each baby should have a tape-measure cut to the length of the endotracheal tube as a guide for measuring the depth of suction, allowance will be made for the holder of the tube. The suction catheter is gently but swiftly passed to the measured depth. If the catheter meets any obstruction it should be withdrawn 0.5 cm, to prevent mucosal damage, before suction is applied.

Size and type of catheter

A catheter with a side eye should be used as those with the hole at the end cause greater mucosal damage. A catheter of too large a size can result in negative pressure being generated during suction and completely occluding the airway for the duration of the suction (Young 1995). Too small a catheter will not remove the secretions efficiently (Table 4.4).

Table 4.4 Suggested sizes of suction catheter.

Endotracheal tube size	Catheter size
2.5–3.5 mm	6 Fr
4–5 mm	8 Fr

Pressure and duration of suction

The suction catheters should be attached to negative pressure suction ideally with a Y connection. This will ensure that the end is not occluded until the catheter is being withdrawn from the suction area.

The recommended pressure is no more than 50–100 mmHg (Hodge 1991; Young 1995) to prevent mucosal damage. It has not been demonstrated that raising the pressure increases the volume of the secretions removed.

The length of time for which the baby is removed from the ventilator, while the catheter is introduced into the endotracheal tube, suction is applied and the catheter withdrawn, should be as short as possible. The actual duration of the negative pressure during the insertion is recommended as no more than 15 seconds (Runton 1992).

Irrigation of the endotracheal tube

Many NNUs irrigate the endotracheal tube to facilitate the removal of secretions, most use 0.9% normal saline (Young 1995). It has been claimed that the giving of warmed humidified oxygen makes this practice unnecessary and may be responsible for adverse responses such as hypoxaemia and epithelial damage. However each baby should be assessed to determine whether instillation of saline is required. If secretions are thick and sticky, saline irrigation may be necessary to loosen or dilute them so that they can be removed from the endotracheal tube.

It has not been proved that aseptic technique is an essential pre-requisite of suctioning. Wearing gloves on both hands does, however, reduce the introduction of hand-borne infections into the endotracheal tube and gloves should be worn as part of universal precautions taken against infection.

Maintenance of blood pressure and blood volume

Babies with severe respiratory problems are often hypotensive during the first hours of life. This hypotension may be caused by depression of cardiac function by severe metabolic disturbance and hypoxaemia or due to hypovolaemia. The use of albumin, plasma and inotropic drugs such as dopamine or dobutamine may be required to stabilise the blood pressure and increase blood volume. Disturbances in blood pressure are implicated in damage to renal function and in the increased incidence of intraventricular haemorrhage.

Arterial lines

The insertion of an arterial line is a widely used practice which allows regular blood gas analysis and blood sampling. Blood pressure monitoring can take place on this line if a transducer is fitted. The advantage for the baby is that there does not have to be repeated capillary sampling taken by heel stab.

A peripheral artery or the umbilical artery can be used for cannulation. Both kinds of artery cannulation carry complications and need to be carefully managed.

Peripheral arterial line

If the cord is too dry to use, or is impossible to cannulate, a peripheral artery is used. The usual sites are the radial or tibial arteries, which can be located by palpation or transillumination.

The cannula is inserted until blood flows freely back when the stilette is withdrawn. It can then be gently flushed with saline. If the limb blanches, the catheter should be withdrawn, as peripheral ischaemia can occur, causing damage to the blood supply with possible loss of fingers or toes. When taping an arterial catheter the fingers and toes should always be visible for observation. If any discoloration occurs the line should be removed.

The catheter is connected to a blood pressure transducer for monitoring and a syringe of heparinised saline to keep the artery patent. The catheter should be attached to the infusion line with a tube that has a Luer-Lok seal on it to prevent accidental disconnection as arterial lines pulse in time to the heart beat and blood pumps out when the line is disconnected.

When the line is removed, the heparin infusion should be stopped for at least an hour before removal so that the blood will clot more easily on removal. Manual pressure will be needed for 2 or 3 min after removal to ensure bleeding has stopped.

Umbilical arterial line

This is a more invasive technique, but the line lasts longer than peripheral lines so preventing repeated resitings. One of the umbilical arteries is cannulated using aseptic technique. The base of the cord is tied to prevent blood loss and sliced cleanly above the tie, with a scalpel, to bring the artery clearly into view. A

3.5 or 5 Fr catheter is inserted into the artery and slowly advanced into the aorta (Fig. 4.5). Success occurs when the blood flows freely back up the catheter. The catheter is then secured using a stitch or two into the rim of the umbilical skin. A protective plastic spray is sometimes used to prevent bleeding. The position of the catheter is checked by X-ray. When this has been verified the line is kept patent by a continuous infusion of 0.5–1 ml per hour of heparin and saline. The baby should not be nursed prone as the catheter might loosen and bleed unnoticed.

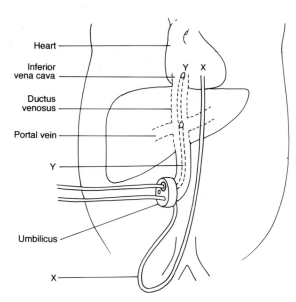

Fig. 4.5 Umbilical catheters *in situ*, arterial X and venous Y. (Adapted from Halliday *et al.* (1989).)

Umbilical artery catheters are thought to be implicated in causing necrotising enterocolitis (NEC). Research to date has resulted in conflicting evidence. There is some thought that if the position of the catheter is too low it may compromise the blood flow in the mesenteric arteries contributing to NEC but this has not been borne out in trials (Kempley *et al.* 1993). Many units are wary of giving a baby with such a line oral feeds because of the risk of infection in the catheter which might cause necrotising enterocolitis (Morgan 1992). The usual practice is to wait until the line is removed to begin feeding.

There is always the risk of thrombosis and infection round the site. Meticulous attention should be paid to the area round the catheter and the perfusion to the lower limbs. If there is reddening or swelling of the abdomen, the catheter should be removed promptly. The legs and feet must be checked the whole time the catheter is *in situ*, for if the artery goes into a spasm the blood supply to the lower limbs could be damaged. This will be indicated by the legs blanching or turning blue. The catheter should be removed immediately to prevent permanent damage.

Removal of catheter

When the catheter is to be removed the heparin infusion should be switched off for at least an hour to encourage clotting in the artery. A ligature is tied around the umbilical stump and when the catheter has been removed the ligature can be tightened. Also the catheter should be withdrawn slowly, and a minute or two should pass before the end is removed – to allow the artery to go into spasm and minimise bleeding.

Nutrition

Providing sufficient calories for growth and to overcome the illness is an important part of neonatal care. An appropriate fluid balance and calorie intake must be maintained so that the infant grows and matures. Oral feeding by nasogastric tube is not contraindicated by ventilation unless the baby is very sick or unstable. A central venous line is sited in very small babies so that sufficient calories can be given for good growth (see Chapter 10).

Drugs

Babies who need high rates and pressures should be sedated and paralysed to maximise lung compliance and prevent complications such as pneumothorax and intercranial haemorrhage caused by the stress of breathing against the ventilator.

Broad-spectrum antibiotic cover should be given to all infants requiring ventilation, after blood cultures are taken, to ensure that the respiratory distress is not caused by a bacterial pathogen. This treatment can be discontinued if the blood cultures are negative for bacterial growth. The choice of antibiotic varies according to unit policy.

Aminophylline is given to prevent apnoea in babies who are being weaned off ventilation. It is given by intravenous infusion at first but when the baby is taking milk feeds oral theophylline can be given. Fentanyl intravenous infusion can be given for pain and sedation during the critical stage of the illness and to combat the anxiety caused by treatment. Pancuronium bromide is used to paralyse babies who are on high rates and pressures. This drug paralyses the muscles but has no analgesic effect and should only be used in conjunction with pain relief.

Positioning and comfort

Ill babies on ventilatory support should be handled as little as possible. Handling often destabilises vital signs and causes valuable resources of calories and oxygen to be used as the baby gets exhausted. Babies take a long time to recover from interactions and need uninterrupted sleep to gain weight, keep oxygen requirements to a minimum and have normal behavioural patterns. The aim should be to do routine hygiene needs, suction and position changes when the baby is awake.

These interventions need only take place at every 6–8 hours to prevent pressure sores and improve flexion and tension movements.

Babies not receiving intravenous pain relief may show signs of distress indicated by an anxious or anguished expression, restlessness, or fixed staring gaze and diminished alertness (Sparshott 1996). Careful positioning and comforting can help settle the baby and oral or rectal drugs can be given to relieve pain.

Care of a paralysed infant

A paralysed baby cannot make any voluntary effort to breathe and will need hand bagging immediately if the endotracheal tube becomes displaced. For the paralysis to have maximum success, the paralysing agent should be given as soon as movement of the eyelids or tongue is noted.

Secretions from the ETT and nasopharynx tend to be copious and thick when using paralysis, so frequent suction is needed. Pain relief must be continuous and adequate for the baby's size and weight. The baby's position will need to be changed 6–8 hourly and attention given to pressure areas. Limbs should be put gently through a series of movements, flexion and tension, to ensure joints are correctly aligned. The baby cannot blink so the eyes must be protected with drops of artificial tears such as hypromellose, to keep the corneas moist. Paraffin gauze can be used to prevent dust entering the eyes.

Supporting parents

Parents are always worried when their baby needs help to breathe and need simple information at first about their baby's illness. The monitors and their functions can be explained to help them orientate themselves, although not all parents wish to know these facts. Some parents worry that if their baby is on paralysing drugs there may be after-effects and they need reassurance. All questions and worries must be answered openly and in non-medical words.

Sometimes the baby will remain ventilated for many weeks with frequent improvements and setbacks. Parents need to talk to senior doctors and nursing staff frequently to discuss treatment and their fears for the future. There may be relationship problems between the parents. The father may have to return to work and the mother may not have transport to visit. There may be problems expressing milk and the mother can get demoralised. Involving parents in the care of their baby is essential though they may be nervous of harming the baby at first. They can be encouraged to touch and talk, choose the clothes for changing, freshen the baby with a top and tail wash at nappy changes. Expressing milk for the baby gives a psychological boost to many mothers.

The emotional behaviour of the parents needs to be carefully monitored so that counselling can be offered if appropriate. Parents sometimes need to talk and air their grievances away from the baby and taken to a quiet area off the unit for a chat with the family support sister. Sometimes parent support groups can help in these cases. These groups usually consist of parents who have been through the same traumas and can understand the day-to-day worries.

Weaning off conventional ventilation

As the blood gases improve, the rate, pressures and oxygen levels on the ventilator are decreased. Paralysing drugs are discontinued and sedation reduced. When the rate is five breaths a minute and the oxygen under 35%

the baby may be extubated to nasal CPAP or head box oxygen (Fleming *et al.* 1991).

Extubation

Before the extubation the baby will be made comfortable and clean and left to rest, to cut down on handling afterwards. Feeds may be stopped for a few hours according to unit policy, some units do this for 4 hours, others for 12 hours. This is done to prevent any abdominal distension from feeding which will embarrass respiratory effort and to prevent vomiting and subsequent aspiration. Intravenous fluids should be used over this period to ensure energy intake and maintenance of blood sugar.

The baby may be progressing to nasal prong CPAP or headbox oxygen so the necessary equipment should be made ready before extubation. If nasal CPAP is to be used, a prong should be cut and set in the holder or the 'piggy' prongs obtained if the baby is very small. If using a head box with humidified oxygen, the head box, humidifier and oxygen analyser should be connected and ready.

Extubation should ideally be carried out by two people so that it can be unhurried and less stressful for the baby. A bag and mask should be ready in case the baby becomes apnoeic and the suction ready. When all is ready the endotracheal tube fastenings are undone and the tube detached from the ventilator. The suction catheter is then introduced, suction applied and the catheter withdrawn bringing the endotracheal tube with it.

If CPAP is to be used the prong is inserted immediately and CPAP commenced or the baby is put into head box oxygen. The baby will be turned prone temporarily to facilitate respiration. The tip of the ETT tube can be kept sterile and sent for culture if this is unit policy. If the baby becomes apnoeic on removal of the tube, re-intubation will take place immediately.

The baby should be left to rest for a few hours after extubation, remaining monitored and carefully observed. If there are apnoeas, bradycardias or rising oxygen requirements blood gases should be checked.

Low flow oxygen

Low flow oxygen is often used in the first few days after extubation instead of head box oxygen to allow the baby to move easily and feel comfortable. Low flow oxygen is also used intermittently with treatment on the flow driver for chronically lung damaged babies. Low flow oxygen therapy is often essential for the chronically lung damaged baby and may be needed for months or years.

Oxygen is given through a commercial nasal cannula and tube set, or a number 8 feeding tube with strategic holes cut at the nostrils. The end is attached to a low flow oxygen meter which is graduated into parts of a litre so that very small amounts of oxygen can be given. Some babies need just a trickle for weeks others will need it only at feed times or when deeply asleep and breathing shallowly. Most babies cope quite happily with the cannula or tube and can be handled and positioned freely by parents and staff. Bathing and feeding are no problem as long as the oxygen flow is not interrupted.

There are a number of factors to be taken into consideration when using low flow oxygen treatment.

Monitoring
Oxygen should be given in measurable quantities and the results evaluated. Too much oxygen can cause retinopathy of prematurity and possible blindness. Too little will cause hypoxia, worsening the lung problem and contributing to neurological problems. The oxygen given must be monitored and this is done using a saturation monitor. The monitor has a light emitter and a light sensor probe which should be fastened round a hand or foot with the emitter and the sensor opposite each other. If the baby is very small it can be used on the ankle or wrist.

A saturation monitor measures how much haemoglobin has been converted to oxyhaemoglobin. When all haemoglobin has been converted to oxyhaemoglobin it is said to be fully oxygenated or 100% saturated. Though there are no safe limits, it is universally recognised that the saturations should not be consistently allowed to stay higher than 96% or frequently drop lower than 90% (Greenough 1994). If this happens fleetingly when the baby moves there is no need for concern but the trend should be in the range of 90% to 96%. If the baby needs increasing amounts of oxygen to keep the saturations within this range, investigations need to be done to ascertain the cause. It could be due to:

- Infection
- Anaemia
- Worsening lung disease

A chest X-ray will show any worsening of the lung disease. Blood gases will be measured to assess lung function. A full blood count can be done to reveal anaemia. Blood cultures will be taken if infection is suspected.

Treatment will depend on the result of the investigations. There may be a combination of factors that need treatment. A blood transfusion will be given for anaemia and antibiotics given for infection. If the lung function is seriously compromised, the baby may benefit from being intubated and re-ventilated for a time.

Progress

Progress will take place in stages as the baby puts on weight and lung function improves. Less oxygen will be needed until the baby is in air at all times. Sometimes oxygen may be needed only during sucking feeds or when asleep. Continuous monitoring is necessary throughout these stages. When the baby has been in air for a few days monitoring can be discontinued and test runs given at feed times for assessment. The baby needs to be off oxygen for at least a week before discharge is considered.

Parents

The parents who have watched their baby graduate from ventilator to flow driver and from head box oxygen to low flow oxygen will be pleased and happy that at last they can safely handle their baby. The saturation monitor does have its drawbacks for many parents as they tend to be anxious about fluctuations in saturations as the baby moves, most learn to accept these with reassurance and guidance.

An advantage of the development of low flow oxygen treatment is that if there is a community service from the unit, the baby can be discharged while still needing oxygen. The baby will have to be gaining weight and sucking all feeds before discharge, and the community team can set up the equipment in the parents' home and supervise the treatment.

OTHER TREATMENTS FOR RESPIRATORY PROBLEMS

Improvements in the technology of ventilators and the management of ventilation have greatly contributed to the survival rate of the sick newborn baby. There is, however, often a cost to the baby. The development of bronchopulmonary dysplasia and chronic lung disease is directly linked to barotrauma from artificial ventilation. Methods which aim to mitigate or prevent this are constantly being researched.

High frequency oscillatory ventilation (HFOV)

There will inevitably be some babies who will not make progress on conventional ventilation and those who will deteriorate. High rates and pressures cause physiological and morphological changes in the lung due to the over distension of the alveoli. High frequency oscillatory ventilation appears to have the potential for altering the outcome for these severely ill patients.

High frequency ventilation is being increasingly used in neonatal units for cases of respiratory failure. The effective gas exchange at a lower tidal volume and peak inspiratory pressure is thought to reduce long term lung trauma, air leaks and the development of bronchopulmonary dysplasia seen when using conventional ventilation (Martin 1995).

High frequency oscillatory ventilation is a method of mechanical ventilation that uses supraphysiological breathing rates and tidal volumes. It prevents further collapse of the alveoli and improves poorly aerated areas of the lung in sick babies especially those with respiratory distress syndrome (HFOV Study Group 1993).

The breaths are delivered by a vibrating diaphragm which provides both positive inspiration and active exhalation. Frequency of breathing is expressed in hertz (Hz). One Hz equals 60 breaths a minute. Commonly used frequencies are 10–15 Hz which give

600–900 breaths a minute. Hertz rate is responsible for enhancing gas distribution in the lungs (Avila *et al.* 1994).

Mean airway pressure (MAP) is used to recruit and maintain lung volume. Mean airway pressure directly affects oxygenation by improving lung volume and is reduced as the baby improves. Alterations to this parameter are made by adjusting the expiratory valve or the oxygen flow rate.

Oscillatory amplitude, also called the delta pressure, determines peak and trough pressure and the tidal volume delivered to the baby. The relationship between the oscillatory amplitude and hertz, controls carbon dioxide elimination (Avila *et al.* 1994). Oscillatory amplitude is increased when levels are high and decreased when low. The I:E ratio is normally left at 1:2. There are no limitations on oxygen administration. MAP improves oxygenation and this should be increased rather than the oxygen except in emergency. If there is lung hyperinflation on X-ray, oxygen should be increased rather than the MAP to prevent pneumothorax.

Making changes in HFOV

The expanded lung volume is assessed by counting the ribs above the diaphragm on X-ray. Adequate expansion is suggested by a diaphragm at or below the eighth rib (Trotter & Carey 1992). Oxygen levels and X-ray assessment of lung volume are used to guide adjustments to ventilator settings (Table 4.5).

Nursing a baby on HFOV

The physical assessment of a baby on HFOV presents different aspects to the nurse. New skills and an alteration of those learnt from using conventional ventilation are necessary. The baby will have the same type of endotracheal tube and connectors as for conventional ventilation but different assessments will be made about chest wall movement, behavioural state and colour.

During this ventilation, vibrations of the chest wall must be even to give good gas exchange. The Sensor Medics ventilator has a centring light that can be checked after turning or moving the baby for X-ray. Small changes in symmetry and rates of vibration are critical and can result in significant alteration in ventilation if left unchecked.

Chest auscultation is difficult because of the vibrations. It can be done when necessary by putting the ventilator alarm on standby for 5–10 seconds and switching off briefly to

Table 4.5 Parameters and their management in high frequency oscillatory ventilation.

Parameters	Management
Hertz (breathing frequency)	Constant 10–15
MAP (mean airway pressure)	Increase to improve PaO_2 and lung expansion
Oscillatory amplitude	Increase to reduce $PaCO_2$ levels
I:E ratio	Constant 1:2
FiO_2 (inspired oxygen)	Increase if PaO_2 low with good lung expansion

listen. This should not be done frequently as the alveoli may recollapse when the ventilator is off.

The need for suctioning can be assessed as for conventional ventilation by gauging oxygen saturations, blood gases or secretions in the ETT. Suctioning can be done by using an ETT indwelling catheter so that the ventilator does not have to be disconnected. This type of suction has to carried out with care. If the catheter is not fully retracted after suction, it can block the airway (Avila *et al.* 1994).

Positioning and comfort

Some babies will be nursed on the Sensor Medics high frequency oscillatory ventilator which has a long rigid arm from the ventilator to the endotracheal tube so more attention needs to be paid to positioning. The rigid arm must be kept straight and slightly tilted downwards to the ventilator so that circuit condensation can flow away from the baby. Moving the baby for X-ray and position changes on this ventilator needs the assistance of two or three people to prevent accidental ETT dislodgement.

Sedation and paralysis are given following an assessment of the baby's condition. Not all babies need sedation and paralysis on this type of ventilation and appear relaxed and comfortable. There are no contraindications to feeding a baby who is able to tolerate nasogastric feeds.

Weaning off HFOV

Eight-hourly chest X-rays and blood gas measurements allow assessment of lung function. When this starts to improve changes can be made in mean airway pressure, amplitude and oxygen rates. Any alteration in settings must be made very gradually involving only one setting at a time to avoid significant fluctuations in blood gases.

When the amplitude, which determines the tidal volume delivered to the baby, has been reduced to zero and the mean airway pressure to 12 or below, the baby is effectively on CPAP and can then be extubated and put on head box oxygen.

Complications of HFOV

The most common complication is lung overinflation. This may result from inappropriate settings or from failure to make changes in the settings when improvement occurs. Chest X-ray will confirm this but decreases in blood pressure, poor perfusion, colour changes, increases or decreases in heart rate may herald the problem. There may be decreased cardiac output if the mean airway pressure is high (HFOV Study Group 1993) which will cause hypotension needing colloids and inotropic support.

Parents

A baby nursed on HFOV is usually very sick and may have proceeded from head box oxygen, CPAP and conventional ventilation. The parents will quite naturally be distressed at the disasters that seem to be happening to their baby and need support and reassurance. It may be difficult for them to understand this type of ventilation and open communication is essential as usual. Parents must always be involved in treatment and encouraged to participate as they feel able in hygiene and comfort needs.

Extra-corporeal membrane exchange (ECMO)

ECMO is a life support system whereby the patient is placed on cardiopulmonary bypass for an average of 10–14 days using thoracic cannulation. It was introduced into the UK in 1989 from America (UK ECMO trial group 1996). It is an expensive treatment requiring a team of highly trained staff for each baby.

ECMO is used to provide temporary oxygenation for babies in respiratory distress who fail to respond to current methods of ventilation. They are usually term babies and need to be over 2 kg to be able to withstand the treatment (Miller 1995). The babies are always gravely ill with meconium aspiration, respiratory distress, persistent pulmonary hypertension, diaphragmatic hernia, or sepsis.

To meet the criteria for ECMO at the current time, babies must be over 34 weeks gestation, in acute respiratory failure and with no evidence of cerebral haemorrhage or life-shortening congenital anomaly (Davenport & Homes 1995).

When the treatment has been successfully carried out the baby is transferred back to the regional centre on conventional ventilation until the lungs recover sufficiently for extubation.

Five centres took part in a randomised trial from 1993 to 1995 to find out if ECMO was cost effective (Davenport & Holmes 1995). Babies who needed this treatment were recruited from regional hospitals and transferred to one of these centres. The result of the ECMO survey was that this kind of support should be actively considered for neonates with severe but potentially treatable respiratory failure (UK ECMO Trial Group 1996). The outcome for surviving babies is good with no developmental problems associated with the increased survival, in America, at one year follow-up (Underman Boggs 1993). The UK trial bore this out and will follow up their patients to school age and beyond.

Nitric oxide

This should not be confused with nitrous oxide used for anaesthetic purposes. Nitric oxide (NO) is a highly diffusible, colourless gas with a sweet sharp odour. It has a vapour density similar to air. Nitric oxide is present in human exhaled gas and this prompted researchers to study all aspects of it. Nitric oxide is produced naturally in the vascular endothelium and acts as a vasodilator when needed. In some diseases such as persistent pulmonary hypertension of the newborn (PPHN) there appears to be a decreased ability to produce this substance (Mitchell 1996). This results in constriction of the pulmonary arteries and a severe hypoxia, which is difficult to treat.

The advantage of giving NO over other forms of vasodilator is that it selectively acts on the lungs and is quickly inactivated leaving no systemic effect. NO acts as a localised pulmonary vasodilator when introduced into the alveoli diffusing directly across the alveolar cell walls, acting on and reducing pulmonary vascular resistance. It is easy and cheap to administer through ventilator tubing and giving NO with the ventilator gases dilates the pulmonary arteries improving oxygenation. Pulmonary shunting is decreased and perfusion enhanced. The treatment has shown great promise for babies suffering PPHN or who are too small for ECMO.

NO can be given with conventional or high frequency oscillatory ventilation, though high frequency ventilation is recommended (Greenough 1995). A cylinder of compressed NO gas is adapted into the ventilator circuit and titrated by a calibrated flow meter into the inspiratory line.

NO combines with oxygen to form toxic nitrogen dioxide, exposure to which can suppress platelet adhesion and aggregation and cause an increase in bleeding time. It must be diluted to the required concentration just before inhalation to limit oxygen contact and is given as near the baby as possible. Expired gas from the ventilator circuit is chemically scavenged to prevent occupational exposure to nitrogen dioxide.

The gas is given for short periods of 24 hours to prevent toxicity and adverse effects as it can inhibit platelet aggregation causing haemorrhagic complications (Miller 1995). Careful weaning is necessary to prevent sudden severe pulmonary vasoconstriction and arterial desaturation. As it has a short duration of action, a back-up device should be available if the cylinder runs out.

This treatment is seen as having immense potential for reducing pulmonary vascular resistance and improving oxygenation and may be the treatment of choice in the future for conditions involving this problem. At the time of writing nitric oxide is only used for clear-cut life saving interventions because of the side-effects and lack of medical quality nitric oxide available (Greenough 1995). A multi-centre trial is in progress at the present time (1997) to decide the best ways of using nitric oxide.

High frequency jet ventilation (HFJV)

The most fundamental difference between high frequency jet ventilation and conventional ventilation is the low tidal gas flow volume of 1–3 ml/kg needed instead of the conventional 6–10 ml/kg. It is used with conventional ventilation which provides the oxygenation and mechanical breaths. During HFJV, inspiratory flow streaming carries more gas into the alveoli and respiratory bronchioles, increasing gas exchange. Inspired gases flow down the centre of the airway while exhaled gases flow closer to the wall of the airway.

The HFJV promotes gas exchange and the removal of carbon dioxide (Allen *et al.* 1995). The ventilator contains a microprocessor that automatically regulates the internal pressure until the desired peak inspiratory pressure (PIP) is reached. It can provide an alternative to conventional ventilation for infants suffering from pulmonary airleaks or as an intermediate step to ECMO. A study done in America found that the use of HFJV in respiratory distress syndrome in very low birth weight preterm babies resulted in more adverse outcomes than in those treated with conventional ventilation (Wiswell *et al.* 1996).

Liquid ventilation

Liquid ventilation is based on introducing oxygenated perfluorochemical liquid (PFC) into the lungs. This liquid is non-toxic, absorbs respiratory gases and minimises surface tension (Greenspan 1993). It provides effective gas exchange and improves lung mechanics at low pressures because elimination of the high surface tension decreases alveolar pressures. This has the potential to reduce or eliminate complications caused by gas ventilation. Potential applications include surfactant deficiencies, persistent pulmonary hypertension, meconium aspiration, diaphragmatic hernia, pneumonia and as a vehicle for drug delivery (Cox *et al.* 1996).

The baby will be intubated and during inspiration, oxygenated PFC fluid is pumped from the fluid reservoir by a cardiovascular pump through a heat exchanger. This oxygenates the liquid and removes carbon dioxide by a counterflow of oxygen/air mixture from a blender. From the gas exchanger the oxygenated PFC is returned to the fluid reservoir and the ventilation cycle is repeated (Cox *et al.* 1996). Any vapour is condensed and returned to the system. The system can work in combination with ECMO or as an alternative.

Liquid ventilation is an exciting new advance in ventilatory techniques but is in the preliminary stages of clinical trials as yet and not generally used in the UK.

COMPLICATIONS OF ALL TYPES OF VENTILATION

Air leaks

Babies who are already very ill with a respiratory disease, ventilated on high rates and pressures are prone to air leaks. An air leak occurs when some of the alveoli collapse letting the air they contained form a collection preventing efficient ventilation and oxygenation. Untreated, more alveoli will be affected, adequate exchange of gases will not be able to take place and the baby may die. It can occur in a ventilated baby, following active resuscitation or CPAP or occur spontaneously.

There are various types of air leak:

- Pneumothorax is the most common, affecting the alveoli of the lungs.
- Pulmonary interstitial emphysema is alveolar over-distension caused by mechanical ventilation and can be seen as bubbles of air throughout the lung on X-ray (Flores 1993).
- Air can leak out of the alveoli and gather around the heart causing pneumopericardium and affecting heart function, or it can collect behind the sternum causing pnuemomediastinum (see chapter 8).

Intraventricular haemorrhage

Sick preterm babies are prone to brain haemorrhage because the fragility of the cerebral vasculature makes it susceptible to changes in oxygenation, temperature and fluid intake (see Chapter 3).

Necrotising enterocolitis

The majority of cases of necrotising enterocolitis (NEC) are seen in sick, low birth weight babies. They have usually been ventilated and have often had arterial lines (see Chapter 5).

Bronchopulmonary dysplasia

Bronchopulmonary dysplasia (BPD) occurs in preterm babies who have needed prolonged ventilation and oxygen therapy. As a result lengthy hospital treatment is needed and often supplemental oxygen at home after discharge.

Aetiology

Bronchopulmonary dysplasia is a multifactorial disease with causes that include barotrauma from ventilator pressures, oxygen toxicity, surfactant deficiency and pulmonary immaturity (Knoppert & Mackanjee 1994). Other factors such as patent ductus arteriosus, pulmonary air leaks, pulmonary oedema, pulmonary infection and poor nutrition are also thought to contribute. The disease is seen more frequently in neonatal units today with the saving of more low birth weight babies. It is estimated that 50% of babies under 1 kg who have been ventilated develop the disease (Roberton 1993b). Many of these babies who are ventilated for a long time for chronic lung disease also have a poor neurological outcome (Wheater & Rennie 1994).

Diagnosis

Bronchopulmonary dysplasia is a chronic, inflammatory lung disease characterised by the need for supplemental oxygen beyond the neonatal period of 28 days. It varies in severity from mild cases that recover in a few months to severe inflammatory lung disease with associated long term morbidity.

If the baby is going to contract BPD there will be clinical and radiological signs by the age of 10–14 days. These signs include:

- The respiratory condition will stop improving or will deteriorate.
- The baby will be permanently dyspnoeic and may go into heart failure.
- Chest X-ray will show areas of collapse, emphysema and cystic formation.

Many babies improve with careful management but others will steadily deteriorate and become ventilator dependent. The definitive diagnosis of BPD is made when the baby has needed supplemental oxygen for more than 28 days, although the Osiris Collaborative Group (1992) suggests that this criterion should be altered to 28 days after the expected date of delivery not the age in days of a preterm baby.

Prevention

Prevention aims at first at averting or mitigating the respiratory problems (Table 4.6).

Steroids
Prenatal steroids will modify the severity of respiratory distress by helping to mature the lungs and improve surfactant production in the baby (Crowley *et al.* 1990).

Surfactant
Surfactant therapy at birth and soon after

Table 4.6 Management of bronchopulmonary dysplasia.

Prevention
  Prenatal steroids
  Surfactant therapy
  Closure of patent ductus arteriosus

Treatment
  Diuretics and fluid management
  Corticosteroids
  Blood transfusions
  Oxygen therapy
  Good nutrition

limits the severity of respiratory problems by increasing surfactant, so decreasing the severity of respiratory distress.

Closure of duct
The second aim of prevention is to treat respiratory problems promptly and aggressively and wean the baby off ventilation as soon as possible. Many small babies will maintain a ductus arteriosus from the fetal circulation, which can cause heart failure, increased oxygen requirements and the continuation of respiratory support. Closure can be effected by treating the heart failure with fluid restriction and diuretics or indomethacin (a prostaglandin synthesase inhibitor). This drug can cause side-effects that include gastrointestinal and intercranial bleeding, prolonged jaundice, decreased platelets and may be contraindicated if the baby is very small or sick (Fleming *et al.* 1991). The earlier the gestation of the baby the less likely the duct is to close on its own (Roberton 1993b) so if medical management fails surgical closure must be considered.

Treatment

Diuretics
Diuretics and restricted fluids help control pulmonary oedema and heart failure.

Corticosteroids
Steroids, in the form of dexamethasone, reduce inflammation in the lungs and shorten the duration of ventilatory support (Knoppert & Mackanjee 1994). The baby may need more than one course of steroids before the inflammation recedes sufficiently for ventilation to be discontinued. Before starting steroids the baby should be free of infection and the ductus arteriosus closed. Short term side-effects may include sepsis, hyperglycaemia, gastric bleeding and hypertension. Babies on steroidal treatment must have blood pressure and blood sugar checked at least twice a day while therapy continues.

At the time of writing a multicentre trial, Open Study of Early Corticosteroid Treatment (OSECT), is taking place to find out whether steroids should be given earlier to prevent or mitigate BPD. Earlier trials have not shown this to be the case but have led to the idea that a larger controlled trial may be more conclusive (Yeh *et al.* 1990; Shinwell *et al.* 1996).

Blood transfusions
Haemoglobin should be kept high with blood transfusions to maximise oxygenation of the blood and so lower inspired oxygen requirements.

Oxygen therapy
Oxygen therapy is important in the prevention of hypoxia and worsening of the lung condition. It is given by low flow cannula and carefully monitored.

Nutrition
Nutrition plays a vital part in the treatment of BPD, encouraging the growth of healthy lung tissue. It is also a major problem as growth is poor for a number of reasons:

- Raised metabolic rate caused by rapid respiration and the babies' characteristically fussy and unsettled behaviour.
- Vomiting thought to be caused by hypoxaemia, anorexia, drugs given, gastro-oesophageal reflux, rapid respiratory rate, poor exercise tolerance.
- Vitamin and mineral absorption may be a problem and mineral supplements such as calcium will be given for good bone growth.
- Fluid restriction may mean that extra calories have to be added to feeds for the baby to gain weight.

Long term prognosis

Often the babies are discharged home on supplemental oxygen and diuretics. Hospitalisations are frequent in the first year with chest infections and failure to thrive and there is a risk of developing fatal cor pulmonale from a combination of pulmonary oedema, intermittent hypoxaemia and lung fibrosis.

Maintaining medical and nutritional stability of these babies helps them to gain weight and achieve growth of new lung tissue. Lung function improves in the second and third year and many children will continue to improve until their eighth year (Hancock 1995). There are often developmental delays and neurological impairments especially for the very low birth weight babies (McCormick *et al.* 1996).

COMMON RESPIRATORY PROBLEMS

Respiratory problems encountered at birth in the neonatal unit are:

- Respiratory distress syndrome
- Birth asphyxia
- Meconium inhalation
- Persistent pulmonary hypertension of the new-born
- Pulmonary hypoplasia
- Congenital pneumonia
- Transient tachypnoea of the new-born (TTN)
- Choanal atresia
- Chronic pulmonary insufficiency of prematurity

Respiratory distress syndrome

Respiratory distress syndrome (RDS) is the most common problem in the NICU. It is a major factor in the morbidity and mortality of the neonatal population and is primarily a disease of the infant born before 36 weeks gestation. Approximately 10% of all preterm infants are affected, with the greatest incidence occurring in those weighing less than 1500 g (3 lb 5 oz) (Klaus & Fanaroff 1993). It warrants assisted ventilation in approximately 25% of infants born at 30 weeks. Susceptibility is believed to depend more on lung maturation than on gestational age (Avery 1994). Factors for some infants at 28 weeks gestation not developing the disease and for others at 38 weeks who do, are not fully understood.

In 1959 Avery and Mead found that respiratory distress syndrome in preterm babies is caused by a lack of pulmonary surfactant. Research and treatments relating to surfactant replacement are based on this discovery.

Antenatal intervention

Advances in neonatal intensive technology, ventilatory support and surfactant replacement therapy together with maternal fetal monitoring have dramatically decreased the incidence of RDS. Most recent preventative measures are the antenatal use of steroids to encourage surfactant production and the prophylactic use of exogenous surfactant. Other important preventative measures are more accurate assessment of gestational age by the use of antenatal ultrasound scanning and early intervention if continuous fetal monitoring is suggestive of fetal distress. The use of surfactant therapy alone has reduced the mortality rate from RDS by 30% to 50% (Roberton 1993b; Schwarz *et al.* 1994).

Delivery

Though respiratory distress syndrome is not always present at birth, it should be anticipated if the baby is preterm. An experienced paediatrician and a neonatal nurse practitioner/neonatal nurse should attend the delivery to resuscitate and ensure the baby is kept warm. A hypoxic preterm baby is immediately at risk of developing respiratory distress syndrome owing to the rapid deterioration in surfactant production caused by hypoxia. Some units give surfactant prophylactically in the labour ward during resuscitation. Others wait for clinical evidence of the disease.

Clinical presentation

The symptoms of RDS may appear immediately following birth or may develop during the first few hours of life. The disease process usually reaches its peak severity at 48–72 hours (Levene & Tudehope 1993).

As the disease progresses, more oxygen is needed due to the increased effort in breathing, tachypneoa, a respiratory rate greater than 60 breaths per minute. An expiratory grunt is a typical sign of respiratory distress and means the baby is breathing against a closed glottis in a physiological effort to prevent the alveoli from closing. There is chest recession and nasal flaring bringing in the accessory muscles of respiration. Central cyanosis is usually present. Auscultation of the chest reveals decreased air entry.

The chest X-ray is usually a characteristic 'ground glass' appearance showing under-aeration of one or both lungs. Lung compliance is reduced and large areas of the lungs are not perfused. Gases will show hypoxia, hypercarbia and acidaemia (low pH).

Management

RDS is a self-limiting disease. The goal of treatment is the maintenance of alveolar ventilation to provide adequate pulmonary perfusion and normal gas exchange while ensuring minimum damage until the disease has run its course.

Treatment with surfactant

Surfactant is natural protein produced in the lungs, which helps maintain constant alveolar pressure and lower surface tension. If the baby is deficient in surfactant because of prematurity, pharmacologically prepared preparations can be given to improve lung function. Surfactant preparations can be divided into two main groups.

Natural surfactants

- Calf lung surfactant extract (CLSE) prepared by washing surfactant out of the lungs of dead calves.
- Porcine surfactant (poractant alpha, Curosurf) is derived from minced pig lungs which is then purified by washing.
- Beractant (Survanta) is derived from homogenised cow lungs.
- Human amniotic fluid surfactant is produced by collecting clean amniotic fluid at elective Caesarean sections for term deliveries.

Artificial surfactants

- Colfosceril palmitate (Exosurf) was patented by Dr Clements in 1982 (Guthrie 1988). This is a mixture of dipalmitoylphosphatidylcholine, hexadecanol (cetyl alcohol) and tyloxapol.
- Artificial lung expanding compound (pumactant, Alec) was devised in Cambridge from two pure sterile phospholipids.

Indications for surfactant

All preterm babies below 1500 g (3 lb 5 oz) who need to be ventilated at birth should be given at least one dose of surfactant soon after birth. Another dose may be given 12–24 hours later if the baby has not improved or has worsened.

The Osiris Collaborative Group (1992) found that giving surfactant immediately after delivery before the initiation of mechanical ventilation is beneficial, resulting in better distribution of surfactant during the period of absorption of lung fluid. They also compared the current standard schedule of administrating two doses of surfactant (colfosceril palmitate) 12 hours apart with the option of giving up to two additional doses. If RDS persisted or recurred at least 24 hours after the first administration, extra doses could be given. The extra doses were associated with 60% more reports of poorly tolerated administration. The group concluded that there was no evidence to justify giving a third or fourth dose having already given the usual two doses.

Babies who present with RDS 4 hours or more after birth can be given a surfactant dose as rescue therapy. This has not proved as successful as giving it prophylactically though it does decrease the severity of the disease (Roberton 1993b).

Administration of surfactant

Each make of surfactant is given by a slightly different method though all are given through the endotracheal tube.

- CLSE is administered by introducing a size 5 Fr feeding tube, which has been cut 1 cm shorter than the ET tube, into the ET tube. The dose is delivered as a single bolus within a few seconds and IPPV is continued as soon as the feeding tube is withdrawn.
- Poractant alpha (Curosurf) administration needs the ET tube to be disconnected momentarily while the surfactant is introduced from a syringe.
- Beractant (Survanta) is administered in much the same way as CLSE although it is delivered in four parts and the baby is positioned differently each time. This is to ensure that the surfactant preparation is evenly distributed throughout the lungs. Between the introduction of the different parts, the feeding tube is removed and the baby is manually ventilated.
- Colfosceril palmitate (Exosurf) is introduced by direct installation into the trachea through a special side-ported ET tube adaptor. There is no interruption from

mechanical ventilation. Half the dose is given over a 1–2 minute period and the patient is turned 90° to one side for 30 seconds. The second half of the dose is then given and the patient is turned to the other side.
- Pumactant (Alec) is introduced into the trachea in a similar way to poractant alpha.

Effects of administration

Bose (1992) states that adverse events during dosing may occur in up to 30% of infants. It is necessary to be aware of the complications. The position of the endotracheal tube must be ascertained, to give adequate air entry into both lungs. Suction should be performed before administration to ensure the tube is patent. In many instances there is a rapid decrease in the amount of oxygen required after surfactant administration so the FiO_2 may have to be turned down rapidly. There may be bradycardia during administration and the risk of cerebral haemorrhage may be increased due to a fluctuating pattern of cerebral blood flow (Wiseman & Bryson 1994). Positioning is an important aspect of care, especially during the administration of particular surfactant preparations.

Other problems with RDS

The baby with RDS may be very sick and unstable for a few days. Inotropic drugs that improve cardiac output, and colloid such as fresh frozen plasma, may be needed to control blood pressure. HFOV may be required if pressures on conventional ventilation exceed 35 mmHg and rates are over 60. There may be gross oedema from leaking capillaries and renal failure if there has been severe hypotension or acidaemia. This may need treatment with peritoneal dialysis to improve kidney function. Paralysis and sedation are usually needed for babies who are moderately to severely affected.

Complications of RDS

The majority of babies do not die of RDS, but rather of a complication related to it. These complications may be allocated into two groups, acute and chronic. Acute complications include the development of a pneumothorax; air leaks; pulmonary interstitial emphysema; patent ductus arteriosus; intraventricular haemorrhage and necrotising enterocolitis. Chronic complications include the development of bronchopulmonary dysplasia.

Birth asphyxia

This affects preterm and full term babies and has a high mortality and morbidity rate. It is characterised before birth by a poor cardiotocograph (CTG) trace, meconium staining or a fetal scalp pH of >7.20. After birth a low Apgar score and the length of time taken to establish respirations and heart beat, will give an indication of the severity of the asphyxia. The baby may have to be delivered quickly by an emergency Caesarian section if there is fetal distress. Problems with oxygen starvation of the brain will not be immediately apparent but become evident in the degree of encephalopathy the baby suffers.

The mildest symptoms will cause the baby to appear wide awake, jittery and restless with poor feeding abilities. This is treated by minimal handling and mild sedation and will resolve in 2–7 days (Fleming *et al.* 1991).

Moderate encephalopathy will cause the baby to be lethargic and hypotonic, with poor feeding attempts. There may be some seizures which need to be controlled with drugs and the symptoms are usually resolved by 7 days. Half the babies with this mild type will have a poor outcome.

The severely asphyxiated baby will need immediate ventilation. There will be profound unresponsiveness with absent reflexes and difficult to control seizures. With this severe type of asphyxia 75–100% die or have severe impairments (Fleming *et al.* 1991).

Treatment

Treatment aims to limit the damage by controlling cerebral oedema and preventing raised intercranial pressure. This is done by restricting fluids, keeping the electrolytes and blood chemistry stable and controlling seizures.

The prognosis for these babies is variable but usually poor. Research is ongoing to prevent the cerebral damage being incurred and to improve the outcome. It is thought that magnesium sulphate given soon after birth may help asphyxiated babies. Magnesium sulphate blocks the *N*-methyl-*D*-aspartate receptor which is the ion channel thought to be responsible for excessive and harmful calcium entry into the neurones following asphyxia (Evans 1996). Magnesium sulphate is administered soon after birth to these babies and reduces secondary neuronal injury and subsequent neurological impairment.

A multi-centre trial, the Randomised Asphyxia Study (RAST) was started in 1995 to ascertain the therapeutic value of treatment with magnesium sulphate soon after the birth of an asphyxiated baby. There is a risk that magnesium sulphate may cause apnoea and because of this the trial has been suspended to find a safer concentration of the drug. It is hoped that after further review the trial will continue (Evans 1997).

Meconium aspiration syndrome

Meconium staining of the amniotic fluid occurs in 8–10% of deliveries and most commonly affects the baby born between 36 and 41 weeks (Moore 1994). It is not known why babies pass meconium *in utero* but they may do so in response to fetal hypoxia, as a normal physiological function related to gut maturity or to increased vagal activity *in utero* (Houlihan & Knuppel 1994).

Thin meconium staining with a normal fetal heart rate is thought to be low in risk compared with thick meconium (Mahomed *et al.* 1994). It is thought that fetal gasping in response to hypoxia is responsible for the meconium entering the lungs. The meconium causes partial or complete airway obstruction and inflammation of the airways and alveoli. Suctioning of the oropharynx as soon as the head is delivered has been a critical factor in the prevention of meconium aspiration syndrome (Fertsch 1995). This stops the baby inhaling the meconium with the first breath.

Many babies with this syndrome will be hypoxic during labour from gasping due to uterine stresses, and subsequent inhalation. At birth they will be cyanosed, grunting and shocked and may have a barrel shaped chest from gas trapping and alveolar distension. The chest X-ray will show typical diffuse patchy irregular densities, hyperinflation at the bases of the lungs and areas of consolidation (Flores 1993). The severity of the condition will depend on the amount of inhalation and hypoxia at birth.

Treatment

Treatment aims to reduce the inflammation in the lungs. This is carried out by ventilating the baby and antibiotics to prevent infection. The babies are usually difficult to ventilate efficiently and require paralysis and sedation. Persistent pulmonary hypertension is common and drugs such as tolazoline and epoprostenol (prostacyclin) may be needed to induce pulmonary vasodilation. Pneumothorax is common because of the inflammation and damage to the alveoli. If there has been birth asphyxia there may be a degree of renal failure so fluid overload is to be avoided until the kidneys are processing urine. Some units give a dose of surfactant as rescue therapy (Robertson 1996). Nitric oxide has been shown to be helpful in decreasing pulmonary hypertension. ECMO treatment for suitable babies has been successful.

Persistent pulmonary hypertension of the newborn

Persistent pulmonary hypertension of the newborn (PPHN) is also known as persistent fetal circulation. It usually occurs in term babies and is triggered by perinatal hypoxia, infection, diaphragmatic hernia or lung tumours, meconium aspiration syndrome, congenital heart disease, polycythaemia, indomethacin treatment of the mother antenatally or any condition that predisposes to high pulmonary vascular resistance (Prullage & Melichar 1993). To understand the mechanics of the disease it is necessary to look at the changes that occur at birth to the neonatal circulation.

At birth, gas exchange is transferred from the placenta to the lungs with the first breath, this causes lung expansion leading to:

- Decreased pulmonary pressure.
- Increased pulmonary blood flow.
- Increased blood return to left atrium.
- Increased left atrial pressure.
- Closure of foramen ovale.

- Increased arterial oxygen tension (PaO_2) constricts the ductus arteriosis.

In PPHN the foramen ovale and the ductus arteriosis remain open causing a right-to-left shunt in the circulation. This induces severe hypoxia and delays the normal fall in pulmonary vasculature.

The condition is not present at birth, symptoms usually develop in the first 24 hours triggered by other medical problems such as meconium aspiration. The baby will be pale with laboured respirations grunting and severe sternal recession. There is poor perfusion of the tissues and low blood pressure with little response to increased oxygen levels.

Treatment is aimed at keeping the baby stable until the pulmonary vasculature returns to normal. High ventilator rates and pressures are necessary and high frequency oscillatory ventilation is often used. Studies have shown that nitric oxide used in the ventilator circuit acts as a vasodilator and contributes to a normal transition from fetal to adult circulation (Miller 1995) so relieving the condition. Hypovolaemia is treated with plasma infusions and a dilution exchange given if there is polycythaemia. Tolazoline and epoprostenol (prostacyclin) infusions are used as vasodilators.

The baby will be critically ill and need extensive respiratory, haematological and pharmacological support to survive. The mortality rate for this condition is approximately 40% (Prullage & Melichar 1993).

Pulmonary hypoplasia

In this condition the lungs have not developed fully before birth and so cannot function efficiently to sustain life. Oligohydramnios, where there is little or no amniotic fluid, is often associated with it and other conditions such as diaphragmatic hernia or genetic malformations are sometimes present. Respiratory failure is severe and persistent pulmonary hypertension of the new-born commonly occurs.

The baby will be ventilated from birth and may need treatment with ECMO therapy which will be used if there is no major genetic life-limiting disease. The lungs may eventually expand sufficiently to sustain the baby but those who do not have, or develop, sufficient lung tissue to sustain life will, inevitably, die.

Congenital pneumonia

This can occur at any gestation and is usually caused by group B streptococcus. Premature rupture of membranes during pregnancy may have allowed infection into the uterus or infection may occur during the passage through the vaginal canal at birth. The condition mimics respiratory distress syndrome and may appear from 3 to 48 hours after birth. The onset may be sudden with the baby having symptoms of severe shock. Survival depends on intensive medical and nursing support and early antibiotic cover.

Transient tachypnoea of the new-born

This is more common in term babies who have been delivered by Caesarian section. They have missed out on the mechanical squeezing of the chest wall, which removes excessive lung fluids, during the descent through the birth canal. At birth the baby will have mild grunting, sternal recession and a raised respiratory rate, cyanosis may be present. If the symptoms are not marked at birth, the baby may present a few hours later with hypothermia and inspiratory grunting. The chest X-ray shows typical streaking.

The lungs begin to clear within 10–12 hours and by 72 hours will appear normal (Flores 1993). The baby will be given warmed humidified head box oxygen and may need this for 3–4 days.

Choanal atresia

This is caused by a bony or membranous obstruction between the nasal cavity and the oropharynx which may affect one or both nostrils. Babies are nose breathers in the early weeks and this condition causes airway obstruction and cyanosis. Diagnosis is confirmed by the failure to pass a nasal catheter and by X-ray.

Cyanosis is relieved when the baby cries or the mouth is opened. The use of an oral airway taped into the mouth provides life-saving though temporary treatment. Surgical correction is carried out as soon as possible.

Chronic pulmonary insufficiency of prematurity

This is seen in some low birth weight babies who have not had RDS but who become breathless and start apnoeic attacks from the second to fifth week of life. Oxygen therapy is usually needed with theophylline, to stimulate the respiratory centre, and sometimes CPAP. The baby may need long term oxygen therapy and follow-up treatment as if for bronchopulmonary dysplasia.

REFERENCES

Allen PD, Turner DT, Brinck MJ. (1995) Ground transport of an infant on high frequency jet ventilation. *Neonatal Network*, **14** (6), 39–43.

Avery GB. (1994) *Neonatology; Pathophysiology and Management of the Newborn*, Fourth Edition. Lippincott, Philadelphia.

Avery M, Mead J (1959) Surface properties in relation to atelectasis and hyaline membrane disease. *American Journal of Diseases of Children*, **95**, 517–523.

Avila K, Mazza L, Morgan-Trujillo L. (1994) High frequency oscillatory ventilation. *Neonatal Network*, **13** (5), 23–28.

Beck F, Moffat DB, Davies DP. (1985) *Human Embryology*, 2nd edn. Blackwell Scientific Publications, London.

Blease J. (1997) Nursing care issues in NCPAP. *Journal of Neonatal Nursing*, **3** (1), centre pages.

Bose G. (1992) Surfactant replacement. Issues relating to currently available preparations. *Neonatal Network*, **11** (4), vii–xii.

Cox CA, Wolfson MR, Shaffer TH. (1996) Liquid ventilation – a comprehensive overview. *Neonatal Network*, **15** (3), 31–43.

Crawford D, Morris M. (1994) *Neonatal Nursing*. Chapman and Hall, London.

Crowley P, Chalmers I, Keirse MJNC. (1990) The effects of corticosteroid administration before preterm delivery: An overview of the evidence from controlled trials. *British Journal of Obstetrics and Gynaecology*, **97** (1), 11–25.

Davenport M, Holmes K. (1995) Current management of congenital diaphragmatic hernia. *British Journal of Hospital Medicine*, **53** (3), 95–101.

Evans D. (1996) Neuroprotection following intrapartum asphyxia. The Randomized Asphyxia Study (RAST). *Journal of Neonatal Nursing*, **2** (3), 14–21.

Evans D. (1997) Update on the randomised asphyxia study. *Journal of Neonatal Nursing*, **3** (1), 24.

Fertsch D. (1995) A neonate with meconium aspiration syndrome and severe respiratory distress. *Current Opinion in Paediatrics*, **7** (2), 152–155.

Fleming P, Speidel B, Marlow N, Dunn PM. (1991) *A Neonatal Vade Mecum*, 2nd edn. Edward Arnold, London.

Flores MT. (1993) Understanding neonatal chest X-rays. *Neonatal Network*, **12** (8), 9–15.

Greenspan JS. (1993) Liquid ventilation: A developing technology. *Neonatal Network*, **12** (4), 23–28.

Greenough A. (1994) Pulse oximetry. *Current Pediatrics*, **4**, 196–199.

Greenough A. (1995) Nitric oxide – clinical aspects. *Care of the Critically Ill*, **11** (4), 120–122.

Guthrie RD. (1988) *Neonatal Intensive Care*. Churchill Livingstone, London.

Halliday HC, McClure G, Reid M (1989) *Handbook of Neonatal Care* 3rd edn, Baillière Tindall, Philadelphia.

Hancock J. (1995) The effects of prematurity on long term outcome. *Paediatric Nursing*, **7** (10), 16–20.

HFOV Study Group. (1993) Randomised study of high frequency ventilation in infants with severe RDS. *Journal of Pediatrics*, **122** (4), 609–619.

Hodge D. (1991) Endotracheal suctioning and the infant; a nursing care protocol. *Neonatal Network*, **9** (5), 7–15.

Houlihan CM, Knuppel RA. (1994) Meconium stained amniotic fluid. *Journal of Reproductive Medicine*, **39** (11), 888–898.

Kempley ST, Bennett S, Loftus BG, Cooper D, Gamsu HR. (1993) Randomized trial of umbilical arterial catheter position – clinical outcome. *Acta Paediatrica*, **82**, 173–176.

Klaus MH, Fanaroff AA. (1993) *Care of the High Risk Neonate*, 4th edn. WB Saunders, Philadelphia.

Korones SB, Lancaster J. (1986) *High Risk Newborn Infants*, 4th edn. C.V. Mosby Co., St Louis.

Knoppert DC, Mackanjee HR. (1994) Current strategies in the management of BPD. *Neonatal Network*, **13** (3), 53–60.

Levene MI, Tudehope D. (1993) *Essentials of Neonatal Medicine*, 2nd edn. Blackwell Scientific Publications, London.

Martin LD. (1995) New approaches to ventilation in infants and children. *Current Opinion in Paediatrics*, **7** (2), 250–257.

Mahomed K, Nyoni R, Masona D. (1994) Meconium staining of the liquor in a low risk population. *Pediatric and Perinatal Epidemiology*, **8** (3), 292–300.

McCormick M, Workman-Daniels K, Brooks-Gunn J. (1996) The behavioural and emotional well being of school-age children with different birthweights. *Pediatrics*, **97** (1), 18–25.

Merenstein GB, Gardener SL. (1993) *Handbook of Neonatal Intensive Care*, 3rd edn. Mosby, St Louis.

Miller C. (1995) Nitric oxide therapy for persistent pulmonary hypertension of the newborn. *Neonatal Network*, **14** (8), 9–15.

Mitchell A. (1996) Persistent pulmonary hypertension of the newborn. *Journal of Neonatal Nursing* **2** (3), 5–10.

Morgan JB. (1992). Nutrition of the very low birthweight infant. *Care of the Critically Ill*, **8** (3), 122–124.

Moore CS. (1994) Meconium aspiration syndrome. *Neonatal Network*, **13** (7), 57–60.

Osiris Collaborative Group. (1992) Early versus delayed neonatal administration of a synthetic surfactant – the judgment of Osiris. *Lancet*, **340** (8832), 1363–1369.

Prullage S, Melichar C. (1993) Stabilisation and transportation of the infant with PPHN. *Neonatal Network*, **12** (7), 45–51.

Roberton NRC. (1993a) *Textbook of Neonatology*, 2nd edn. Churchill Livingstone, Edinburgh.

Roberton NRC. (1993b) *A Manual of Neonatal Intensive Care*, 3rd edn. Edward Arnold, London.

Robertson B. (1996) New targets for surfactant replacement therapy: experimental and clinical targets. *Archives of Disease in Childhood, Fetal and Neonatal Edition*, 75, 1–3.

Robertson NJ, McCarthy LS, Hamilton PA, Moss ALH. (1996) Nasal deformities from flow driver continuous positive airway pressure. *Archives of Disease in Childhood, Fetal and Neonatal Edition*, **75**, 209–212.

Runton N. (1992) Suctioning artificial airways in children. Appropriate technique. *Pediatric Nursing*, **18** (2), 115–118.

Schwartz RM, Luby AM, Scanlon JW, Kellogg RJ. (1994) Effect of surfactant on morbidity, mortality and resource use in newborn infants weighing 500–1,500g. *New England Journal of Medicine*, **330** (21), 1476–1480.

Shinwell ES, Karplus M, Zmora E, *et al.* (1996) Failure of early postnatal dexamethasone to prevent chronic lung disease in infants with respiratory distress syndrome. *Archives of Disease in Childhood, Fetal and Neonatal Edition*, **74**, 33–37.

Sparshott MM. (1996) The development of a clinical distress scale for ventilated newborn infants. *Journal of Neonatal Nursing*, **2** (2), 5–10.

Trotter C, Carey B. (1992) Assessment of respiratory effort. *Neonatal Network*, **11** (8), 61–63.

UK Collaborative ECMO Trial Group. (1996) UK collaborative randomised trial of neonatal extracorporeal membrane oxygenation. *Lancet*, **348** (9020), 75–82.

Underman Boggs K. (1993) Family adaptation and infant developmental outcomes one year after ECMO. *Neonatal Network*, **12** (7), 68.

Wheater M, Rennie JM. (1994) Poor prognosis after prolonged ventilation for bronchopulmonary dysplasia. *Archives of Disease in Childhood, Fetal and Neonatal Edition*, **71**, 210–211.

Wiseman LR, Bryson HM. (1994) Porcine-derived lung surfactant – a review of the therapeutic efficacy and clinical tolerability of a natural surfactant preparation (Curosurf) in neonatal respiratory distress syndrome. *Drugs*, **48** (3), 386–403.

Wiswell TE, Graziani LJ, Kornhauser MS, *et al.* (1996) High frequency jet ventilation in the early management of respiratory distress syndrome is associated with a greater risk for adverse outcomes. *Pediatrics*, **98** (6), 1035–1043.

Yeh TF, Torre JA, Rastogi A, *et al.* (1990) Early postnatal dexamethasone therapy in premature infants with severe respiratory distress syndrome: A double blind controlled study. *Journal of Pediatrics*, **117**, 237–282.

Young J. (1995) Endotracheal suction and the intubated neonate. *Journal of Neonatal Nursing*, **1** (4), 23–28.

5 Nursing Management of Babies Requiring Neonatal Surgery

LEARNING OUTCOMES

When this chapter has been read and understood the reader should be able to:

- ○ Discuss antenatal measures that can help a baby with a surgical condition.
- ○ Describe the preoperative and postoperative care of a baby.
- ○ List the common types of surgical condition seen in NICU.
- ○ Compare the treatment and outlook for gastroschisis and exomphalos.
- ○ Describe the care of a baby with diaphragmatic hernia.
- ○ Identify the predisposing causes of necrotising enterocolitis.

NEONATAL SURGERY

Neonatal surgery has been carried out in this country for more than 40 years. The provision of specialist surgical units and more efficient antenatal scanning has meant the success and morbidity rate for conditions requiring neonatal surgery have dramatically improved in the last decade. Babies that used to die or have significantly impaired quality of life can now be treated successfully in these units (Roberton 1993b).

Babies who need surgery in the neonatal period often have congenital conditions that cause life-threatening problems. Many of the common problems can now be picked up on ultrasound scanning in pregnancy. This will alert doctors so that a high definition scan can be done to reveal the exact parameters of the baby's problem (Proud 1994).

Antenatal diagnosis

Antenatal clinics now offer routine scans to pregnant women at about 16 weeks gestation. Women are not always aware that the main purpose of the scan is to find out if the baby has an anomaly (Smith & Marteau 1995). They need to be informed intelligently and sensitively of this possibility so that they can be prepared for a possible adverse outcome.

The discovery of an anomaly can enable doctors and parents to plan the course of the pregnancy and allow for choices of treatment. No parents should be hurried into a termination for a fetal anomaly without knowing all the options for treatment and the prognosis of the condition. It has been found that the antenatal team are not always aware of the good prognosis for some anomalies and may advise termination unnecessarily (Fisher *et al.* 1996). It is important that there is counselling in these matters before any decision is taken, though not all hospitals have this facility available (Marteau 1990).

SATFA (Support Around Termination For Abnormality) can help and parents in this predicament should be encouraged to contact them for advice. The organisation offers support, advice and information and is making itself known in many hospitals throughout the country.

Fetal intervention

Early antenatal diagnosis gives increased opportunities for medical intervention such as termination or fetal surgery. Alternatively the time and place for delivery could be planned so that suitable facilities are available.

Fetal interventions consist of measures to prevent continuing damage to organs threatened by the build-up of fluids. Hydrocephalus, lung effusions and build-up of backflow urine in kidneys can be controlled by drainage tubes. This is done by putting in appropriate shunts under ultrasound scan direction (Roberton 1993a) so that the excess fluid runs into the amniotic sac. The surrounding organs can then develop without being compressed by the extra fluid. The intervention may cause a miscarriage and this

should be explained to the mother before deciding on treatment.

In America intrauterine fetal surgery for diaphragmatic hernia has been carried out. The success rate was not encouraging with the majority of pregnancies ending in the death of the fetus (Harrison *et al.* 1993). Research is ongoing to find suitable methods to intervene in surgically correctable fetal defects but this needs to address the aspects of fetal rights and fetal pain which will open up new ethical minefields for this type of surgery (Carter 1990).

Although at the moment these interventions have limited success, research and advances in technology make safe fetal surgery more than a possibility in the near future.

NURSING A BABY WHO NEEDS SURGERY

Parents who decide to continue their pregnancy will be referred to the care of a neonatal surgeon. The mother will be delivered in a unit with neonatal surgical facilities. In appropriate cases Caesarian section or induction of labour is planned earlier than the mother's expected date of delivery in an attempt to minimise the damage of the defect. It may also be done to ensure that the mother does not go into labour and deliver in a hospital without surgical facilities for her baby (Fisher *et al.* 1996).

The neonatal unit will be notified when the mother is admitted so that parents can meet the staff who will look after their baby. They will be given any written material available and shown around the unit if they wish. The mother is asked to consider expressing her breast milk at this stage even if she had not intended to breast feed. Breast milk can often be given and absorbed earlier than formula milk and helps counteract infections with the immunoglobulins it provides. The milk is frozen until the baby is ready for it.

At birth

After birth the baby is admitted to the neonatal surgical unit. Babies born with a defect needing surgery, at a hospital without such facilities will be referred to the appropriate unit after consultation with the surgeons.

On admission the surgical team will see the baby to assess the condition and order any diagnostic tests needed to plan the operation. They will speak to the parents and explain the treatment involved and may at this stage ask them to sign a consent form. It is helpful if the nurse is present when the surgeons speak to the parents so that any information given can be reinforced later if necessary (Farrell & Frost 1992).

If the baby has come from another hospital, the mother may not be well enough after the delivery to be transferred and the father might prefer to stay with the her. In these cases the doctor from the referring hospital or the doctor on the transport team can explain the treatment and obtain a signed consent form for surgery.

Nursing assessment on admission

Weight, baseline temperature, apex beat, respiration, blood pressure and blood sugar levels need to be recorded on admission so that any problems can be corrected immediately. The baby will be nursed in an incubator and kept warm, the most efficient way to ensure this is to use the servo-controlled temperature mode on the incubator. This will adjust the incubator to bring the baby's temperature within normal limits. It is important that the baby does not become cold, as this lowers blood pressure, impairs circulation and destabilises blood sugar.

Preoperative care

In the past babies were rushed to the surgical unit and taken straight to theatre for surgery as soon as possible after birth. It is now considered better management to stabilise blood pressure, blood gases, temperature and blood chemistry before theatre (Davenport & Holmes 1995). In order to improve the baby's condition for surgery, assessment and stabilisation should involve:

- Respiratory status
- Haematological status
- Blood pressure
- Fluid balance

Respiratory status

The baby may need ventilation because of the defect, or may be electively ventilated before going to theatre. Blood gas assessment will be taken to ensure that ventilation is efficient. Nursing care will include continuous monitoring of the baby's vital signs, oxygen requirements and airway management (Chapter 4).

Haematological status

The baby may be shocked as a result of the delivery, the surgical problem or respiratory distress syndrome which will cause the blood pressure to fall. Colloid infusions of fresh frozen plasma or human albumin will be given to improve perfusion and help raise blood pressure. Blood electrolytes will be assessed and any imbalance be corrected.

Haemoglobin level and a full blood count will be taken; if there is anaemia a transfusion will be given before theatre. Maternal blood will be needed for cross-matching of blood for the baby during surgery. Most units give intramuscular vitamin K before theatre to decrease the risk of bleeding.

Blood pressure

Blood pressure can be assessed by cuff pressure or by an electrode fitted into an arterial line. Umbilical arterial catheters should be avoided as they may interfere with the operation site. Peripheral arterial blood pressure measurement is accurate and has the advantage of making blood sampling for gases and other tests easier and less painful for the baby. The disadvantages are, that it is an invasive procedure and profuse disastrous bleeding can occur if the cannula is accidentally disconnected or dislodged. The arterial line should be labelled and connected to a monitor with an alarm system. To prevent a spasm that could impair the circulation, no drugs except heparin and saline must be given into the artery.

Fluid balance

The baby will be given an intravenous infusion of 10% dextrose with electrolytes, as soon as a vein can be cannulated, to prevent dehydration and blood sugar problems. Intravenous fluids may be needed to replace fluids lost by drainage from nasogastric tubes or defects such as gastroschisis or exomphalos. Urine output should be recorded. Antibiotics are given prophylactically and many surgeons like the first dose of an antibiotic to be given before theatre.

Parents reactions

It is very distressing for parents to watch helplessly as their baby is prepared for surgery. If the condition was diagnosed before birth the parents will know the likely treatment and prognosis, though will still be very anxious and stressed.

If the defect was not diagnosed *in utero*, the shock of having an ill baby needing emergency surgery and possible transfer to a hospital away from family and friends, adds to their distress. They will still be recovering physically and mentally from the delivery at this vulnerable time, especially if this is their first baby. The added stress of having an ill baby can make the adjustments necessary to become parents, seem almost insurmountable (Orford 1996). Nursing staff are aware of these difficulties and can help by being sensitive, tactful, listening to their worries and keeping them informed of the baby's progress.

The surgeons will see parents as soon as possible after admission to explain the operation and answer any questions they may have. The consent form will be explained and the parents asked to sign it when they have understood the operation.

Mothers will be encouraged to express their milk for the baby if they have not already been approached about this. The benefits to the baby need to be explained, namely that the milk is easier for the baby's delicate gut to absorb and it contains antigens that help the baby fight infection.

Parents may want a christening or other religious ceremony performed before the operation and this can be arranged. They may want a clergyman from their church or faith or other religious adviser and to have members of their family present.

If the mother is a patient the father will usually be allowed to stay with her on the postnatal ward. When the mother has been discharged, parents should be given accommodation in the hospital if they live more than a few miles away.

Preoperative checks

Most theatres have a check list that is used on the unit before transferring the baby for surgery. This will include:

- Checking details of armbands.
- Covering of any metal parts with sticking plaster to cut down on static electricity in theatre.
- Giving the premedication drug if ordered.
- Collecting notes, X-rays, current ward charts.
- Ensuring consent form signed and accompanying the baby.
- The latest temperature, heart rate and respiration for baseline checking.

Fluid lines should be patent with no swelling or redness: if this is noted a new line must be sited before going for surgery. Equipment that is battery operated must be fully charged to last through the operation and recovery periods. Emergency resuscitation equipment should go with the baby in the incubator drawer.

Hospital corridors will be colder than the neonatal unit and unless the incubator is battery operated it will be unheated for the journey. It is important not to let the baby get cold during transfer as this may destabilise blood sugar and raise oxygen needs, so a blanket sized piece of Gamgee tissue and/or bubble plastic should cover the baby in the incubator. An oxygen saturation monitor must be attached to the baby and able to give a continuous reading during the journey.

When the baby is ready for theatre, experienced nursing and medical staff should accompany the baby to observe and treat any change in condition during the journey. Porters will be needed for moving the incubator, drip stands, manipulating doors and operating lifts. The parents may accompany the baby to the anaesthetic room if they wish. It will be upsetting for them when they have to leave, wondering if the baby will survive. Sensitive, sympathetic treatment from nursing staff helps now as they are shown to a quiet waiting room and told approximately how long the operation will take. Parents can be assured that as soon as the baby is out of theatre, staff will let them know.

The nurse accompanying the baby usually returns to the ward after checking the baby with theatre staff and handing over. Continuity of care should be maintained at the handover and the neonatal nurse will check that the incubator is plugged into the mains during the operation to keep it heated for the return journey.

Postoperative nursing care

After surgery the baby will usually remain ventilated for at least 24 hours for the effect of the anaesthetic gases to wear off and for opioid pain relief to be given. Continuous cardiorespiratory monitoring will be carried out and temperature, blood sugar levels and blood pressure will also be assessed. The wound site must be checked frequently for bleeding and the dressing should be in view at all times. Drainage from wounds will need to be measured and colour and content noted. The fluid drained may need to be replaced with intravenous fluid to prevent electrolyte imbalance.

Stabilising

Blood will almost certainly have been given in

theatre or the surgeons may wish it to be given on return to the ward. Haematological status is monitored by blood pressure readings and intravenous colloids such as fresh frozen plasma and blood will be given to keep blood pressure and haemoglobin stable. Parenteral maintenance fluids will be continued as prescribed and blood sugar monitored carefully until stable. High sugar readings may indicate stress or pain which can be relieved. Low blood sugars indicate cold stress or shock and may lead to neurological damage if not promptly corrected.

A central venous line will often be sited in theatre and may need to be X-rayed on the unit to ensure it is in the correct position (Reid & Frey 1992). When the position is satisfactory the maintenance fluids can be started through this line, using aseptic precautions to connect the central line to the giving set tubing and fluid bag.

Pain relief

Pain management is essential and its effects should be monitored so that the baby remains comfortable. Continuous intravenous opioid pain relief, such as fentanyl, gives the best analgesic cover. Ventilatory support is usually given after major surgery to allow intravenous pain relief to be given more freely (Cote *et al.* 1991). The depressing effect on the respiratory system makes many clinicians wary of giving opioid drugs to unventilated babies.

Pain relief can be gradually reduced as the baby tolerates it and paracetamol suppositories substituted when ventilation is discontinued (Andrews & Wills 1992). The aim is to assess the baby's pain and treat it and to ascertain whether pain relief or comfort measures can help. Often position changes, non-nutritive sucking or just a friendly voice may

help the baby settle when a few days have passed after surgery (Sparshott 1989).

Parents

Parents should be informed as soon as the baby reaches the ward after theatre and allowed to visit as soon as possible. At this stage the baby should not be disturbed and though they will have been prepared for the surgery they may be upset to see the baby looking so pale, still and possibly ventilated. The surgeon who has carried out the operation or the unit doctor will speak to the them as soon as possible to explain the operation, the findings and what they can expect over the next few hours.

The nurses' role with the parents will consist of explaining the surgery, if they have not understood from the surgeon, and letting them know what to expect over the next few hours as the baby wakes up from the anaesthetic. Some parents may want to discuss the implications of the surgery especially if the baby has had a colostomy or gastrostomy. Knowledge and experience on the part of the nurse plays a vital role here in giving parents realistic, positive information. Not all parents wish to talk about the future at this stage preferring their baby to recover from the surgery first. All parents will be relieved that their baby has returned safely to the unit but anxious about the survival over the next few days.

Progress

When the baby is weaned off the ventilator and is stable, there will be a transfer out of the intensive area into a high dependency area where monitoring will take place for a few more days. Though this move is a boost for most parents as a sign their baby is improving many will worry whether their baby will get the same good care. There are fewer nurses in this area and parents still see their baby as very sick. Nurses need to understand that this is a common reaction and no reflection on their care. Constant reassurance is needed for the first few days the baby is out of intensive care.

Feeding

When the surgeons are satisfied that there are good bowel sounds indicating that intestinal function has returned and that nasogastric aspirates are very small, oral feeds will be started providing there are no other contra-indicatory factors. Some units begin with clear fluids, such as oral rehydration salts (e.g. Dioralyte), for 4–6 hours then use breast milk if available. Others start with small hourly amounts of milk, preferably expressed breast milk, or semi-elemental osmolar preparations such as Pregestimil, as this is more easily absorbed than formula milks.

If oral feeding is tolerated without vomiting or abdominal distension then it is increased slowly, say 1 ml 6-hourly depending on the baby's condition. Intravenous fluids are decreased as oral fluids increase. The process of weaning to full feeds can take weeks and malabsorption problems can be troublesome in conditions such as gastroschisis or exomphalos (Lister & Irving 1990).

Promoting the toleration of milk feeds

All mothers of babies undergoing surgery should be encouraged to express their milk even if they do not intend to breast feed later. Breast milk is easier to digest and also has anti-infective properties that help the baby's response to infection. It has been shown that expressed breast milk empties from the stomach twice as fast as formula milk in babies (Ewer *et al.* 1994). It has also been found that tilting the baby's tray with the head uppermost and nursing prone speeds up gastric emptying (Dellagrammaticas *et al.* 1991). This means that the amount of milk feed given to the baby can be increased more quickly without incurring vomiting.

When the baby is on full oral feeds the intravenous fluids will be discontinued. The feeds progress from one hourly to two hourly then three hourly. At any of these stages the mother can try breast or bottle feeding if the baby wants to suck.

Parents

As the baby's condition improves the parents can do more, bathing, cuddling and feeding. Some conditions may require an extensive period of time in the neonatal unit and this often makes parents feel frustrated (Affonso *et al.* 1992). After the drama of the birth and the operation, the long, dragging days of recovery can put great strain on them, their family and the nursing staff. Giving the parents more control over caring for their baby often helps in these situations. If the baby is otherwise well, families appreciate being able to go out with the baby in a pushchair around the hospital grounds. Intravenous lines can be capped for an hour or so and the fluid requirement made up later. This gives the family a chance to be together without the unit staff.

Financial help may be needed from Social Services if travelling causes financial problems. Ideally parents of long stay babies, benefit from staying in hospital accommodation and caring for their baby. This is especially helpful for them if the baby is to go home with a central line for intravenous feeding or has a tracheostomy or colostomy.

Staying with the baby may be difficult if there are other children who need the mother's attention.

Discharge planning will begin early and parents will be taught to care for their baby. If the baby has a tracheostomy or bowel stoma parents will be taught the care needed. Parents always worry about being able to cope at home and introducing them to a member of the community team or stoma care nurse can reassure them that help and support will continue after discharge. Open communications and understanding of parents' needs, help promote good relations with these long term babies, their families and unit staff (Hickey 1990).

Transfer back to referring hospital

Regional units have a large number of referrals from outside their own area and it is not possible to keep every baby referred until discharge. So that they are prepared for the transfer, parents need to be told early on in their baby's admission that transfer back will take place when the baby is well enough. Arrangements will be made for transfer back as soon as full milk feeds are tolerated and the surgeons are pleased with the progress.

The transfer helps parents who have had difficulties with visiting, but can upset other families if they feel that their own hospital will not be able to cope. Transferring the baby can sometimes denigrate the referring hospital in the parent's eyes and they may apportion blame for some aspect of the baby's illness. Some families feel they have made good relationships with the staff in the regional unit and cannot trust anyone else to care for their baby. Written and oral communications with the referring hospital are essential for continuation of care. Many regional units support nurses doing courses from other hospitals and so form a link with smaller units, which helps with liaison.

Staff need to give as much information as possible to the parents about the care the baby will have on return. Parents will want to know who will accompany the baby and how he will travel (Kuhnly & Freston 1993). Nurses can explain the benefits and changes that the parents will encounter in the home hospital so that the parents will see the transfer as a positive manoeuvre. As the likely time approaches for the transfer it should be made clear to the parents when and how this is going to happen.

Discharge

When the baby is gaining weight and taking all feeds by bottle or breast, the surgeons and paediatricians will arrange follow-up appointments and discharge.

Great Ormond Street Hospital carried out a study of babies who had undergone neonatal surgery. These babies were more difficult to look after in their first year of life, they were more temperamentally exacting than the healthy control babies and had more disturbed sleeping patterns. The disrupted sleep pattern often persisted up to the age of three. This was in spite of parents being in the unit with their baby during the stay. The parents of babies who have had surgery need help and advice for a long time. Units specialising in surgery often have a system by which the parents can be put in contact with other parents, whose babies have had the same problem, for long term advice and support (Ludman 1992).

The above is a general outline of the care a baby will receive in a neonatal surgical unit. Individual preoperative and postoperative care will depend on the particular condition, the assessment of need and the care plan. It is helpful to look in more detail at some of the more common conditions and their treatment and outcome.

COMMON CONDITIONS REQUIRING NEONATAL SURGERY

- Diaphragmatic hernia
- Tracheo-osphageal atresia
- Duodenal atresia
- Exomphalos
- Gastroschisis
- Imperforate anus
- Hirschsprung's disease
- Necrotising enterocolitis

Diaphragmatic hernia

This is one of the most serious and life-threatening neonatal conditions and one that, even with immediate specialist intervention, carries a high mortality rate of 50–80% depending on the severity of the lung damage (Davenport & Holmes 1995). It occurs in 1 in 4000 births and a significant number of miscarried fetuses have been found with the condition.

Embryology

The diaphragm forms between the eighth and tenth week of pregnancy. Defective formation and/or fusion of the pleuroperitoneal membrane results in a gap or weak area. If normal fusion has not occurred by the tenth week when the intestines return to the abdomen from the umbilical cord or if the bowel returns prematurely, herniation into the chest can occur.

Defects vary in size from a comparatively small triangular or oval defect in the diaphragm with well developed diaphragmatic muscle to huge deficiencies with partial absence of the diaphragm. About 80% are posterolateral hernias, left-sided, the right-sided ones are parasternal (Lister & Irving 1990) (Fig. 5.1).

Physiological outcome

The gut migrates through the hernia into the chest, compressing the lungs and preventing development. Babies are born with varying degrees of pulmonary hypoplasia. Pulmonary hypertension is usually present owing to the poor development of the conducting airways and alveoli. It is the extent of the lung hypoplasia and the pulmonary hypertension that determines the mortality and morbidity rate. There is some controversy as to whether the pulmonary hypoplasia and poor pulmonary vasculature would exist whether there was a hernia or not (Moreno & Iovanne 1993a; Davenport & Holmes 1995). Malrotation of the mid-gut and oesophageal dilation are common complications associated with diaphragmatic hernia (Moreno & Iovanne 1993a).

Prognosis

Babies, with the condition, who have no respiratory problems at birth do well because their lung development has not been badly affected. The hernia may only be found some hours or even days later when the baby presents with raised respiratory rate. A chest X-ray will confirm the condition and the diaphragm will be repaired. The baby will usually make a trouble-free recovery with no adverse sequelae. It has been known, though, for these late presenting hernias, if undiagnosed, to result in sudden death from gastric perforation or cardiorespiratory compromise (Moreno & Iovanne 1993a).

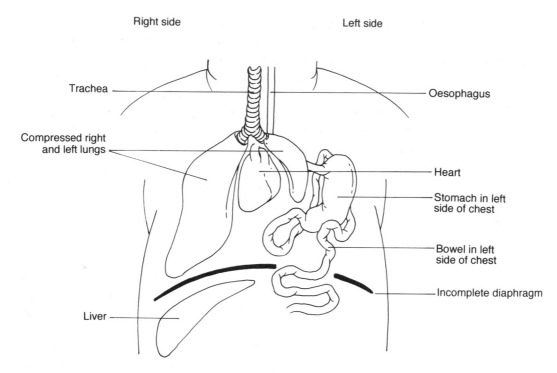

Fig. 5.1 Diagram of left-sided diaphragmatic hernia.

Babies who develop respiratory problems at or soon after birth have impaired lung function and there is a high morbidity and mortality rate. Though the diaphragm is often simple to repair the consequences of the lung hypoplasia and resultant pulmonary hypertension are often severe and there may not be enough lung tissue for the baby to survive.

Antenatal diagnosis

Diagnosis is often made during antenatal ultrasound scanning. Three features are usually present:

- Polyhydramnios
- Mediastinal displacement
- Absence of an intra-abdominal bubble

If these signs are seen, a further high definition scan should be made to look for dia-phragmatic hernia. It is usually possible to tell how seriously affected the baby will be by the size and development of the lungs in relation to gestational age.

Parents of severely affected babies are offered a termination because of the poor prognosis. Those who wish to continue their pregnancy after advice and, ideally, counselling, will be referred to the surgeons on a neonatal unit that carries out surgery. The mother will have her baby at that hospital so that there can be immediate treatment under controlled conditions.

Delivery

If the condition is not detected on ultrasound scan it is often difficult to diagnose immediately. The baby might be well at birth but collapse with secondary apnoea after a few minutes. This is because the gut in the chest fills with air with the first few breaths and prevents the lungs expanding.

The baby commonly presents with cyanosis, dyspnoea or apnoea and the chest may be larger on one side. Resuscitation is difficult and using a bag and mask worsens the problem by introducing more air into the intra-thoracic gut. An endotracheal tube should be passed on apnoeic babies before bagging, and mechanical ventilation started as soon as possible. Heart sounds will be heard on the right owing to displacement by the gut and the abdomen will probably be scaphoid (concave) from the absence of intestines.

A baby that has been diagnosed antenatally will be intubated immediately and transferred to the neonatal unit.

Preoperative care

On the neonatal unit the baby will be paralysed and sedated quickly to prevent swallowing of air which will inflate the intestines in the chest. Confirmation of the condition is obtained by X-ray of chest and abdomen which will show the mediastinal shift of the heart and loops of bowel in the chest in continuity with intra-abdominal bowel loops.

An 8 Fr nasogastric tube should be passed and aspirated frequently to keep the gut decompressed. The baby is nursed lying on the side of the hernia, if possible, to give the best lung the maximum chance to function. The tray of the incubator should be raised at the head end to encourage the gut to gravitate towards the abdominal cavity.

Ventilatory settings will have rapid rates with minimal pressures to prevent pneumothoraces. A high oxygen percentage is needed for the small inefficient lungs. The blood pH is kept above 7.4 to reduce the severity of the pulmonary hypoxic vasoconstriction. Intravenous tolazoline, a vasodilator,

is often given before and after surgery to reduce pulmonary vascular resistance and achieve adequate oxygenation.

Surgery is delayed until the baby is in a stable condition. The aim is to reduce the associated pulmonary hypertension, maintain adequate blood pressure and optimise oxygenation. It has been found that this delay in surgery can improve the condition in the immediate postoperative period (Davenport & Holmes 1995).

The operation

This involves opening the abdomen, pulling the gut from the chest into the abdomen, and repairing the hole in the diaphragm. In cases where the diaphragmatic defect is large, an artificial patch is stitched over the defect before the wound is closed. The gut is inspected and any malrotation corrected at this time. When the abdomen is closed there may be added pressure on the diaphragm from the abdominal contents. This may compromise respiration and ventilatory requirements may have to be increased. The skin of the abdomen will be tight as the abdominal walls were not stretched *in utero* by the gut. Gaping of the wound may be a problem as healing takes place and may allow infection to take hold. There may also be paralysis of the gut because of the pressure in the abdomen.

Postoperative care

The first few days, sometimes weeks, are critical because of the hypoplastic lungs and the resultant pulmonary hypertension. The baby relies on ventilatory support and it is often difficult to reduce the rate and pressure. Pneumothoraces are common and nursing care is aimed at astute assessment of vital signs in order to recognise and minimise complications. The baby will be paralysed and sedated for 48–72 hours, and in some cases for longer, to maximise oxygenation.

Gradually ventilator pressures and rates are reduced but the oxygen requirements can remain high for longer. Over the first week the lungs will expand but still only partially fill the thoracic cavity. Physiotherapy is given to keep the lungs clear of mucus. Aspirates from the nasogastric tube should be replaced, if copious, with intravenous electrolyte solutions.

It is generally accepted that these babies will always have a higher than normal carbon dioxide level because of the inefficient lungs. This means that ventilatory treatment should not attempt aggressively to reduce the carbon dioxide levels at the expense of lung damage from high pressures and rates.

Intravenous parenteral nutrition is given until the baby's condition improves, oral feeds can be started when bowel sounds are heard, if the condition is stable. Milk will be given in slowly increasing amounts through the nasogastric tube. The gut, which has been handled at operation, is still delicate and often adhesions and sometimes further malrotation can develop (Moreno & Iovanne 1993b).

Progress

When the baby is weaned off the ventilator CPAP (continuous positive airway pressure) may be needed and then humidified head box oxygen. There may be episodes of cyanosis during bouts of agitation as the tiny lungs struggle to provide efficient gas exchange. Periods of reventilation might be necessary and chest infections are common.

Eventually a third of these severely affected babies will go home. The rest will succumb either to overwhelming infections as a result of antibiotic resistance or to pulmonary hypertension leading to pulmonary interstitial emphysema and heart failure. For the survivors there is a risk of recurrent chest infections and the child will always sound 'wheezy'. The parents of these children have to be constantly aware that colds could develop into chest infections and keep the baby away from obviously infected people. Continuous exposure to smoky atmospheres will worsen problems and parents who smoke should be tactfully advised as to how to protect their baby.

The future

The babies with hypoplastic lungs and almost non-existent lung function have a high mortality rate even in specialist centres. Treatment with low dose nitric oxide gas is gaining success (Davenport & Holmes 1995). This gas can be 'bled' into a ventilation circuit and acts as an endogenous vasodilator. It has no effect on systemic vasculature, only on the lungs, and it reduces the pulmonary hypertension that so severely complicates this defect.

Extra-corporeal membrane oxygenation (ECMO) has now improved the prognosis for these babies. This is currently carried out in five specialised units in the UK. The USA claims 69% survival rate for severely affected babies using ECMO (Davenport & Holmes 1995).

Tracheo-oesophageal atresia and fistula

In this congenital condition there is a structural defect affecting the trachea and oesophagus. The most common cases consist of the oesophagus ending before reaching the stomach and fistulating into the trachea. There are other variations, but the most common are shown in Fig. 5.2.

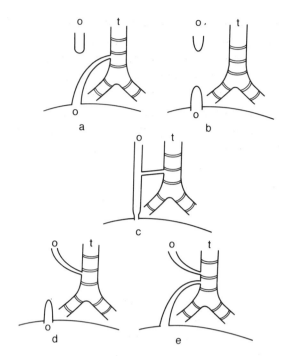

Fig. 5.2 Types of tracheo-oesophageal atresia (o = oesophagus, t = trachea).
(a) Tracheo-oesophageal atresia with distal fistula (most common type).
(b) Oesophageal atresia only.
(c) Tracheo-oesophageal fistula without atresia (H-type).
(d) Oesophageal atresia with proximal fistula.
(e) Both upper and lower oesophagus connect with trachea.

Embryology

It occurs in 1 in 3500 births and although most are in a single member of the family there is a known familial occurrence. The fault occurs in the embryo at about the fourth or fifth week of pregnancy and is thought to be caused by the failure of the pharynx and trachea to separate, leading to webbing between the two (Sadler 1990). The defect may be part of a syndrome with other abnormalities present.

Physiological outcome

The main problem with all types of tracheo-oesphageal atresia is the aspiration into the lungs of oral fluids. Asphyxiation and aspiration will occur when attempts at feeding are made resulting in permanent damage to the lungs and possible death.

Antenatal diagnosis

The condition can be seen on a scan at 16 weeks by the absence of the intra-abdominal bubble, which indicates an obstruction (Proud 1994). Other indications in the mother are polyhydramnios, likely because the fetus cannot swallow the liquor.

At birth

If the baby has been diagnosed antenatally, the mother will be delivered in a hospital with a surgical unit. Undiagnosed cases are suspected at birth if the mother had polyhydramnios and the baby has abundant frothy mucus around the mouth.

The mucus is caused by the baby being unable to swallow saliva and can cause choking attacks and cyanosis. An 8 Fr nasogastric tube should be passed in suspicious cases, before feeding, to see if there is a passage through to the stomach. If the tube cannot be passed into the stomach, then the baby should be X-rayed with a radio-opaque tube passed as far as possible into the oesophagus. If this shows up the blind end of the oesophagus, arrangements should be made with a paediatric surgical team for transfer to a neonatal surgical centre for treatment.

Diagnosis

Most types of the defect can be diagnosed by

chest X-ray. The most difficult to diagnose is the H-type fistula because it is possible to pass a nasogastric tube into the stomach. The fistula from the oesophagus into the trachea can lie anywhere along the length of the oesophagus, allowing milk and saliva to pass across to the trachea. Undiagnosed, this will cause repeated chest infections and choking episodes and often permanent lung damage. It is so uncommon that a number of other conditions may be thought of and followed up before it is eventually diagnosed by bronchoscopy.

The laryngeal cleft has the highest morbidity and it is also the rarest type occurring in one in 10 000 to 20 000 and often accompanies other significant abnormalities which affect the outcome of treatment. The defect consists of an abnormal communication between the trachea, larynx and oesophagus. Treatment is effected by tracheostomy and gastrostomy at first, followed by a difficult staged repair later when the baby has grown (Corbally 1993).

Preoperative care

Once the diagnosis has been made the 8 Fr tube in the oesophageal pouch should be attached to low continuous suction, to prevent saliva from entering the lungs, until the operation has been performed. The oesphageal pouch must be checked frequently to ensure it is draining efficiently to reduce the risk of inhalation and a chest infection before surgery.

The operation

At operation the fistula is located by bronchoscopy and tied off. The ends of the oesophagus are joined in a primary anastomosis if possible. A nasogastric tube will be inserted in theatre passing the site of the anastomosis. This is called the transanastomotic tube and remains in place until the site heals, which takes about a week. The baby can be fed through this within a few days of the operation. Vigilance, ingenuity and firm fixing ensure the tube does not accidentally become displaced as passing a new one could damage the delicate repair. An extrapleural chest drain is inserted to drain off any anastomotic leaks.

If there is a large gap in the oesophagus, a gastrotomy will be fashioned for milk feeds to be given until a full repair can be made. The upper end of the oesophagus is then brought out onto the skin surface of the neck so that saliva can drain. This operation allows sham feeds to be given to the baby so that normal sucking mechanisms and feeding behaviour can develop.

Postoperative care

After surgery the baby will be given pain relief and will remain ventilated to ensure that intubation, which could damage the repair, will not be needed. After 24 hours ventilation and opioid pain relief are discontinued and rectal paracetamol is given regularly for the first few days. The chest drain will stay in for a week until the anastomosis has healed (Cote *et al.* 1991). Oral suction must be done with care to prevent disturbing the anastomosis and should not stimulate the cough reflex. The catheter should be inserted into the mouth for 2–3 cm (1–$1\frac{1}{4}$ inches) only.

Progress

Feeding is commenced, in small amounts, through the transanastomotic tube in the first few days after the operation. The stomach will be smaller than normal because there was no swallowing and filling of the stomach with amniotic fluid in fetal life. When the baby is a week old, the chest drain is removed and milk feeds are given orally by breast or bottle. Some surgeons like a barium X-ray at this stage to see if the anastomosis has healed.

Feeding will be a problem for some time as the normal reflex mechanism of the oesophagus is disturbed by the defect. Feeds should be given slowly to prevent reflux, overspill into the lungs and vomiting. Parents will also be told that should these signs worsen at home, their baby should be brought to hospital for a dilatation and that this could be a frequent event in the early years. These babies often have a brassy cough which may last about 18 months. Babies who do not have a primary repair will have their second operation at about a year to give the ends of the oesophagus some time to grow. A small piece of the colon is used to join the two ends of the oesophagus.

Parents should be given the address of a support group to contact when they are ready. The TOFS group is based in Nottingham but can put parents in touch with a local group nearer their home (Appendix 1).

The future

Very few babies die with uncomplicated tracheo-oesophageal fistula. Effective surgical intervention and good nursing care ensure that damage from leaks and pneumonia is minimised.

Duodenal atresia

Duodenal atresia is a congenital narrowing or blockage of the duodenum, the first part of the small intestine just below the stomach (Fig. 5.3). The atresia causes a build-up of fluids in the stomach so that the baby vomits oral feeds. Duodenal atresia is the most common form of congenital neonatal bowel obstruction.

Embryology

Duodenal atresia is caused by an error of development which occurs at around 30–40 days of fetal life (Lister & Irving 1990). This discovery was made when a high proportion of children with duodenal atresia was found in mothers who had taken thalidomide in the first month of their pregnancy in the 1960s. The incidence is 1 in 6000 births (Roberton 1993b).

There are two types of duodenal atresia:

Intrinsic

Normally around 30–40 days there is a proliferation of the mucosal cells in the gut which completely plug the duodenum. Before the 60th day a recannulisation of the gut occurs. If this is incomplete a membranous atresia could result. The most common site is the curve on the C of the duodenum called the ampulla of Vater. There may be a complete atresia, partial atresia or a stenosis (Lister & Irving 1990).

Annular pancreas

Normally the two halves of the embryonic pancreas fuse and rotate around the duodenum. In this defect, the right portion of the ventral bud migrates along its normal route but the left part goes in the opposite direction. The duodenum is thus surrounded by pancreatic tissue. This often causes constriction of the duodenum leading to complete obstruction.

Diagnosis

Duodenal atresia can be diagnosed easily in the late second and third trimester of pregnancy by ultrasound scan. Fluid in the baby's upper abdomen each side of the obstruction gives a typical double bubble picture.

Some 30% of babies with trisomy 21 have

duodenal atresia and other babies who have additional major gut abnormalities often have duodenal atresia (Roberton 1993b). The scanner operator will look closely at the rest of the baby for associated problems when a diagnosis of duodenal atresia is made.

At birth

The typical baby will be growth retarded, under 2500 g and deliver prematurely to a mother who has hydramnios. It is not certain whether the growth retardation results from nutritional deprivation or from the inability to absorb nutrients from the amniotic fluid (Lister & Irving 1990).

If the duodenal atresia is not picked up on a scan, the baby appears well at birth. Vomiting usually starts within a few hours of birth and for most babies this will be copious and bile stained. Abdominal distension will not be marked as only the stomach and the proximal duodenum can extend. Distension will often subside after gastric aspiration. Meconium is not normally passed in cases of intestinal obstruction but it is not uncommon for it to be passed in this condition, the reason for this not being clear (Lister & Irving 1990). A plain abdominal X-ray will reveal the double bubble of duodenal atresia.

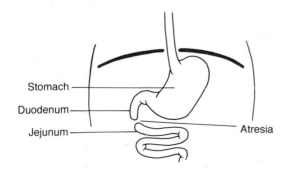

Fig. 5.3 Diagram of duodenal atresia.

Preoperative care

An X-ray will confirm the diagnosis. An 8 Fr infant feeding tube will be passed and aspirated hourly for gastric decompression. An intravenous infusion of dextrose and electrolytes will be started and if the baby is more than a few hours old, blood samples will be taken to estimate urea and electrolyte balance, which may be abnormal from the vomiting. This will then be corrected if necessary before theatre.

If the baby is to be referred to a surgical centre, it is not essential that surgery is performed immediately. As long as the baby is kept well hydrated and the nasogastric tube on low suction for gastric decompression, the operation may be delayed for up to 24 hours.

The operation

The surgeon makes a transverse abdominal incision, just above the level of the umbilicus, extending from the right flank almost to the midline (Lister & Irving 1990). This gives easy access to the duodenum. At the site of the atresia, the surgeon will effect a repair by suturing each side of the atresia then cutting it and opening the narrowed part. The two parts are then joined together. An oral trans-anastomotic tube is passed in theatre, bypassing the site of the anastomosis, and is left *in situ* for at least 7 days until the stitches have healed. The abdominal wound is then sutured.

A central venous line may be inserted in theatre, so that the baby can be given high energy parenteral nutrition until oral feeding is established. These babies are likely to develop a postoperative ileus and some take weeks to get established on full milk feeds.

Postoperative care

The main problem these babies are going to have after they have recovered from the anaesthetic is the establishment of oral feeds. When bowel sounds are heard, clear fluids, then breast milk are introduced gradually into the transanastomotic tube bypassing the atresia site. Some units pass a nasogastric tube so that the stomach can be aspirated to ensure the milk is not pooling there. In these cases where the baby has a tube in both nostrils, careful observations for respiratory difficulties must be made as babies are nose breathers. If problems occur the nasogastric tube should be removed.

The transanastomotic tube is left in for about a week to ensure the sutures in the anastomosis have healed. Milk can then be given through the nasogastric tube into the stomach. The amounts of milk are increased until full oral requirements are tolerated. This stage is sometimes prolonged if the baby produces excessive bile or if there is recurring abdominal distension and vomiting. The feeds may have to be stopped and restarted after 24 hours many times before the baby can tolerate full milk feeds.

Exomphalos

Exomphalos (omphalocele) is a congenital defect where normal abdominal wall development has not taken place. The contents of the abdomen herniate, through the umbilical ring, which has failed to close, into the base of the umbilical cord. Exomphalos can vary in size from a tiny gap of less than 5 cm (2 inches) containing a small amount of intestine, to a huge hernia covering the whole abdominal wall and containing all the abdominal contents (Fig. 5.4).

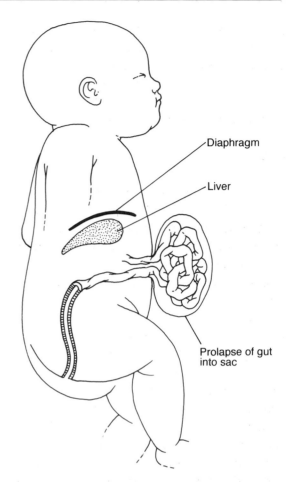

Fig. 5.4 Diagram of exomphalos. Large umbilical defect with viscera protruding from abdominal cavity into transparent moist sac.

Incidence figures are quoted at between 1 in 6000 and 1 in 7500 births (Fisher *et al.* 1996) and in 67% of cases, it is associated with other abnormalities (Lister & Irving 1990). Early diagnosis and examination of other anomalies can help predict the mortality rate. This can be as high as 75% for those with severe abnormalities and counselling of parents about the advisability of continuing the pregnancy in these cases, may be necessary (Fisher *et al.* 1996). Treatment in a specialist unit is essential immediately after birth to give the baby the best chance of survival.

Embryology

The way the defect occurs *in utero* is not exactly known. The problem is that a similar condition, gastroschisis (where the contents of the abdomen herniate through a cleft in the abdominal wall) also occurs around this time. It seems that both defects occur around the 52nd day of gestation in the fetal sac when the oblique and abdominus rectus muscles form. Exomphalos is a herniation of the gut into the umbilical ring. Gastroschisis is the herniation of the gut through a cleft in the abdominal wall. Embryologists cannot determine whether the one leads to the other or which develops first.

The defect

It differs from common umbilical hernia in that the protrusion is not covered by skin but by a translucent, avascular membrane. This consists of peritoneum inside and avascular membrane outside which is separated by a layer of the Wharton's jelly that makes up the cord. The rupture of the sac *in utero*, during labour or after birth is a common complication. The exposed gut is then at risk of infection, trauma, heat and water loss. This will cause problems with temperature and electrolyte stability and possibly peritonitis after surgical repair.

Diagnosis

Ultrasound scanning during pregnancy now means that most babies with exomphalos are diagnosed *in utero* and the defect accurately assessed. It is very important that this defect is distinguished from gastroschisis on scan before any advice is offered the parents. Exomphalos carries a far higher risk of other anomalies and so has a poorer outcome.

When the diagnosis of exomphalos is made, high definition scanning may reveal heart defects or other problems. The mother may be given an amniocentesis to check for chromosomal abnormalities at this stage. This condition is more common in boys so the family history is also checked, as there can be sex-linked inheritance. If a chromosomal abnormality or familial tendency is found the parents will be referred to the genetic team for advice, counselling and prognosis.

If the defect is high it is associated with congenital heart disease and defects of the diaphragm. If it is low, it is associated with cloacal extrosophy, spinal abnormalities and imperforate anus (Merenstein & Gardner 1993). Babies with exomphalos can have the defect as part of a syndrome which may be Beckwith–Wiedemann syndrome, trisomy 13 (Patau's), trisomy 18 (Edwards') and trisomy 21 (Down's) (Roberton 1993b).

At birth

Caesarian section is the usual method of delivery, especially if there is a large exomphalos, to prevent the sac rupturing. The condition is usually obvious at birth but occasionally a very small exomphalos that is covered by Wharton's jelly might be overlooked. This may not be diagnosed until the cord separates and some bowel prolapses. Sometimes a very small defect may be clamped accidentally with the cord, causing a fistula or intestinal obstruction. All babies with small or large exomphalos should be examined for other defects.

At birth the covering sac is translucent, soft and pliable and the organs inside are identifiable. After a few hours it becomes opaque and white and in 24 hours, if not treated, the sac will crack, allowing bacteria to enter; or the sac may rupture spilling the abdominal contents. The skin of the abdomen may merge into the membrane at the neck of the sac or reach up the sides for a short distance (Lister & Irving 1990).

Preoperative care

The baby will be taken to the neonatal unit and nursed in an incubator for warmth. There is rapid heat loss from the exposed gut so clear plastic wrap is used to cover the sac which will be supported in an upright position to allow the contents to settle into the abdomen as much as possible.

An 8 Fr nasogastric tube will be passed and kept on continuous low suction to prevent abdominal distension from swallowed air. Intravenous electrolyte dextrose will be started immediately and colloids such as fresh frozen plasma or human albumin, given to stabilise the baby for theatre. Antibiotics will be started (Yeo 1996).

Management

The method of treatment is dependent on the size of the exomphalos. Defects of less than 5 cm can be closed by surgical primary closure under anaesthetic (Levene *et al.* 1987). The amniotic sac is excised and the protruding viscera are reduced into the peritoneal cavity. The skin is incised around the neck of the sac leaving a 1-mm wide strip attached to the amniotic membrane which is then closed over the defect. The intestines are carefully inspected for malrotation and congenital bands which are then corrected.

If the defect is large, reduction causes too much pressure on the diaphragm. This embarrasses respiration and could lead to intestinal ischaemia, renal failure and haemodynamic instability (Langer 1996). A Silastic pouch is sutured to the abdominal wall to cover the area of the exomphalos which is gradually reduced by the surgeon over a period of 3–5 days. Once the viscera are all in the abdomen the Silastic pouch is removed and the abdominal wall closed (Langer 1996).

When the defect is enormous, conservative management is often the treatment of choice. If infection and rupture of the sac can be prevented the skin of the abdominal wall will slowly grow over it leaving a ventral hernia. The sac will be supported upright and may gradually reduce till it reaches a manageable size for surgery. The advantage of this method is that it can be used in cases where the baby is in poor condition or has other anomalies requiring more urgent surgery. The disadvantage of conservative treatment is that the gut is not inspected for anomalies and the baby may need surgery to correct malrotation or congenital bands later.

Postoperative care

Ventilatory support is always needed as the pressure of the abdominal contents may prevent adequate lung expansion. Babies with Beckwith–Wiedemann syndrome, who are often very large at birth, will have problems with hypoglycaemia and hypocalcaemia.

Central venous lines are essential for parenteral nutrition as there may be a long period of paralytic ileus. When bowel sounds are heard, oral fluid is commenced very slowly, starting with clear liquids.

If there is a Silastic covering, feeding is not usually started as infection is a constant hazard. Strict aseptic techniques must be used when re-dressing the sac or handling the central line. If there is infection, other antibiotics are added to those already being given, according to bacteriological findings. Nystatin is given as prophylaxis for *Candida* colonisation from prolonged antibiotic use.

Progress

Oral fluids can be started when bowel sounds are heard. The progression to full milk feeds may take weeks as the damaged intestine settles down.

Complications

Malrotation of the gut is a common complication and if an obstruction is caused surgery will be required. Babies who have had skin flap repairs will have a large ventral hernia which will require surgery at about 12–18 months of age. Corrective cosmetic surgery is done at about 2 years of age to give the child a realistic looking umbilicus and to tidy up the scar left by the original operation. Syndrome-related cases may need corrective treatment for other defects.

Prognosis

The survival rate for babies with exomphalos used to be poor with only 25% of babies reaching their first year (Fisher *et al.* 1996). Antenatally this prognosis is still valid but the exclusion, by termination, of many babies with lethal malformations has increased the one year survival figure to 80% (Fisher *et al.* 1996).

Gastroschisis

Gastroschisis is a congenital defect of the abdominal wall that occurs in 1 in 6000 to 7500 births (Fisher *et al.* 1996). There is no family incidence and additional malformations are uncommon apart from those affecting the gut.

In this condition the contents of the abdo-men herniate through a full thickness cleft in the abdominal wall near the umbilicus (Fig. 5.5). The defect itself is often small compared with the actual size of the viscera protruding. Immediate treatment and repair is needed to minimise the damage to the intestines. The blood supply to the intestines is often seriously impaired causing strangulation and gangrene of the gut.

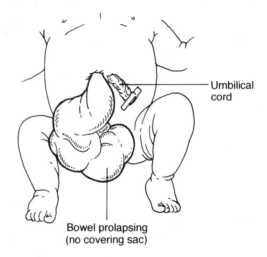

Fig. 5.5 Diagram of gastroschisis. Abdominal wall defect to right of midline.

Embryology

The precise embryogenesis of gastroschisis is not clear. Exomphalos, where abdominal contents herniate into the base of the umbilical cord, occurs at the same embryological time. The difficulty comes in deciding how each has developed in the fetus. It seems likely that both defects occur around the 52nd day when the oblique and rectus abdominus muscles form.

The defect

Gastroschisis literally means cleft belly. It is a defect of the muscle of the abdominal wall which allows the contents to extrude. Though usually fairly small it can vary from a few centimetres, to a gap extending from the sternum to the pubic symphysis. It occurs next to the umbilicus and most often to the right of it. Occasionally only a short length of gut protrudes but more commonly all the small intestine and much of the colon are eviscerated. Stomach, testes or uterus, gall bladder and urinary bladder are sometimes included. There is no membrane covering the eviscerated gut which is usually dilated, thickened and showing evidence of fetal peritonitis owing to the irritant action of the amniotic fluid. The intestine is sometimes shortened with atresias and malrotations.

Diagnosis

Ultrasound scanning during pregnancy now means that all but the smallest gastroschisis defects are diagnosed *in utero*. It is very important that gastroschisis is properly diagnosed, as exomphalos, which appears similar on a scan, carries a high incidence of chromosomal and other abnormalities. The scan will be carefully studied before the results are given to parents. Some hospitals offer termination for this abnormality in spite of the good results from surgery and this may be because it is confused with exomphalos (Fisher *et al.* 1996).

When gastroschisis is diagnosed the mother will be given advice on the condition and the prognosis, she should be referred to a maternity hospital, which has a neonatal surgical unit, for her delivery. The surgical team of the receiving hospital should be notified when the scan diagnosis is made. Scan assessment is carried out frequently to estimate the amount of dilatation and thickening of the bowel wall. The irritant effect of the amniotic fluid and restriction from the defect can cause irrepar-

able damage to the eviscerated gut (Nicholls *et al.* 1993). If the blood supply to the gut is threatened, gangrene of the bowel could mean that most of the gut has to be removed at birth with a poor outcome for the baby. Delivery will be induced at 36–38 weeks depending on the results of the scans (Pryde *et al.* 1994).

At birth

Surveys have shown that mothers of these babies are likely to be under 20 years old and the baby is likely to be their firstborn (Lister & Irving 1990). There are usually no complications of the pregnancy but birth weight is likely to be as low as 2500 g (5 lb 8 oz) at term. The defect is obvious at birth and the intestines may show evidence of fetal peritonitis. Impaired circulation to the bowel from pressure exerted by the small hole through which it has herniated is common and sometimes the bowel is gangrenous.

Preoperative care

Surgery should be performed as soon as possible to prevent further damage to the gut. Hyperthomia and dehydration as a result of the heat and water loss from the exposed gut can be prevented by wrapping the intestines in clear plastic film. This is easy to handle and allows the gut to be seen at all times. Some units place the lower half of the baby in a draw string 'intestinal bag' that covers the defect while leaving it visible.

An 8 Fr nasogastric tube is passed and aspirated continuously on low suction to keep the bowel decompressed. Large amounts of bile-stained fluid will be excreted from the damaged gut and this fluid should be replaced intravenously by an electrolyte solution. Intravenous electrolyte dextrose is started as soon as possible to prevent hypoglycaemia and fresh frozen plasma or human albumin are given to replace fluid loss from the gut and to correct perfusion for theatre. Intravenous antibiotics are commenced (Yeo 1993).

The operation

The clear plastic film or protective bag should be left in place until the baby is anaesthetised in theatre. Throughout the operation care is taken to keep the exposed intestines warm and well perfused. The bowel is cleaned with aqueous chlorhexidene and milked gently to help decompression. The hole in the abdominal wall often has to be enlarged before the gut can be returned. The abdominal wall is thoroughly stretched by the surgeon working over the skin with fingers, the thumb inside the abdomen. This is to increase the capacity of the abdomen to allow it to accommodate the large amount of bowel. The gut is inspected from end to end for atresias and rotations. Any gangrenous bowel is resected before the abdomen is closed.

Postoperative care

Most babies are electively ventilated after surgery as respiration is compromised by the tense abdomen after closure. Ventilatory support is usually only necessary in the first 48 hours except in cases where the closure is very tight. The abdomen is kept decompressed by continuous low suction on the nasogastric tube. This is to help prevent swelling of the gut and to remove the copious secretions that occur.

A long period of paralytic ileus can be expected because of the damage to and handling of the gut. Intravenous antibiotics are given and continued for 7 days to sterilise the bowel after the handling before and during surgery. A central venous line is used so that a concentrated formula of total parenteral nutrition can be given.

The wound will be very tense and may gape as healing occurs. Careful observation for signs of infection is necessary. When bowel sounds are heard and the bile secretions diminish, continuous suction is stopped, clear solutions of oral fluid in small hourly amounts are given. If the baby tolerates this without vomiting or abdominal distension, the mother's breast milk can be started in the same amounts after 12–24 hours.

Progress

The process of weaning from intravenous nutrition to oral feeding takes from a week to a few months.

Outcome

The outcome for gastroschisis is very good. Babies who have had only a skin closure will have a ventral hernia which is closed at 12–18 months. Male babies who have had Silastic pouches often develop inguinal hernias which also need surgical repair. If there are no problems at discharge the parents can expect no further sequelae.

Imperforate anus

This occurs in 1 in 2500 births (Roberton 1993b) and is usually discovered during the first examination after birth. There are a number of types of imperforate anus:

- A membrane covering the anus.
- A low or high atresia of the rectum.
- An opening which ends after a centimetre or so.

Often there is a fistula from the rectum into the urethra or vagina through which meconium will be passed.

Diagnosis

Imperforate anus is unlikely to be diagnosed on a scan unless other anomalies are noted. Imperforate anus often accompanies other defects of the gastrointestinal tract such as tracheo-oesophageal fistula and problems coming under the heading of VATER complex which covers Vertebral, Anal, Tracheal, Oesophageal, Renal/Radial anomalies and syndromes. The higher the atresia of the rectum the more complicated the condition is likely to be (Figs 5.6 and 5.7).

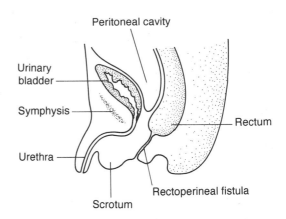

Fig. 5.7 High imperforate anus or rectal atresia. The rectum has failed to develop. Often a rectoperineal fistula is present. (Adapted from Sadler (1990).)

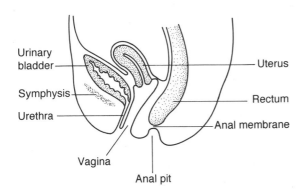

Fig. 5.6 Low imperforate anus. The anal membrane forms a diaphragm between upper and lower portions of anal canal. (Adapted from Sadler (1990).)

Preoperative care

A baby with a simple imperforate anus is not usually an immediate emergency. An intravenous dextrose infusion is started and nothing given orally, the surgery can then be delayed up to 24 hours. If transfer to a surgical unit is needed this can be delayed until a convenient time, such as the next morning if the baby is born at night. When the baby arrives at the unit an examination and X-ray will be taken to assess the extent of the problem and indicate the type of treatment needed.

The operation

If the problem is a simple membraneous obstruction, the procedure is an uncomplicated one often done on the unit under local anaesthetic. The rectal membrane will be cut with a scalpel. The baby must be carefully observed over the next few days to see if meconium is passed vaginally or urethrally; thus indicating a fistula into the bladder or vagina that will need to be repaired.

Correction of other types of imperforate anus is done in three stages:

(1) The formation of a colostomy.
(2) The formation of a new anus when the bowel is pulled down to the anus, usually undertaken when the baby is 9–14 months old.
(3) The closure of the colostomy after the new anus is working efficiently.

Postoperative care

The baby will be well after surgery and should not need ventilating unless the imperforate anus is complicated by another condition. The colostomy may pour out meconium as soon as it is fashioned, so a stoma bag will need to be fitted early to prevent continually disturbing the baby.

The parents need a great deal of nursing input and support to come to terms with their baby's colostomy and learn how to cope with it. They will need careful teaching and practice to gain the physical skills and confidence necessary. The community stoma service will be contacted and parents will be introduced to the district stoma nurse. When they leave the unit the parents should feel confident about looking after their baby with the colostomy, obtaining supplies and about future plans. There are a number of societies that give help and information to parents (Appendix 1).

Hirschsprung's disease

Hirschsprung's disease or congenital intestinal aganglionosis occurs in 1 in 5000 births (Roberton 1993b). Four males will be affected for every female and there may be a family history. The baby will normally be full term and well at birth but meconium is not passed and abdominal distension and often vomiting occur.

The disease is caused by a lack of nerve cells in a segment of the bowel and it prevents peristalsis so causing abdominal distension and obstruction from delayed movement in the bowel. The lower half of the colon is usually affected although, rarely, the whole of the colon and even some of the small intestine may be involved. An abdominal X-ray will show dilated loops of bowel. The definitive

diagnosis is by rectal biopsy which shows the aganglionic section.

A colostomy will be fashioned at 1–2 days of age, with surgery to resect the aganglionic bowel section performed at 4–12 months when the infant is thriving. As with imperforate anus the baby will be well after surgery and the parents will need nursing support and input to come to terms with and cope with their baby's colostomy. The most important nursing input at this stage, is the informative and practical attitude fostered by the nurses to give parents a positive outlook.

Necrotising enterocolitis

Necrotising enterocolitis is a potentially lethal condition characterised by ischaemic changes and necrosis of the gastrointestinal tract frequently leading to perforation. It is the most common surgical emergency in the neonate and carries a 30–50% mortality rate (Parker 1995). It is a major cause of mortality and morbidity in neonatal units and affects 12% of babies whose weight is under 1.5 kg (3 lb 5 oz). Though it usually affects preterm babies it can occur at any gestation and 3–5% of all babies nursed in the neonatal unit will be affected.

It occurs most commonly between the third and tenth day of life but may occur as early as the first 24 hours or as late as 3 months. Most full term babies are affected in the first week of life suggesting that they were affected *in utero* (Rescorla 1995). Early recognition and treatment of the disease is associated with decreased mortality.

Causes

There is no proven causative factor for the condition but is thought to be associated with injury to the bowel mucosa and with bacterial invasion. This damage may be caused by a number of factors. Mucosal injury is thought to be the most important factor and can be attributed to ischaemic events, decreased blood flow states, umbilical vessel cannulation, antenatal indomethacin (Gordon & Samuels 1995) and maternal cocaine use. These events can be caused antenatally, at birth or neonatally (Table 5.1).

feeds, increase in aspirates, vomiting, mild abdominal distension and sometimes blood in the stool, or reducing substances are detected by use of sugar analysis reagent tablets.

The nurse caring for the baby will notice a difference in usual behaviour and will alert the paediatrician. This is a vital observation and may save the baby

---

Table 5.1 Events and factors thought to increase the risk of necrotising enterocolitis.

Before birth
   Placenta abruption causing poor blood supply to the baby
   Prolonged rupture of membranes leading to infection
   Maternal cocaine use, though the reason is not known
   Indomethacin given to the mother to prevent preterm labour

At birth
   Low Apgar scores and apnoea causing hypoxia
   Respiratory distress syndrome causing hypoxia, shock, stress
   Polycythaemia where the blood is thick and sluggish

After birth
   Umbilical arterial catheter could introduce infection or cause trauma to the bowel
   Exchange transfusion
   Early feeding

Diagnosis

As there are so many possible causative factors, it is impossible to predict which babies will succumb but early recognition and treatment improve the mortality and morbidity of this disease. Continuous vigilance by neonatal nurses may prevent the disease developing into the fulminating stage.

The disease has three stages:

(1) The first stage consists of vague symptoms and may resemble other common conditions in preterm babies. Symptoms include temperature instability, lethargy, apnoea, bradycardia, loss of interest in

from developing the full-blown disease. Necrotising enterocolitis should always be suspected and treated if there is any doubt about diagnosis.

(2) The symptoms are more definite with severe abdominal distension and frank blood in the stools and nasogastric aspirate. X-rays will show pneumatosis intestinalis which consists of submucosal cysts filled with gas.

(3) The baby becomes acutely ill, shocked and collapsed. Immediate surgery, to remove the gangrenous, perforated gut, is necessary. This stage has a 60% mortality rate.

Treatment

The management depends on the stage of the disease. The surgical team should be consulted for all infants with suspected necrotising enterocolitis. Stage 1 can be managed conservatively with septic screening and monitoring of blood chemistry, platelets, gases and urinary output. Broad-spectrum antibiotics are given intravenously and continued for at least 14 days. If the baby is small, some units give immunoglobulin G to boost the immunity if surgery is required (Rowe *et al.* 1994). Nothing is given orally and parenteral nutrition commenced by a central line if necessary. Frequent X-rays check if the gut is perforated.

In the more advanced stage the baby may need to be ventilated because abdominal distension restricts respiration. The baby will be very sick at this stage and may need inotropic drugs and plasma infusions for hypotension, decreased perfusion and acidosis.

The timing of surgical intervention is difficult. The goal is to resect the necrosed area before perforation but not to perform a resection in a baby who would have recovered without surgery (Rescorla 1995). Most surgeons operate when there is pneumoperitoneum and portal vein air seen on X-ray (Rescorla 1995).

At operation the gangrenous bowel and perforations are resected and if a short segment is involved, a primary anastomosis will be performed. Often there is extensive necrosis which may require a colostomy or ileostomy. Sometimes there may be insufficient bowel left to survive if resection takes place. In these cases many surgeons do not resect the bowel and allow the child to succumb from the natural process of the disease (Rescorla 1995).

Once the acute stage has passed, feeding is not recommenced immediately. Most units will have a policy varying from 3 days to 3 weeks to allow the gut to heal. There have been no studies done and when feeding can start will be based on the surgeon's clinical judgement (Parker 1995).

Sequelae

Often these babies, even the ones who have not had surgery, may present later with strictures of the bowel from healed lesions. This is characterised by abdominal distension and vomiting and may require further surgery. Sometimes strictures will recur in other parts of the bowel and can become a long term problem.

Babies who are left with a short bowel may need intravenous therapy for years. Cases have been reported of babies with as little as 11–13 cm of small intestine though this is unusual (Rescorla 1995).

The future

As the number of very low birth weight infants surviving increases so the incidence of this disease increases. There seems no advance in the prevention of the disease though many theories abound. No studies have yet shown a clear indication of what is necessary to prevent this disease. Studies trying non-nutritive sucking to improve gut motility; delaying or hastening milk feeds; positions of umbilical catheters, have not proved any conclusive benefits (Kempley *et al.* 1993; Pickler 1994).

Corticosteroids given to mothers in preterm labour to help the maturation of the baby's pulmonary system have been found to have a positive effect on the maturation of the gastrointestinal system. Corticosteroids given to the baby postnatally may also improve the clinical outcome. These interventions may be shown in later surveys to be beneficial in the prevention of necrotising enterocolitis (Rescorla 1995).

REFERENCES

Affonso DD, Mayberry LJ, Hurst I, Haller L, Lynch ME, Yost K. (1992) Stressors by mothers of hospitalised infants. *Neonatal Network*, **11** (6), 63–70.

Andrews K, Wills B. (1992) A protocol for pain relief in neonates. *Professional Nurse*, **8** (8), 528–532.

Carter BC. (1990) Fetal rights – a technologically created dilemma. *Professional Nurse*, **5** (11), 590–593.

Corbally MT. (1993) Laryngo-tracheo-oesophageal cleft. *Archives of Disease in Childhood*, **68**, 532–533.

Cote JJ, Morse JM, James SG. (1991) The pain response of the postoperative newborn. *Journal of Advanced Nursing*, **16**, 378–387.

Davenport M, Holmes K. (1995) Current management of diaphragmatic hernia. *British Journal of Hospital Medicine*, **53** (3), 95–102.

Dellagrammaticas MD, Kapetanakis J, Papadimitreiou M, Kourakis G. (1991) Effect of body tilting on physiological functions in stable very low birthweight neonates. *Archives of Disease in Childhood*, **66**, 429–432.

Ewer AK, Durbin GM, Morgan MEI, Booth IW. (1994) Gastric emptying in preterm infants. *Archives of Disease in Childhood*, **71**, 24–27.

Farrell MF, Frost C. (1992) The most important needs of parents of critically ill children. *Intensive and Critical Care Nursing*, **8**, 130–139.

Fisher R, Attah A, Partington A, Dykes E. (1996) Impact of antenatal diagnosis on incidence and prognosis in abdominal wall defects. *Journal of Pediatric Surgery*, **31** (4), 538–541.

Gordon MC, Samuels P. (1995) Indomethacin. *Clinical Obstetrics and Gynaecology*, **38** (4), 697–705.

Harrison MR, Adzick NS, Flake AW, *et al.* (1993) Correction of congenital diaphragmatic hernia in utero – hard earned lessons. *Journal of Pediatric Surgery*, **28**, 1411–1412.

Hickey M. (1990) What are the needs of families of critically ill patients? *Heart and Lung*, **19** (4), 401–415.

Kempley ST, Bennett S, Loftus BG, Cooper D, Gamsu HR. (1993) Randomized trial of umbilical arterial catheter position – clinical outcome. *Acta Paediatrica*, **82**, 173–176.

Kuhnly JE, Freston MS. (1993) Back transport: exploration of parents feelings regarding the transition. *Neonatal Network*, **12** (1), 49–56.

Langer JC. (1996) Gastroschisis and omphalocele. *Seminars in Paediatric Surgery*, **5** (2), 124–128.

Levene MI, Tudehope D, Thearle J. (1987) *Essentials of Neonatal Medicine*, 2nd edn. Blackwell Scientific Publications, London.

Lister J, Irving I. (1990) *Neonatal Surgery*, 3rd edn. Butterworths, Oxford.

Ludman L. (1992) Emotional development after major neonatal surgery. *Paediatric Nursing*, **4** (4), 20–22.

Marteau TM. (1990) Reducing the psychological costs. *British Medical Journal*, **301** (7), 26–29.

Merenstein G, Gardner S. (1993) *Handbook of Neonatal Intensive Care*, 3rd edn. Mosby, St Louis.

Moreno CN, Iovanne BA. (1993a) Congenital diaphragmatic hernia; Part I. *Neonatal Network*, **12** (1), 19–27.

Moreno CN, Iovanne BA. (1993b) Congenital diaphragmatic hernia; Part II. *Neonatal Network*, **12** (2), 21–27.

Nicholls G, Upadhyaya V, Gornall P, Buick RG, Corkery JJ. (1993) Is specialist centre delivery of gastroschisis beneficial? *Archives of Disease in Childhood*, **69**, 71–73.

Orford T. (1996) Crisis and crisis intervention. Psychological support for parents whose children require neonatal intensive care. *Journal of Neonatal Nursing*, **2** (1), 11–13.

Parker LA. (1995) Necrotizing enterocolitis. *Neonatal Network*, **14** (6), 17–26.

Pickler RH. (1994) Non-nutritive sucking and necrotizing enterocolitis. *Neonatal Network*, **13** (8), 15–18.

Proud J. (1994) *Understanding Obstetric Ultrasound*. Books for Midwives Press, Cheshire.

Pryde PG, Bardicef M, Treadwell MC, *et al.* (1994)

Gastroschisis: can antenatal ultrasound predict infant outcomes? *Obstetrics and Gynaecology,* **84** (1), 505–510.

Reid S, Frey A. (1992) Techniques for the administering of intravenous medication/parenteral fluids in NICU. *Neonatal Network,* **11**, 6.

Rescorla FJ. (1995) Surgical management of necrotising enterocolitis. *Current Opinion in Paediatrics,* **7**, 335–341.

Roberton NRC. (1993a) *Textbook of Neonatology,* 2nd edn. Churchill Livingstone, Avon.

Roberton NRC. (1993b) *Manual of Neonatal Intensive Care,* 3rd edn. Edward Arnold, London.

Rowe MI, Reblock KK, Kurkchubasche AG, Healey PJ. (1994) Necrotizing enterocolitis in the extremely low birth weight infant. *Journal of Pediatric Surgery,* **29**, 987–991.

Sadler TW. (1990) *Langman's Medical Embryology.* 6th edn. Williams and Wilkins, London.

Smith DK, Marteau TM. (1995) Detecting fetal abnormality serum screening and fetal anomaly scans. *British Journal of Midwifery,* **3** (3), 133–136.

Sparshott M. (1989) Pain in the special care baby unit. *Nursing Times,* **85**, 1.

Yeo H. (1993) Expert care at a critical time. Surgical repair of gastroschisis. *Child Health,* **1** (2), 74–78.

Yeo H. (1996) Surgical intervention for the repair of exomphalos. *Professional Nurse,* **11** (4), 226–228.

6 | Nursing New-born Babies with Congenital Heart Disease

LEARNING OUTCOMES

After reading this chapter and studying the contents the reader will be able to:

○ Compare fetal and neonatal circulation.
○ List the causes of neonatal congenital heart disease (CHD).
○ Describe the current diagnostic and surgical techniques.
○ Demonstrate a knowledge of neonatal heart failure and its treatment.
○ Identify common heart conditions and treatments in the neonatal period.
○ Discuss support needed by the baby's family.

PHYSIOLOGY OF THE HEART

Embryology

The cardiovascular system is the first system to function in the embryo. Blood begins to circulate by the middle of the third week after conception to provide the rapidly growing embryo with nutrients and to dispose of waste products.

Between the 22nd and 28th day, the heart tube thickens and coils. The critical period for developmental faults occurs at approximately the 28th day when the major chambers are evolving. At this time blood is flowing through the heart and septation of the heart and great vessels occurs (Sadler 1990).

Fetal circulation

The heart of the fetus beats throughout pregnancy but the placenta supplies oxygen and nutrition, and removes carbon dioxide through the umbilical vessels. These vessels follow a system of short cuts through the fetal heart, bypassing the lungs and making the blood-flow from the placenta through the heart more efficient.

Oxygenated blood from the placenta goes to the fetal inferior vena cava by the umbilical vein and is directed through the foramen ovale between the atria. Oxygenated blood is then pumped by the left ventricle into the aorta and up to the brain. Deoxygenated blood from the upper body flows into the right ventricle which pumps it into the pulmonary artery. The ductus arteriosus between the pulmonary artery and the aorta restricts the blood flow to the lungs so that most of the blood goes down the aorta to the fetal abdomen where the umbilical arteries lead to the placenta (Fig. 6.1). The pulmonary arterioles, which are constricted and hypertrophied, are resistant to blood flow to protect the lungs as they develop and grow.

At birth

At birth systemic vascular resistance greatly increases when the first breath is taken, as the

lungs now need a much bigger blood supply. The first breaths of the baby increase oxygen tension, which dilates the pulmonary arterioles so increasing pulmonary blood-flow. This extra blood-flow causes the left atrial pressure to increase and close the foramen ovale. Circulating fetal prostaglandins are reduced as a result of increased pulmonary blood flow and this together with the increase of oxygen initiates the constriction of the ductus arteriosus. The ductus does not close immediately at birth taking a few days or even weeks in some babies (Table 6.1). Once these changes take place, the newborn circulation resembles that of an adult.

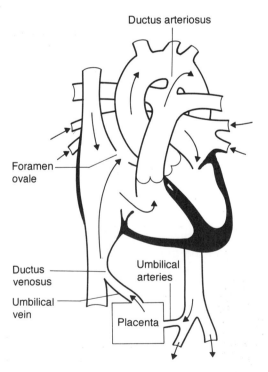

Fig. 6.1 Diagram of circulation before birth. (Unless otherwise referenced figures in this chapter are adapted from Rees *et al.* (1989).)

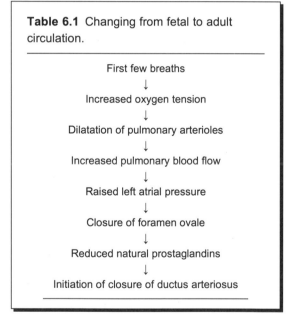

Table 6.1 Changing from fetal to adult circulation.

First few breaths
↓
Increased oxygen tension
↓
Dilatation of pulmonary arterioles
↓
Increased pulmonary blood flow
↓
Raised left atrial pressure
↓
Closure of foramen ovale
↓
Reduced natural prostaglandins
↓
Initiation of closure of ductus arteriosus

Normal heart circulation

To understand the abnormal heart it is important to be familiar with the normal heart and circulation. The heart can be considered as two pumps connected by a series of valves to stop the blood flowing back. Pressure generated by the left ventricle drives the blood through the systemic circuit. The purpose is to pump oxygenated blood round the body to all the organs and back through the lungs where it will pick up oxygen and then recirculate (Fig. 6.2).

Deoxygenated blood returns from the body in small veins which eventually join together to form two large veins, the superior vena cava from the upper body and inferior vena cava from the lower trunk and limbs. These empty into the right atrium then through the tricuspid valve into the right ventricle. When the right ventricle contracts this valve closes and the pulmonary valve leading to the pulmonary artery opens. Blood is then pumped via the pulmonary artery to both lungs where it is reoxygenated and pumped through the pulmonary vein back into the left atrium. The mitral valve opens into the left ventricle and blood flows through the aortic valve into the aorta which takes the oxygenated blood round the body. The heart beats at 70–150 beats a minute, depending on the age of the person, throughout life.

CAUSES OF CONGENITAL HEART DEFECTS

Congenital defects of the heart affect about 6 in every 1000 live born babies (Wren 1996). Out of this at-risk population about one-third will develop life-threatening symptoms carrying a high mortality rate, in the first few days of life (Paul 1995). In the 1990s with improvement in diagnostic, medical and surgical techniques 60% of babies with critical heart malformations survive to their first birthday. Congenital heart defects have a recurrence risk of 3% for the next baby born to the same parents whatever the cause (Proud 1994).

Potential causes

The causes of congenital heart defects are not clearly known and are thought to be influenced by a number of factors.

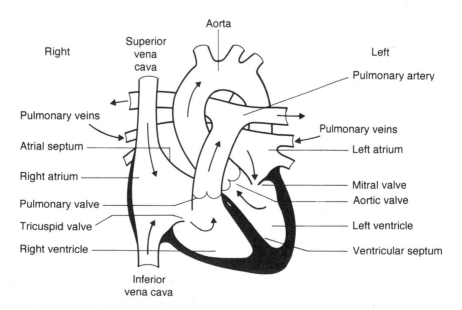

Fig. 6.2 Diagram of a normal heart and circulation.

Chromosomal abnormalities

There are several known chromosomal abnormalities which often include congenital heart disease such as Turner's syndrome, DiGeorge syndrome and trisomies 13, 18 and 21.

Viruses

Exposure to certain viruses (e.g. rubella and cytomegalovirus) during pregnancy may cause fetal abnormalities.

Drugs

Some drugs may affect the cardiac development of the fetus. These include anticonvulsants (such as phenytoin and phenobarbitone), antidepressants (such as lithium), the contraceptive pill and alcohol.

Maternal ill health

A mother with diabetes mellitus carries a 5% risk of having a baby with congenital heart defects. Transposition of the great vessels, ventricular septal defect, patent ductus arteriosis and cardiomyopathy, a disorder of the heart muscle, are the most common defects (Park 1991). Phenylketonuria and systemic lupus erythematosus (SLE) in the mother are also known to cause congenital heart defects in the baby.

Exposure to teratogens

Teratogens are substances capable of disrupting fetal growth and producing malformations. Exposure to radiation, chemicals or any substance that has an adverse effect on fetal development can cause problems if exposure takes place very early in pregnancy.

Fetal arrhythmias

These are abnormal heart sounds in the fetus and some are associated with structural heart disease.

Fetal hydrops

In this condition the baby is grossly oedematous. There are a number of causes including severe rhesus disease, thalassaemia and congenital infections. There will be a cardiac abnormality in 25% of cases (Allan & Baker 1993).

ANTENATAL DIAGNOSIS OF CONGENITAL HEART DISEASE

Ultrasound scanning

Many heart defects are now diagnosed on ultrasound scan, though minor defects can be missed on routine scan. Major heart defects can be identified by the 18th week of pregnancy by an experienced ultrasonographer (Wren 1996). A follow-up scan is arranged in these cases to look at the heart of the baby in more detail. After diagnosis the mother is usually advised to undergo amniocentesis to exclude a genetic disease. Babies are often referred for fetal echocardiogram if another anomaly is found.

Counselling of parents

Parents may be encouraged to seek termination of the pregnancy if the heart condition is lethal or complicated by genetic abnormalities. Few children with congenital heart disease are severely disabled in the long term but approximately 55% of pregnancies with a fetal heart defect are terminated. The decision is justified on the grounds of the surgery and mortality risk (Wren 1996).

The parents' decision will depend on the information provided by the cardiologist and advice from the obstetrician. Time should be allowed for consultation with other family members or counsellors before they decide on a course of action.

Antenatal care

Early diagnosis makes little difference to the outcome of most forms of CHD. If the pregnancy is to continue parents are advised to have the delivery in a hospital with neonatal cardiac facilities where the baby can be assessed and treated after birth. Indications for antenatal treatment may be fetal arrythmia such as supraventricular tachycardia which can lead to hydrops or death. The mother is treated with digoxin which improves the chance of the baby's survival (Wren 1996).

POSTNATAL CARE OF A BABY WITH CONGENITAL HEART DISEASE

Nursing a neonate with a congenital heart defect requires careful assessment and early recognition of clinical signs that may affect the outcome of the condition. If the baby has a defect that obstructs normal circulation, life will depend on the fetal ductus arteriosus remaining open.

When the duct starts to close 24–48 hours after birth, the baby will have minor symptoms which include dyspnoea, tachycardia or failure to complete feeds. If these signs go unnoticed and untreated the baby may deteriorate suddenly into cardiac failure, shock and possibly die.

Babies diagnosed in the neonatal period are sent to a neonatal cardiac unit for assessment. Admissions generally fall into four categories.

Babies diagnosed at early maternal discharge or at home

In these days of early maternal discharge and the small but steady increase in home births, the diagnosis may not be made until the baby is examined for discharge or when at home. A murmur may be heard on auscultation of the chest during the examination. A soft systolic murmur is common in new-born babies due to the remains of fetal circulation and this disappears later. A loud systolic murmur is a reason for immediate cardiac investigation so the baby is admitted to the neonatal unit for assessment. After the relief and excitement of a safe delivery of a well baby, parents suddenly have to re-adjust to having an ill baby who could need major surgery or even die.

Babies born in hospitals with no cardiac unit

The regional unit will be contacted and a team comprising a registrar and an experienced nurse, or nurse practitioner, will arrange to collect the baby as soon as possible. It is important to establish the exact condition of the baby before the team leaves the regional hospital, to ascertain whether the referring hospital needs to start treatment immediately. When the team arrives at the referring hospital they will be given a full report on the treatment already given. The team will then stabilise the baby for the return journey by establishing the following: secure airway, good intravenous access for drugs and fluid, satisfactory thermal condition and stable blood sugar. This will ensure the baby will travel safely and arrive in the best condition possible at the receiving unit.

If the parents are not able to accompany the baby, they must be told of the possible need for emergency surgery and what the surgery will entail. A signed consent form should then be obtained. It may be impossible to tell the parents exactly what the operation will entail until the baby has been properly assessed on the cardiac unit. Ideally one or both parents should accompany the baby, the mother will be accommodated on the postnatal ward at the receiving hospital and the father can usually stay with her.

Undiagnosed babies born in maternity units with specialist units

Hospitals with neonatal cardiac facilities are often in large maternity or children's hospitals. Even with scans performed by experienced ultrasonographers, babies with heart problems sometimes remain undiagnosed and are admitted to the postnatal wards with their mothers. After a day or two they get breathless and distressed as the ductus arteriosus closes. When these clinical symptoms appear the baby is sent to the neonatal unit for investigation.

Babies scheduled to be born at the regional unit

Diagnosis of a major cardiac problem on ultrasound scanning means that the mother will be referred to and delivered at a hospital with neonatal cardiac treatment facilities. After birth the baby is transferred to the unit where assessment and further diagnostic tests are carried out. Parents may have been to the unit before the birth, met the staff and seen the equipment. After the diagnosis, they will be prepared for problems and this will help them

to understand what is happening, but does not mean they will find the course of their baby's illness and treatment any easier to bear. Staff on the unit will always offer support, information and involvement with their baby's care throughout the stay.

Admission

Most babies diagnosed in the prenatal period will be well on admission. It is only as the ductus arteriosus starts to close and the heart labours to overcome the defect that symptoms occur. In life-threatening defects that depend on the patency of the ductus arteriosus for a complete circulation, heart failure may be sudden in onset when the duct closes. This mimics the symptoms of a severe infection such as septicaemia, pneumonia or meningitis and may lead to a delay in diagnosis.

Nursing care on admission

The current treatment of a baby with a congenital heart disease aims to anticipate and treat heart failure so as to prevent permanent damage to the heart and lungs before surgery is undertaken. This is done by monitoring vital signs, observing the baby, managing fluid balance, giving good nutrition and administering drug treatment to strengthen and stabilise circulatory function.

The baby is weighed on admission so that drug doses, fluids and nutritional needs can be calculated on this weight. Baseline observations of heart, respiratory rate, oxygen saturation, central and peripheral temperature, and blood pressure are taken. Continuous cardiorespiratory monitoring is carried out during assessment and diagnosis. A blood pressure reading is taken on each of the baby's limbs to aid diagnosis, as some conditions can cause upper and lower limb pressures to be different, depending on the site of the circulatory obstruction.

Maintenance of patent intravenous lines for drugs and nutrition is vital especially if the baby is dependent on drugs to keep the ductus arteriosus open. Attention should be given to provision of adequate energy for growth, as the baby is usually fluid restricted to prevent pulmonary and peripheral oedema caused by the failing circulation.

Observation and monitoring of anticipated cardiac failure

Heart failure occurs when the heart is unable to pump sufficient blood to meet the metabolic requirements of the body. This needs prompt treatment to prevent damage to other organs such as the kidneys, brain and gut, which function poorly or fail when blood supply is diminished. The baby's condition is monitored in the following manner and treatment initiated on the symptoms.

Tachycardia
Many babies with congenital heart defects will have a fast or irregular heart beat. The heart beats faster in an effort to pump the blood round the body and this can cause the metabolic rate to rise and uses valuable energy. The baby will perspire in an effort to stay cool, though the feet often remain cold because of the poor circulation. The core and toe temperatures should be monitored as a difference of more than 3°C is indicative of reduced cardiac function. To ensure the baby's comfort, even when the core temperature is satisfactory, bootees and mittens should be worn.

Cyanosis
Congenital heart disease is divided conventionally into acyanotic and cyanotic lesions. Cyanosis is the result of blood shunting from the pulmonary circulation to the systemic circulation without having been reoxygenated by the lungs. In acyanotic conditions the lung perfusion and blood oxygenation may not be affected.

If cyanosis is present it may be central and the baby is very pale or blue with cyanosis of gums and mucous membranes. Peripheral cyanosis, blueness of the hands and feet, can be due simply to poor circulation. Some newborn babies have blueness of the palms of the hands and soles of the feet, called acrocyanosis, which clears spontaneously and has no cardiac disease implications.

Respiratory effort
Increased respiratory effort may be the result of pulmonary congestion or decreased pulmonary blood flow. The baby may be breathless and tachypnoeic with chest retraction and reduced air entry on auscultation. Mechanical ventilation may be necessary to control the blood gases. Diuretics are given to relieve pulmonary congestion and oedema. If the baby is not ventilated, breathing may be easier if the incubator mattress is raised at the head end.

Raised oxygen requirements
Oxygen should be used with caution as it produces pulmonary vasodilation and hypertension encouraging closure of the patent ductus arteriosus which may be keeping the baby alive. Oxygen requirements are monitored using pulse oximetry or transcutaneous monitoring. Acceptable pulse oximetry readings for babies with cardiac problems, where there is mixing of oxygenated and deoxygenated blood, will be much lower than for a baby with a normal heart. Readings below 80% saturated arterial oxygen

may be accepted if the baby is well perfused and not distressed or tachypnoeic.

Oedema

Fluids are restricted so as not to overload the system, which cannot efficiently deal with it. An accurate fluid balance should be kept and urinary output monitored to check for fluid retention or anuria. If the baby is producing less than 1 ml/kg per hour, the urine is concentrated (as shown by a high specific gravity on ward testing), or there are signs of oedema, then renal function is poor. Reduced renal function is a reliable indicator of reduced cardiac function because a diminished blood supply, particularly to the renal artery, causes renal failure. Daily weighing is necessary to assess success of diuretics and fluid management.

Nutritional problems

The high metabolic rate induced by the tachycardia means that the baby uses extra calories at a time when fluids are restricted. Poor cardiac function will impair gastric performance causing slower emptying and vomiting. Attention must be paid to the provision of adequate calories for growth and recovery. If intravenous parenteral nutrition is used the baby should have a central line and high energy fluids, which include fats, proteins and glucose, should be used.

If the baby will tolerate oral feeds these are given to diminish the complications that may arise from administering intravenous fluids, such as infections in the line, gut stasis and choleostatic jaundice. Breast feeds or expressed milk can be given if the baby is tolerating oral feeds. Tube feeding may be necessary if the baby is unable to cope with sucking all feeds. Extra energy in the form of protein or carbohydrate powder may need to be added to milk feeds to ensure good growth.

Treatment and prevention of cardiac failure

The prevention of cardiac failure depends on maintaining an adequate circulation for the baby's metabolic needs. The aim is to strengthen the heart beat and maintain the circulation by using a combination of fluid restriction, diuretics and cardiac support drugs. Commonly used cardiac drugs include:

- Prostaglandin E_1
- Adrenaline
- Frusemide
- Dopamine
- Dobutamine
- Digoxin
- Indomethacin
- Tolazoline
- Fentanyl

Prostaglandin E_1

Many congenital heart defects depend on the patency of the ductus arteriosus to keep the circulation intact. Prostaglandin E_1 is given as a continuous infusion to keep the duct open while diagnosis and assessment of the defect is taking place. Prostaglandins are endogenously produced lipids that have a variety of effects in the body. Artificial prostaglandin E_1 acts on the smooth muscle of the duct keeping it open. It must be given in a continuous infusion as it is rapidly metabolised and as soon as the infusion stops the duct starts to close (Rikard 1993). It is essential to give it through a large vein, peripherally or centrally, and to maintain the patency of the line. Some units advocate having a second peripheral line ready for use in case one fails. It is used in a variety of heart malformations (Table 6.2).

Prostaglandin should only be given in units where there are full resuscitation facilities as this drug has the potential to cause apnoea

Table 6.2 Congenital heart defects for which prostaglandin E_1 is used.

Pulmonary atresia
Pulmonary stenosis
Transposition of the great arteries
Tetralogy of Fallot
Interrupted aortic arch
Coarctation of the aorta
Hypoplastic left heart syndrome
Aortic stenosis

and heart rhythm disturbances. The baby should have full cardiopulmonary monitoring while undergoing this treatment. If there are adverse effects such as apnoea, the baby will be ventilated but the drug must not be stopped as closure of the duct could cause death. Other side-effects to watch for include flushing and high temperature, blood pressure fluctuations, hypoglycaemia, gastrointestinal disturbances and renal insufficiency (Rikard 1993).

Adrenaline

This is a vasoconstrictor used for heart failure and it also increases blood pressure. It is usually given intravenously but can be given as a bolus through the endotracheal tube or through the heart with a long needle in an emergency arrest situation. It can cause tachycardia, vasoconstriction and impaired renal function if not monitored carefully.

Frusemide

Frusemide acts by preventing reabsorption of sodium in the kidneys and so prevents fluid retention. It thus controls oedema and eases the load on the heart. It can cause electrolyte imbalance so serum electrolytes need at least daily assessment.

Dopamine

This is an inotropic drug that acts on the heart muscle. It decreases vascular resistance and increases blood flow to the organs by improving the strength of the heart beat. It is used to raise the blood pressure in the treatment of shock and hypotension associated with heart surgery. A low dose improves renal function. It is given by continuous infusion and as there may be blanching of the skin over a peripheral site, it is best given by a central line.

Dobutamine

This inotrope is a synthetic preparation of dopamine which is given to augment the action of other inotropic drugs. It is given as a continuous infusion to increase cardiac output and blood pressure thus stabilising arrhythmias and improving tissue perfusion.

Digoxin

This is an inotrope which improves the heart rhythm and controls arrhythmias. It is given in divided doses orally or intravenously. It causes slowing of the heart so if the apex beat falls below 120 the next dose is omitted. Digoxin can reach toxic levels in the blood which may precipitate ventricular fibrillation and high blood pressure so serum levels must be monitored.

Indomethacin

This is used to close the ductus arteriosus and can be given intravenously or orally in a divided dose bolus. It blocks the actions of naturally circulating prostaglandins, which help to keep the duct open, by inhibition of prostaglandin synthesis. Electrolyte imbalance and hypoglycaemia, gastrointestinal bleeding and renal damage are side-effects.

Tolazoline

This is a vasodilator that often greatly improves oxygenation, though it can cause hypotension. It is given in a continuous infusion and may cause red tracking along the vein so should be given through an intravenous line with no other drugs.

Fentanyl

Pain relief and sedation should be given to keep the baby comfortable and relaxed, as crying increases the strain on the heart and lungs. Fentanyl, a systemic opioid, is used in many units as a continuous infusion for pain relief. It is usually only given if the baby is ventilated as it tends to depress the respiratory centre but can be given cautiously, in small doses, in unventilated babies.

Parents

A heart defect is seen by most people as very serious and life-threatening and parents need to talk over the problems of treatment, surgery and eventual outcome. Events usually move fast in the early days when the baby is undergoing tests and being prepared for surgery and parents may feel confused and frightened. Many of the cardiac defects carry a high mortality and morbidity rate even with major surgery and this needs to be clearly explained to the parents. If the baby has a congenital abnormality such as Down's syndrome, the parents may not wish their baby to have surgery. This is not their choice as the law now stands (Children's Act 1992) and treatment is undertaken with the baby's best interest in mind. If the surgeons decide the baby will make a good recovery with a reasonable quality of life after the surgery, it will be carried out. Nurses will necessarily bear the brunt of any decision and may find working with the parents in this situation

difficult. If there is a hospital counsellor available to the parents, he or she may help diffuse the situation. Parents and staff work best in partnership planning and carrying out the baby's care together.

Parents are encouraged to help with the hygiene needs of the baby and to give feeds. Accommodation is arranged where possible and if the mother is expressing her milk while staying at the hospital, this can usually be done on the unit.

Many units transfer babies, who are to have surgery using cardiopulmonary bypass, to a cardiac intensive care unit and re-admit them when stabilised after surgery. Although this is the best treatment for the baby it tends to be disruptive for the parents who have to get used to new staff.

Cardiac team

After admission, the paediatric cardiology team see the baby as soon as possible for assessment. The cardiac team will consist of a cardiac surgeon, a cardiologist and an experienced cardiac anaesthetist. This combination of expertise along with skilled nursing staff has been shown to give the best and most cost-effective results for the baby (Jonas 1995).

Diagnostic techniques

Radiology

A chest X-ray often gives clues to the diagnosis though heart changes may occur as a result of a traumatic delivery such as birth asphyxia (Kelnar *et al.* 1995). Some heart shapes may be diagnostic, such as the boot shaped heart of Fallot's tetralogy; the oval, egg shaped heart of transposition of the great vessels; or the square shape of tricuspid atresia (Paul 1995).

Electrocardiogram (ECG)

This is a tracing of the heart's activity. The normal ECG consists of a series of waves. The P wave occurs at the beginning of each contraction of the atria, the QRS complex occurs at the beginning of each contraction of the ventricles, the T wave occurs as the ventricles recover and prepare for the next contraction. The period between these waves is the retractory period. To detect abnormalities of heart rhythm a five lead ECG is performed to obtain all aspects of cardiac activity and a printout used to help with a definitive diagnosis.

Cardiac ultrasound (echocardiography)

Cross-sectional echocardiography has become established as a reliable technique for the detection of most congenital heart malformations. This is a major tool in the diagnosis of congenital heart defects when used by an experienced cardiologist. It is non-invasive and can be performed at the baby's bedside. Cross-sectional studies provide a two dimensional picture of the heart while Doppler echocardiography uses the principle that moving objects alter the frequency of sound waves. Thus the sound of the blood flow through a ventricular septal defect can be detected and diagnostic measurements made. Some scanning machines allow echoes and Doppler flow patterns to be simultaneously shown, with the flow in different colours. This is called colour-coded Doppler-flow imaging. The diagnostic accuracy of echocardiography has taken away the need for cardiac catheterisation in many cases.

Cardiac catheterisation

Cardiac catheterisation, used as a diagnostic tool, enables the cardiologists to record pressure measurements within the cardiac chambers and great vessels, obtain blood samples to analyse their oxygen content and inject radio-opaque dye to visualise the anatomy and function of the heart, great vessels and coronary circulation.

Cardiac catheterisation is mainly used for interventional procedures such as balloon septostomy or Rashkind's procedure (Fig. 6.3) to increase mixing of circulatory blood. It is being increasingly used to treat some cardiac problems such as tricuspid atresias and pulmonary stenosis instead of traditional surgery (Qureshi 1993). A balloon catheter is inflated in the blocked vessels to widen or push through them. Success appears good and in the future there may be an increasing number of defects treated this way.

Cardiac catheterisation is a major procedure for a new-born baby especially if small or sick. It is an invasive procedure necessitating the use of a general anaesthetic. A radio-opaque catheter is inserted into the femoral vein either by venipuncture or by cut-down. The catheter is then threaded up into the heart under X-ray guidance so that the four chambers of the heart can be visualised.

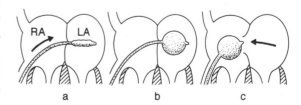

Fig. 6.3 Rashkind's atrial septostomy.
(a) A catheter is pushed into the right atrium (RA) and through the foramen ovale into the left atrium (LA).
(b) The balloon at the tip of the catheter is inflated.
(c) The catheter is withdrawn sharply tearing the atrial septum allowing improved oxygenation of the circulation. (Adapted from Kelnar, Harvey and Simpson (1995).)

Before catheterisation

If the baby is to have the procedure undertaken in theatre, blood pressure should be stable and haemoglobin satisfactory. Oral feeds are stopped for about 4 hours before the procedure. Intravenous fluids, at the appropriate volume for age, weight and condition should be started to ensure the baby does not become dehydrated and hypoglycaemic before or during the catheterisation. If there is severe congestive cardiac failure, infection, pyrexia or arrhythmias the operation should be postponed until the problems have been treated.

The baby should be put in an incubator for transport to ensure warmth for the journey, dressed in a simple easily removable gown and covered with a quilt of Gamgee tissue. Armbands must be checked and a premedication drug given if needed. The incubator should have a supply of oxygen and emergency resuscitation equipment such as bag, mask and airway. A ventilated baby will be accompanied to theatre by a doctor and nurse. Current ward charts, X-rays and a signed consent form for treatment should accompany the patient.

The procedure is explained to the parents and any written literature given to them. The complications that might occur should be talked through before the consent form is signed. They can usually accompany the baby to the anaesthetic room if they wish. Cardiac catheterisation takes anything from 1 to 3 hours and this time will seem endless as parents wait to hear their baby's diagnosis.

After cardiac catheterisation

On return of the baby to the unit, heart, respiratory rate and oxygen saturations are monitored for 4–6 hours. Potential complications include haemorrhage from the femoral site, heart rhythm disturbance and embolus. The catheter entry site should be checked for bleeding half hourly for 4–6 hours and then 1 hourly as the condition indicates. The pulse at the ankle in the limb used must be checked half hourly for 4–6 hours. If the pulse cannot be felt there could be an occluding clot in the vessel. Colour and warmth of the foot should be noted at the same time for the same reason. Any problems with the circulation are promptly dealt with by the use of intravenous anticlotting agents such as streptokinase, to prevent emboli with possible loss of toes or foot.

Feeds can be restarted after a few hours and intravenous fluids can be stopped. Parents are contacted when their baby comes back to the unit and the cardiac team will explain their findings as soon as possible.

Treatment of the defect

Once the diagnosis has been made there may be a number of options open to the cardiac team and parents.

Palliative surgery

In cardiac terms, palliative surgery means an operation to help improve heart function but not completely correct the problem. Palliative treatment is carried out on neonates, where the condition allows, as a temporary measure until they are strong enough to withstand major heart surgery. This type of treatment includes:

- Shunts
- Banding
- Balloon atrial septostomy

Shunts

The aim of these procedures is to ensure an effective route for systemic blood flow and to provide a controlled volume of pulmonary blood flow at low pressure. There are various types of shunt and the one used depends on the heart problem. A patch of Gore-Tex may be grafted on to one of the main vessels or the vessels may be anastomosed to give an effective circulation. These shunts usually have to be renewed as the baby grows.

Banding

Where a defect allows too much blood to be directed to the lungs, pulmonary damage will occur. The damage is caused by the large blood flow from the pulmonary arteries overloading the left ventricle. The heart has to pump harder and faster to keep up with the supply, tires and goes into failure. The lungs then get logged with blood and respiratory problems are caused. Putting a stricture or band on the pulmonary artery, narrows it, allowing less blood through. It is a temporary procedure buying time for the baby to grow before major surgery is attempted.

Balloon atrial septostomy

This is done to make an artificial hole in the heart when there is an incomplete or inefficient circulation (Fig. 6.3). It is called a 'Rashkind procedure' or balloon septostomy, and is sometimes done as an emergency when the duct has closed completely and the baby's circulation is failing. In these cases it is carried out on the neonatal unit under echocardiograph control. This procedure is sometimes done at the time of a diagnostic cardiac catheterisation, if necessary.

The catheter is inserted into the femoral vein and fed up into the heart under X-ray guidance as in cardiac catheterisation. A polythene balloon catheter is used and when it

reaches the correct place in the heart, is briefly but forcefully inflated with a dilute contrast solution. It is then pulled through the atrial septum from left to right creating a large atrial septal tear. This improves blood flow in conditions such as transposition of the great arteries, total anomalous pulmonary venous return, tricuspid atresia, pulmonary atresia (Park 1991).

Surgery

Surgery is usually carried out when the baby is relatively well and free from infection. Cardiac surgery in the new-born is divided into two categories, closed heart and open heart procedures.

Closed heart procedures are performed for extra-cardiac anomalies such as patent ductus arteriosus, or for palliative procedures such as pulmonary artery banding.

Open heart procedures involve the use of the cardiopulmonary bypass (CPB) machine with deep hypothermia and cardiac arrest techniques. They are used to repair ventral septal defects, tetralogy of Fallot, transposition of the great arteries and other anomalies. The improvement in managing babies before and after surgery now means that wherever possible the defect is corrected in one stage using cardiopulmonary bypass techniques (Jonas 1995).

Cardiopulmonary bypass

Cardiopulmonary bypass allows the surgeon to work on a still and bloodless area. The action of the heart is taken over by a mechanical pump using an oxygenating and heat exchanging device (Acari 1992). The procedure uses extra-corporeal circulation so that oxygenation of the vital organs can continue. The chest is opened via a median sternotomy and the pericardium is opened to expose the heart. The ascending aorta and the right atria are the usual sites to be cannulated and these are then connected to the cardiopulmonary bypass circuit. Heparin is used to prevent blood clotting in the circuit.

The baby is cooled, using the heat exchanging device on the bypass machine, to moderate hypothermia (28–32°C) or deep hypothermia (18–22°C) depending on the length of circulatory arrest needed for the operation. This hypothermia reduces metabolic demands and minimises hypoxic damage to the brain and major organs.

The heart contracts normally until the surgeon reaches the point in the operation where the heart must be still. The aorta is cross clamped near the cannula and a cardioplegic solution is infused into the heart to induce cardiac arrest. At 18–22°C the circulation may be safely interrupted for 35–40 minutes (Jonas 1995). While the baby is on bypass, the circulation is managed and treated by perfusionists who are experts in this care.

After surgery is completed the sternum may be left 'open' with just a skin flap covering the wound for easy access to the heart in case of haemorrhage or arrest. The baby is warmed using the heat exchange mechanism on the machine and the circulation returned to normal.

Complications after cardiopulmonary bypass surgery

When the operation is completed the baby is sent back to the intensive care unit for appropriate postoperative nursing and medical care. After cardiopulmonary bypass all the baby's systems will be unstable and need meticulous minute by minute correction with drug and fluid management for the first few hours.

Metabolic acidosis

This can occur from an accumulation of carbon dioxide and lactic acid in the blood. The baby will be pale and shocked and blood gases will reveal a high carbon dioxide level and a high base excess. Untreated this can lead to severe hypoxia and brain damage. The cause may be too rapid warming after the surgery, inefficient ventilation and/or poor perfusion of the tissues. Treatment needs to be prompt with adjustments in ventilation and infusions of fresh frozen plasma to improve acidosis and perfusion.

Haematological complications

There may be bleeding from the operation site in the heart which can cause cardiac tamponade. This is bleeding round the heart into the pericardium which will obstruct heart function. It will be recognised by sudden onset of bradycardia, the baby will be pale and clammy and there may be facial or nuchal (neck) oedema. Treatment consists of re-opening the chest and draining the pericardium.

Disseminated intravascular coagulation (DIC) is a common complication causing abnormal clotting and haemorrhage. Haemolysis takes place in the blood vessels as a result of damage to blood cells during the procedure. Coagulopathy is linked to the heparin given in theatre to prevent clotting.

Clotting factors will be replaced by transfusions of fresh frozen plasma. Vitamin K is given to help prevent bleeding. Severely affected babies or those not responding to fresh frozen plasma may be given an exchange transfusion of blood not less than 48 hours old which has retained maximum clotting factors. Blood will have been cross-matched before surgery so that it is ready for urgent use.

Pulmonary problems

Hypoxia will be treated with high oxygen levels and increased ventilation. Pulmonary oedema results from the long period of anaesthesia and stasis. Decreased compliance of lungs is due to reduced levels of surfactant, after being 'washed out' during bypass. Pulmonary hypertension is a common complication causing ventilator dependence and instability of vital signs. Research in the USA has shown that nitric oxide gas given with ventilator gases after operation, reduces pulmonary hypertension by acting as a pulmonary vasodilator when introduced into the lungs (Jonas 1995).

Renal problems

Kidney failure may be transient or permanent owing to poor blood supply to the renal artery. Peritoneal dialysis will be started, as soon as the urine output falls below 0.5 ml/kg an hour, to prevent kidney damage and stimulate renal function.

Neurological damage

This may be caused by emboli, hypoxia, hypoglycaemia or decreased perfusion. The baby may have convulsions and sometimes the damage is long term with hemiplegia or paraplegia. Studies have shown that the length of the circulatory arrest during bypass is directly related to the likelihood of neurological abnormalities. This was noted at a one year of age follow-up (Jonas 1995).

Advantages of using cardiopulmonary bypass

The advantages of cardiopulmonary bypass greatly outweigh the disadvantages. The risk of mortality from the bypass procedure is much less than that of untreated congenital heart defects (Park 1991). Continuous improvements in operating techniques and the advent of specialist perfusionists reduce the complications and mortality rates. Without this technique many heart disorders could not be surgically treated with safety and heart transplants could not even be attempted.

Parents

The sight of their baby after cardiac surgery is always traumatic. There are many wires and tubes surrounding the baby as well as a large wound in the centre of the chest. The tense atmosphere as the staff treat the baby at this critical stage will be obvious. There will be very little parents can do in the immediate postoperative period except talk to the staff when they are able. The uncertainty as to the outcome of the surgery and their baby's survival means they are in great need of supportive care from the staff.

As the days go by and the baby improves, they can resume changing the nappy and attending to hygiene needs. The cardiac team will let them know what the future holds for their baby and the follow-up treatment needed. The baby may be transferred back to the neonatal unit or to the paediatric cardiac ward a few days after the operation.

Nursing management after heart surgery

The baby's systems take time to recover from the cardiopulmonary bypass procedure and the heart and major vessels have to adjust to the corrective surgery.

Fluid balance

Retention of fluid is common because of

decreased renal blood supply, possibly as a result of shock from the surgery or bypass procedure. If fluid retention is untreated it will cause a return of heart failure, so diuretics are given to encourage excretion of fluid and a continuous intravenous dopamine infusion is given to improve renal function. Daily weighing is essential to monitor fluid retention.

Drug treatment

Digoxin may be needed to control tachypnoea. Low flow oxygen therapy may be needed for some time after surgery while the baby's lungs recover and should be monitored carefully to prevent hypoxia or hyperoxia. Antibiotics will be given prophylactically, often for life, to prevent infections that could cause a strain on the heart.

Nutrition

The relationship between congenital heart disease and poor nutrition is well known (Sinden & Sutphen 1995). Babies who have congestive heart failure, pulmonary hypertension and cyanotic heart disease such as Fallot's tetralogy usually have significant nutritional problems. This is attributed to high metabolic consumption as a result of the heart disease and further complicated by tachypnoea, chronic fatigue, hypoxia and malabsorption. Diarrhoea and vomiting may be troublesome and are caused by malabsorption and slow gastric emptying as a result of poor cardiac function. Other contributing factors to poor nutrition can be intrauterine growth retardation, prematurity and other congenital abnormalities that often affect these babies.

Fluid requirements are based on the degree of cardiac compromise and diuretic therapy, coupled with the losses from vomiting or diarrhoea. Sodium intake needs to be monitored as excessive sodium exacerbates renal overload causing oedema (Sinden & Sutphen 1995). A high energy intake of 500–590 kJ (120–140 kcal) per kilogram a day is needed for good growth (Sinden & Sutphen 1995). After surgery the baby will continue to be given intravenous nutrition containing carbohydrates, protein and fats for growth. As soon as medically feasible, enteral feeding should begin, by continuous or bolus tube feeding. Enteral nutrition has advantages over parenteral feeding in that it is more economical and safer to administer and promotes the physiological function of the gastrointestinal tract. Prolonged use of parenteral nutrition may result in gastrointestinal tract atrophy and erosion of the mucosal barrier, leading to bacterial infection and possible necrotising enterocolitis, perforated gut and peritonitis.

Breast milk does not generally have enough energy for the requirements of these babies but can be enhanced with carbohydrate supplements. Breast feeding can be alternated with high energy formulas to ensure a good energy intake. Formula milks with low sodium to prevent fluid retention can be used and energy supplements added if necessary. If growth remains poor, fats can be added to the milk.

If the baby cannot take enough milk by bottle or breast feeding because of breathlessness, tube feeding can be implemented at night. This ensures that normal feeding and speech development from sucking and social interaction can take place, as well as providing the extra energy. Babies with severe vomiting and failure to thrive that is likely to be long term, may need to be fed by a jejunostomy or gastrostomy tube.

Problems of growth and failure to thrive can persist well into childhood. A period of trial and error is often needed to find the right combination of milk and drugs on which the baby will grow adequately and stay healthy.

Behaviour

Babies with congenital heart conditions are often restless and fussy from the high metabolic rate which causes tachycardia, sweating and breathlessness. They may vomit frequently and refuse feeds, presenting a challenge to nurses and parents. Keeping the baby comfortable often reduces vomiting and fussy behaviour, helping the baby to thrive. Cool cotton clothing should be used though often mittens and socks are needed for cold hands and feet from the poor circulation. Raising the head of the cot or sitting the baby in a chair, often helps to prevent vomiting as well as helping the baby to breathe more easily. Interventions and disturbances should be kept to a minimum and then carried out when the baby is awake.

Parents will be involved in their baby's care from birth, learning to understand reactions and needs. They will learn how to give the drugs needed and to be alert for signs of recurring heart failure gaining confidence to assume responsibility after discharge.

Discharge

The baby will be discharged on diuretics and any other drugs needed to control heart failure. Some will require prophylactic antibiotic cover for life as heart disease predisposes the patient to the development of bacterial endocarditis from normally harmless infections. The baby will be followed up as an outpatient and may be referred to dieticians, physiotherapists and occupational therapists to help attain maximum potential.

Parents will be advised to let their baby be immunised at the correct times and to keep people with coughs and colds away to reduce the risk of bronchiolitis or whooping cough. These can be life-threatening in a baby with cardiac disease owing to reduced lung compliance, lung damage and abnormal gas exchange caused by the cardiac defect and nursery school attendance is not advised for this reason. Dental hygiene advice will be important later to prevent the teeth being a source of infection.

Coping at home

Parents with a baby suffering from a congenital heart condition, are never free from anxiety and the possibility of further problems. If the baby has had major surgery they will worry about coping with the responsibility of caring. They may not be sure about future health and there may be further operations to come. Every change in behaviour will be attributed to the condition and they may forget that other babies get restless and fretful. The baby may be a poor feeder, falling asleep in the middle of the feed and waking up screaming later. Weight gain can be poor and often there is a reluctance to give the fat-rich milks advised in case of causing thickening of the arteries in the damaged heart and the worry that a weight gain could cause strain on the heart (Sinden & Sutphen 1995). They need to understand fully the purpose and aims of their baby's diet, which is to improve growth rate and physiological functions so that the baby can grow into a healthy child.

There will be periods when they feel overwhelmed with the baby's needs and treatment. Follow-up may be intense at first then tail off. Parents may then want to join a parent support group that can help and to meet people with similar experiences who will listen to their problems and give advice if asked.

The Department of Social Security gives various allowances depending on the income of the family and the disablement of the baby. The Social Services will help by advising the parents on facilities in their area and the financial help to which they are entitled.

The child may always have decreased tolerance to exercise and tire easily but most will be able to attend school, play games and enjoy life.

COMMON DEFECTS SEEN IN THE NEONATAL UNIT

The lesions which account for 80% of all cases are listed below in order of commonest incidence:

- Patent ductus arteriosus
- Ventricular septal defect
- Atrioventricular canal
- Fallot's tetralogy
- Pulmonary stenosis
- Coarctation of the aorta
- Aortic stenosis
- Transposition of the great arteries
- Hypoplastic left heart syndrome

It is interesting to look at some of the more common defects seen in the neonatal unit so that some knowledge of the treatment needed and outcome for the baby is gained.

DEFECTS CAUSING LEFT-TO-RIGHT SHUNTING

The most common heart problems in the neonatal unit are caused by left-to-right shunting of the blood through the heart. Conditions in which this occurs have an inefficient circulation as blood is syphoned off through abnormal openings in the heart. The most common of these defects are patent ductus arteriosus, ventricular septal defect, atrial septal defect and atrioventricular canal. These are not dramatic or life-threatening conditions and often do not need surgery in the immediate neonatal period but they may cause a degree of heart failure needing treatment.

Patent ductus arteriosus

Patent ductus arteriosus is the most common cause of heart failure in the neonatal unit. It is not a congenital heart defect but a failure of the heart to adjust to normal circulation after birth. The duct which lies between the aorta and the pulmonary artery of the heart is a normal part of fetal circulation which should close soon after birth (Fig. 6.4).

It closes in response to high oxygen blood levels, reduction in natural prostaglandin and lowered pulmonary resistance that occurs when the baby is born. It often remains open in babies with respiratory distress syndrome, where oxygenation is variable and oxygen tension is low preventing the fall in pulmon-

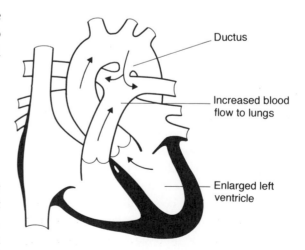

Fig. 6.4 Diagram of patent ductus arteriosus.

ary vascular resistance. When the pulmonary vascular resistance eventually falls, the baby is left with a left-to-right shunt and from the aorta into the pulmonary artery. This results in a mixing of oxygenated and deoxygenated blood which increases cardiac output and leads to heart failure.

There is a high incidence of patent ductus arteriosus in preterm and very low birth weight babies. Often the duct closes without treatment but the lower the birth weight the less likely the ductus is to close naturally. Babies below 1 kg (2 lb 3 oz) have a 75% incidence of patent ductus (Fleming *et al.* 1991).

Clinical presentation

The baby is usually preterm, of low birth weight and has had a respiratory illness needing ventilation. Attempts to wean from the ventilator are unsuccessful and at a few weeks of age the baby is ventilator dependent. Weight gain is poor, there is tachycardia and copious endotracheal secretions. There will be a bounding pulse and a heart murmur heard on examination.

Diagnosis

Investigations are instigated when a murmur is heard on a preterm ventilated baby who is not improving. The chest X-ray will show an increased heart size and pulmonary plethora (Roberton 1993). A definitive diagnosis of patent ductus is made by echocardiography.

Treatment

Before an attempt is made to close the duct, the baby should have reached at least 33 weeks gestation to allow time for natural closure. Treatment before this involves preventing heart failure by providing adequate ventilatory support, preventing hypoxia, restricting fluids and diuretic therapy.

Medical closure is attempted first with a course of indomethacin, which acts by blocking naturally occurring prostaglandins. If the duct does not close following this treatment, then surgical ligation is considered.

Provided any chest infection or heart failure is treated medically before the operation, surgical ligation of the duct is uncomplicated. The operation entails entering the chest by a thoracotomy and tying off the duct. The baby will need intensive skilled treatment for the first few hours after the operation but recovers quickly. Once the duct has been ligated and the baby recovers from the operation there should be a significant improvement in condition.

Ventricular septal defect (VSD)

This is the most common form of congenital heart defect and involves 20–25% of babies with congenital heart defect (Park 1991). It is often associated with coarctation of the aorta. There is a gap in the ventricular septum caused by imperfect septal division during early fetal development. It may vary in size from a small hole which causes no problems to a complete absence of the septum (Fig. 6.5).

Clinical presentation

A small ventricular septal defect does not cause any problems of growth or development. A moderate one will cause tachypnoea, poor feeding, failure to thrive and repeated chest infections.

A large defect may cause congestive heart failure and will usually be repaired in infancy. Congestive cardiac failure can develop at

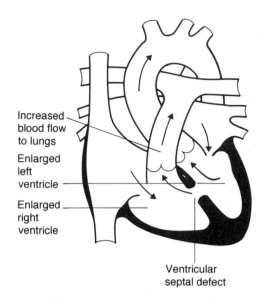

Increased
blood flow
to lungs

Enlarged
left
ventricle

Enlarged
right
ventricle

Ventricular
septal defect

Fig. 6.5 Diagram of a ventricular septal defect.

about 4–6 weeks in babies with larger defects because blood will shunt from the left ventricle into the right ventricle and into the pulmonary circulation causing pulmonary hypertension. Increased pressure in the right ventricle, resulting from shunting and pulmonary resistance, can cause the right ventricle to hypertrophy and the right atrium to enlarge to accommodate the increased work. This will cause pulmonary vascular resistance to rise causing heart failure which will need treatment with diuretics and digoxin.

Diagnosis

A murmur will be heard on chest auscultation and a chest X-ray will reveal a cardiomegaly of varying degree with enlargement of the right atrium. Echocardiography will provide an accurate diagnosis of the position and size of the defect.

Treatment

Some 30–40% of small ventricular septal

defects close naturally in the first year of life and moderate ones tend to become smaller as the baby grows (Walker 1991).

Surgical treatment

Palliative banding of the pulmonary artery may be needed to reduce the volume and pressure of pulmonary blood flow to the lungs and relieve congestive cardiac failure. If the congestive cardiac failure does not respond to medical treatment surgical intervention is required early. If heart failure is well controlled direct closure of the defect will be done using cardiopulmonary bypass when the child is 12 months to 4 years of age and growth has diminished the size of the defect. If the VSD is large, a prosthetic patch may be needed (Park 1991). If there is aortic insufficiency, an aortic valvoplasty may be performed when the septal defect is repaired.

Atrioventricular canal

This defect accounts for 2% of cardiac defects and occurs in approximately 30% of Down's syndrome babies. In this defect there are partial atrial septal defects and sometimes complete absence of the ventricular septum. The mitral and tricuspid valves are split making this condition appear as cleft or canal through the middle of the heart (Fig. 6.6).

Clinical presentation

The baby may become blue on crying, there will be failure to thrive and repeated chest infections. A loud murmur or 'thrill' will be heard on auscultation. Congestive heart failure occurs at 1–2 months of age. Babies who do not have surgery usually die in their second or third year from heart failure.

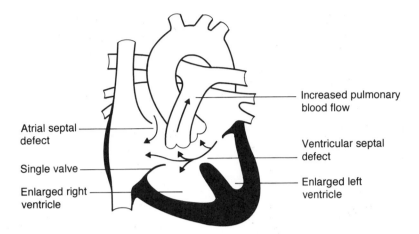

Fig. 6.6 Diagram of complete atrioventricular defect (AV canal).

Diagnosis

There will be a loud murmur heard and the chest X-ray will show an enlarged heart with pulmonary vascular markings (Park 1991) from the large amount of blood going through the pulmonary arteries. Echocardiography will reveal the extent of the defect.

Treatment

Surgical correction is difficult and complicated because of the deficiency in atrial and ventricular tissue and the deformities of the valves. Medical treatment is used to control heart failure in the neonatal period. In suitable cases palliative banding of the pulmonary artery is done to decrease the blood flow to the lungs. Corrective surgery using cardiopulmonary bypass is carried out, when the child is a few months to several years of age depending how well the heart failure can be controlled and depending on the cardiac unit policies.

Surgery

During surgery the septal defects are closed and a valvoplasty performed to make the atrioventricular valves as competent as possible (Walker 1991). Surgery carries risks, especially for symptomatic babies whose hearts may have been damaged by congestive cardiac failure. Postoperative complications include congestive cardiac failure, haemorrhage and respiratory failure. Further surgery may be needed later to replace an incompetent mitral valve.

DEFECTS CAUSING RIGHT VENTRICULAR OUTFLOW OBSTRUCTION

Defects causing right ventricular outflow obstruction. These are defects affecting the right side of the heart and include:

- Pulmonary stenosis
- Tetralogy of Fallot

Fallot's tetralogy

This is a defect causing a right ventricular outflow obstruction (Fig. 6.7). The condition usually consists of four anatomical defects. These are:

- Ventricular septal defect
- Aorta that overrides the pulmonary outflow tract
- Pulmonary artery obstruction or stenotic pulmonary valve
- Right ventricular hypertrophy

The severity of this lesion depends on the degree of pulmonary valve stenosis (Walker 1991).

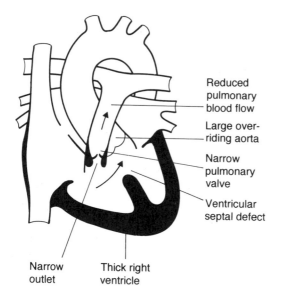

Fig. 6.7 Diagram illustrating Fallot's tetralogy.

Clinical presentation

Cyanosis is present as deoxygenated blood is forced through the septal defect into the aorta, being unable to pass through the pulmonary artery. The degree of cyanosis will be related to the severity of the pulmonary obstruction.

Hypertrophy of the right ventricle results from blood shunting through the septal defect. Paroxysmal hypoxic 'spells' are common and are thought to be the result of an increase in the right-to-left shunting causing a spasm of the right ventricular outflow tract. They start typically at about 2 months of age. The baby will have a period of rapid deep breathing followed by a prolonged bout of irritable crying. There will be increasing cyanosis during this time and decreased heart sounds. A severe attack may cause limpness, unconsciousness cerebrovascular accident or even death. These 'spells' are an indication for surgery.

Clubbing of fingers and toes develops as the baby grows. Chronic arterial denaturation causes polycythaemia which could result in strokes or brain abscesses. Bacterial endocarditis is commonly associated with tetralogy of Fallot.

Diagnosis

The definitive diagnosis is made by echocardiography on a symptomatic baby.

Treatment

Medical treatment focuses on prevention of heart failure, polycythaemia and infection until surgical repair is performed.

Surgery

The surgical treatment is governed by the size of the pulmonary arteries (Allan & Baker 1993). In cases with mild pulmonary stenosis, close medical follow-up treatment will prevent complications and elective surgery is usually performed between the ages of 18 months and 5 years.

Palliative surgery may be needed if the pulmonary valve is severely stenosed and the pulmonary arteries are small. A modified Blalock shunt is carried out where the subclavian artery is anastomosed to the pulmonary artery. This improves the blood supply through the pulmonary arteries and encourages them to grow. The shunt is taken down when corrective surgery is performed.

Recently non-surgical catheter treatment of pulmonary valve stenosis has been used where a balloon catheter is guided through an artery in the groin up to the heart. When it reaches the stenosed area it is opened to dilate the valve (Qureshi 1993). This treatment has far fewer risks for the baby than major surgery and follow-up at 12 months shows that the dilatation is maintained.

Total correction requires the use of a cardio-pulmonary bypass. The ventricular septal defect is repaired and the right ventricular outflow tract is reconstructed.

DEFECTS CAUSING CYANOSIS

Cyanotic lesions occur where there is mixing of oxygenated and deoxygenated blood and include:

- Transposition of great arteries
- Tricuspid atresia

Transposition of the great arteries (TGA)

This is a cyanotic lesion where there is mixing of oxygenated and deoxygenated blood. TGA is a life-threatening condition in which the aorta arises from the right ventricle and the pulmonary artery from the left ventricle. The

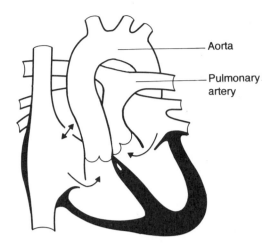

Fig. 6.8 Diagram of simple transposition of the great vessels.

left and right sides of the heart function as two parallel circuits (Fig. 6.9). Mixing of blood between the pulmonary and systemic circulations can occur initially through the ductus arteriosus and foramen ovale but when these close, there is effectively no circulatory route (Fig. 6.8). When the diagnosis is suspected a prostaglandin infusion should be started to keep the ductus open.

Clinical presentation

The baby will present soon after birth, with deepening cyanosis which does not improve

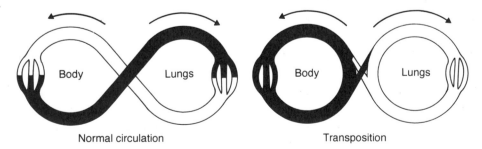

Fig. 6.9 How transposition affects circulation. In normal circulation on the left, the right and left sides of the heart are connected in series. In transposition on the right, they are in parallel and the only effective flow to the lungs is through an atrial septal defect. (Adapted from Jordan and Scott, (1989).)

with oxygen administration. Definitive diagnosis is made by echocardiography.

Treatment

Treatment depends on the surgeon's preference. Most centres perform an early balloon septostomy to improve the mixing of blood, followed by an operation to revert the circulatory systems a week later. The surgery most preferred is the arterial switch procedure which was first used by Gaiters in 1975 (Marsland 1991). The aorta and pulmonary artery are 'switched' back and correct implantation of the coronary arteries made. The most common complication following the switch procedure is pulmonary artery stenosis which can be improved by balloon dilatation. Research results of the 'switch' operation found this operation was successful and gave a good quality of life to children of 8 years of age who had had surgery in infancy (Jonas 1995).

Tricuspid valve atresia

This is a cyanotic lesion where there is mixing of oxygenated and deoxygenated blood. It is often associated with other anomalies such as ventricular septal defect, atrial septal defect or hypoplastic right ventricle. Blood supply to the lungs is poor and if the atresia is complete, there is no outlet to the right atrium except through one of the defects (Fig. 6.10). Survival depends on the size of the defects and a patent ductus.

Clinical presentation

The baby will present with severe cyanosis in the neonatal period as the ductus arteriosus starts to close off the pulmonary circulation. The severity of the cyanosis then depends on

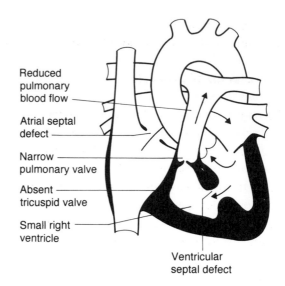

Reduced pulmonary blood flow

Atrial septal defect

Narrow pulmonary valve

Absent tricuspid valve

Small right ventricle

Ventricular septal defect

Fig. 6.10 Diagram of tricuspid valve atresia.

the size of the ventricular defect. Respiratory distress may be present with hypoxic episodes and poor feeding ability.

Treatment

Prostaglandin infusion will be given to keep the duct open until surgery. A balloon septostomy will be done urgently to improve the circulation. The blood flow to the lungs is improved by palliative shunts which may need to be repeated as the child grows. When the child is about 4 years old, if there are good pulmonary vessels with low pressure and an efficient left ventricle, more definitive surgery will be carried out (Park 1991).

DEFECTS CAUSING LEFT VENTRICULAR OUTFLOW OBSTRUCTION

These are defects affecting the left side of the heart and are the commonest cause of heart failure in the first week of life. They include:

- Coarctation of the aorta
- Hypoplastic left heart syndrome

Coarctation of the aorta

The term coarctation describes a constriction in the aorta (Fig. 6.11). This causes left ventricular outflow obstruction. Over half the patients with coarctation have other lesions such as ventricular septal defects, mitral valve abnormalities and aortic stenosis. Survival initially depends on the patency of the ductus arteriosus to maintain the circulation.

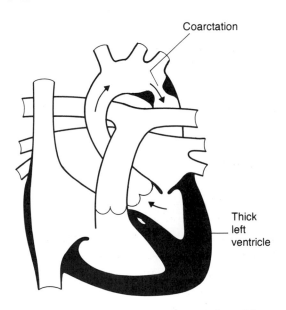

Fig. 6.11 Diagram to illustrate coarctation of the aorta.

Clinical presentation

Symptoms usually present in the second to tenth day of life when the ductus arteriosus starts to close and the circulation of blood is obstructed. There will be poor peripheral circulation, the brachial pulses are palpable initially and the femoral pulses weak, but eventually all the pulses are poor as the ductus closes. Blood pressure is higher in the arms

than in the legs because the blood cannot be pumped adequately through the constriction of the aorta to the lower limbs.

Diagnosis

Severe cases can be detected on antenatal scan. After birth diagnosis is made by echocardiography on a symptomatic baby.

Treatment

Prostaglandin infusion is given to keep the duct open while the baby is prepared for surgery. The ductus needs to be kept patent to ensure a flow of blood to the lower part of the body. Ventilatory support and correction of acidosis and electrolyte imbalance are essential. A dopamine infusion is given to improve renal function as the blood supply to the kidneys is poor and may result in renal failure.

Some surgeons are now beginning to use balloon dilatation to treat selected patients with an otherwise normal aorta. Good results have been acheived but as yet there is no long term follow-up on the patients (Brown & Salmon 1996).

Surgery

The operation is performed using cardio-pulmonary bypass. The surgery of choice nowadays is the subclavian flap operation, whereby the left subclavian artery is ligated and the flap is brought down as a gusset and anastomosed to the aorta (Fig. 6.12). Other defects present are repaired at the same time (Sandhu *et al.* 1995). Whatever the choice of operation recoarctation may still occur. Balloon dilatation is sometimes used to correct

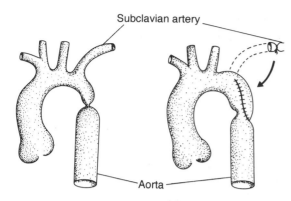

Fig. 6.12 Subclavian flap repair of coarctation of the aorta. (Adapted from Jordan and Scott (1989).)

this but may cause aneurysms of the aorta (Qureshi 1993).

Hypoplastic left heart syndrome

Hypoplastic left heart syndrome (HLHS) accounts for only 1% of congenital heart defects but causes 25% of all cardiac deaths in the first week of life (Sreeram 1996). The condition and its associated cardiac defects were considered fatal until the last decade, with no

choice of treatment. Improvements in technology, knowledge and research have now brought into existence other options which offer a chance of survival, although the mortality rate is still very high.

In the most severe form there is atresia of the aortic valve, the left ventricle is rudimentary and represented by a mere slit and there is an atresia or hypoplasia of the mitral valve and ascending aorta. The left atrium empties through the open foramen ovale or atrial septal defect, into the right atrium and ventricle causing mixing of oxygenated and deoxygenated blood (Fig. 6.13). As these babies have only one effective ventricle they depend on the patency of the ductus arteriosus for their systemic and coronary circulation (Table 6.3).

Clinical presentation

Babies with this condition are usually symptomless at birth and unless diagnosed by antenatal scanning, they are sent to the postnatal ward after delivery. Mothers booked for

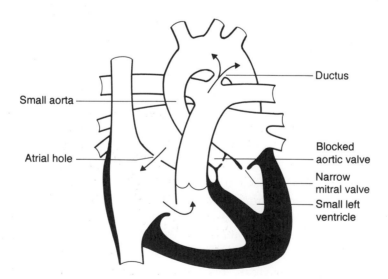

Fig. 6.13 Diagram of hypoplastic left heart with patent ductus arteriosus to illustrate hypoplastic left heart syndrome.

Table 6.3 Primary defects in hypoplastic left heart syndrome.

Diminutive aorta, sometimes aortic atresia
Mitral valve stenosis
Aortic valve stenosis
Mitral valve atresia
Hypoplastic left ventricle

early discharge may take their babies home before any symptoms appear.

Problems arise when the ductus arteriosus begins to close 8–12 hours after the birth or sometimes a few days after delivery. Initially the baby becomes breathless and slightly blue on feeding as the duct begins to close. When it finally closes the condition suddenly deteriorates with symptoms of congestive heart failure which include:

- Poor systemic perfusion
- Tachycardia
- Tachypnoea
- Respiratory distress
- Decreased peripheral pulses
- Decreased urinary output with cool extremities and mottling
- Enlarged liver

Diagnosis

The diagnosis of HLHS may be suspected on examination when the peripheral pulses are found to be absent or faint and the blood pressure equal but low on all limbs. Chest X-ray shows an enlarged globular heart outline with variable pulmonary vascular markings.

The diagnosis is confirmed on echocardiography which demonstrates the small left ventricular cavity and ascending aorta and the nature of both the mitral valve and aortic valves. Cardiac catheterisation is usually only performed in the more complex form to further define the extent of the defect.

Treatment

Prostaglandin is given to keep the duct open while the options for treatment are considered. Surgical correction utilises the one effective ventricle as the systemic pumping chamber by a series of staged surgical repairs involving a number of major operations. The surgery is difficult and complicated and many babies do not survive the first stage. For many babies with this condition the defects of the heart are impossible to correct and they are put on the waiting list for a donor heart transplant as soon as possible.

HEART TRANSPLANTS

Infant heart transplantation has emerged as an effective treatment for babies with severe forms of heart disease in the last few years. An estimated 10% of babies born with congenital heart disease have such complex anomalies that corrective surgery is impossible (Razzouk & Bailey 1995).

Heart transplantation is limited by the number of donor hearts that become available so to ensure optimum use of donor hearts and to improve the success rate of the surgery a rigorous selection procedure is employed. Before being accepted as a candidate for heart transplant a thorough evaluation of the baby's general health and heart condition is undertaken by a medical and surgical team. The baby must be free of life-limiting genetic disease, central nervous system abnormalities, major sepsis and have normal renal function.

Parents

The scarcity of donor hearts makes the assessment of parents essential. If the baby is to have the best chance of a good survival and quality of life, the parents must be prepared for the commitment of years of time-consuming and painful treatments for their child with frequent hospitalisations. They will undergo lengthy counselling so that they know exactly what that commitment will be and if they can cope with it. Family life will be disrupted and the added emotional stress of knowing their child could die at any time will take its toll of everyone.

The donor heart

Infant heart transplantation is a donor-dependent therapy. This necessarily raises emotive issues as prospective donors are infant victims of head injuries, sudden infant death syndrome and birth asphyxia. It is not easy to persuade the parents of such potential donors, in their shock and distress, to allow their child's heart to be removed. The harvesting of donor hearts has to be achieved with sensitivity and understanding.

When the consent form from the donor's parent is signed, the donor heart will be scanned for structural abnormalities, which might render it useless, then the donor's blood is checked for serious infection such as hepatitis or human immunodeficiency virus. When a donor heart becomes available it is carefully matched for tissue type and blood group with the waiting recipient. If there is a good tissue match the chances of rejection are considered to be less of a problem and the transplant will go ahead.

Waiting for a heart

The baby waiting for a donor heart will often need intensive care and close monitoring. A continuous prostaglandin infusion will be essential and if the duct closes in spite of the prostaglandin, a balloon atrial septostomy will become necessary to sustain life. If there is unrestricted pulmonary blood flow it may be necessary to perform pulmonary banding to protect the pulmonary vasculature. Using these management techniques and with good nutritional support and fluid management it has been known for a baby to survive for up to 6 months while waiting for a donor heart (Razzouk & Bailey 1995).

Because of the difficulties of obtaining a donor heart, if a diagnosis of an inoperable cardiac defect is made before birth, a suitable fetus may be considered as potential recipient. If a donor heart then becomes available the baby may be delivered by Caesarian section or induced after 36 weeks and operated on immediately (Razzouk & Bailey 1995).

There will be only a few hours notice when a matched donor's heart has been located. The donor heart will be removed, packed in a transport solution surrounded in crushed ice and taken to the recipient's hospital. Donor hearts have been known to be usable up to 10 hours after removal using this method (Razzouk & Bailey 1995).

Surgery

This is carried out using cardiopulmonary bypass and deep hypothermic circulatory arrest. The new heart is grafted on to the atria and great vessels by continuous suture techniques. Aortic arch reconstruction may be carried out at the same time.

Postoperative complications

The postoperative care is intensive as for other major heart surgery. These babies often make a swift recovery as they now have a normal heart structure and their postoperative period may not be as stormy as with other conditions. The babies used to be nursed in isolation cubicles with a clean air flow for the first few days, to prevent any infection which may cause the new heart to be rejected but are now nursed normally in the cardiac intensive care unit.

Immunosuppressant drugs

The major complication after surgery is that of rejection of the donor heart. This is the most common cause of death in the first 3 months after transplant (Large 1995) and will be a life-long problem for the recipient. Immunosuppressive drugs are vital and finding an efficient drug with few side-effects has proved difficult. The introduction of cyclosporin as an immunosuppressant has greatly improved survival, though side-effects can cause excessive weight gain, excess hair and depression.

Cardiac biopsies are done frequently to check for rejection. If caught in the early stages, rejection episodes can be reclaimed by corticosteroids though retransplantation using another donor heart is a common occurrence. The child may undergo many such episodes which eventually may cause death.

The future of heart transplantation

The most important single issue is that of donor supply. Not every baby survives to receive a transplant as the demand exceeds the supply. Raising public awareness is only part of the answer, re-examination of the criteria for donor hearts and techniques for reactivating 'dead hearts' may improve the supply. At the present time it is considered unethical to keep an anencephalic fetus for use as a donor or to use hearts from babies who have already died. Research into use of animal hearts (xenografting) and mechanical substitutes is being pursued and may bring a solution (Large 1995).

Another important issue is that of tissue rejection. This is usually the cause of death of many of the recipients. In order that recipients survive as long as possible, frequent painful medical procedures, hospitalisations and medication for life are essential. Advances in immunosuppressive drugs have improved the survival rate from rejection and research is active in this area.

THE FUTURE OUTLOOK FOR THOSE WITH CONGENITAL HEART DISEASE

The successful treatment of congenital cardiac defects means that many people who would have been severely restricted by their condition can now live relatively active lives. Many conditions require extensive follow-up and antibiotic and diuretic therapy for life and often there may not be a normal life span owing to vascular complications. Careful medical management means that many more children are surviving into adolescence without surgery and developments in heart transplant techniques and the improvements in immunosuppressant drugs are giving hope to children who might otherwise have died. As babies who are born with cardiac defects increasingly survive into adulthood, they now present a different challenge to cardiologists in the medical and psychosocial aspects of the effects of the defect on adult health. As a result of modern paediatric cardiology a new and growing section of adults need life-long medical care and treatment to maintain their health.

Adult survivors of congenital cardiac disease want advice about contraception, pregnancy and the risk of passing the defect to their children. Oral contraceptives that contain oestrogen increase the risk of polycythaemia, as a result of cyanotic lesions, thus increasing the risk of strokes. Intrauterine devices are associated with the risk of pelvic infection possibly leading to bacterial endocarditis. Many women with congenital heart disease can attempt pregnancy without risk to themselves but there is a high incidence of fetal death because of low oxygen saturations in the mother or because of her anticoagulant treatment (Thorne & Deanfield 1996).

The recurrence risk of heart defects for siblings is about 2%, and when the parent has a defect the risk rises to 5% (Wren 1996). For many lesions the risk is considered to be higher when the mother rather than the father is the affected parent (Thorne & Deanfield 1996).

REFERENCES AND FURTHER READING

Acari M. (1992) Operating the cardiopulmonary bypass machine. *Nursing Standard*, **6** (18), 53–54.

Allan L, Baker EJ. (1993) Prenatal diagnosis and correction of congenital heart defects. *British Journal of Hospital Medicine*, **50** (9), 513–521.

Brown EM, Salmon AP. (1996) Interventional cardiology in practice. *Current Paediatrics*, **6**, 150–155.

Fleming PJ, Speidel BD, Marlow N, Dunn PM. (1991) *A Neonatal Vade Mecum*, 2nd edn. Edward Arnold, London.

Hazinski S. (1992) *Nursing Care of the Critically Ill Child*, 2nd edn. Mosby Year Book, St Louis.

Huggan I. (1992) Invasive techniques in paediatric cardiology. *Nursing Standard*, **6** (18), 51–53.

Jonas RA. (1995) Advances in surgical care of infants with congenital heart disease. *Current Opinion in Paediatrics*, **7** (5), 572–579.

Jordan S, Scott O. (1989) *Heart Disease in Paediatrics*. 3rd edn., Butterworth, Guildford.

Kelnar C, Harvey D, Simpson C. (1995) *The Sick Newborn Baby*, 3rd edn. Baillière Tindall, London.

Large SR. (1995) Cardiac transplantation – the next decade. *British Journal of Hospital Medicine*, **53** (9), 440–445.

Marsland L. (1991) Transposition of the great arteries. *Nursing Standard*, **6** (13), 35–39.

Merenstein G, Gardner S. (1993) *Handbook of Neonatal Intensive Care*, 3rd edn. Mosby Year Book, St Louis.

Park MK. (1991) *The Paediatric Cardiology Handbook*. Mosby Year Book, St Louis.

Paul KE. (1995) Recognition, stabilisation and early management of infants with critical heart disease. *Neonatal Network*, **14** (5), 13–20.

Proud J. (1994) *Understanding Obstetric Ultrasound*. Books for Midwives Press, Cheshire.

Qureshi SA. (1993) Catheter treatment of congenital heart disease. *British Journal of Hospital Medicine*, **50** (9), 523–528.

Razzouk AJ. Bailey LL. (1995) Infant heart transplantation. In: *Moss and Adams Heart Disease in Children and Adolescents*, Volume 1, (eds G.C. Emmanuelides & H.D. Allen), 5th edn. pp. 510–516. Williams and Williams, Baltimore.

Rees P, Tunstill A, Pope T, Kinnear D, Rees S. (1989) *Heart Children: a Practical Handbook for Parents*, Heart Line Association, Biggleswade.

Rikard DH. (1993) Nursing care of a neonate receiving prostaglandin E1 therapy. *Neonatal Network*, **12** (4), 17–22.

Roberton NCR. (1993) *A Manual of Neonatal Intensive Care*, 3rd edn. Edward Arnold, London.

Sadler W. (1990) *Langman's Medical Embryology*. 6th edn. Williams and Wilkins, Baltimore.

Sandhu SK, Beekman RH, Mosca RS, Bove LE. (1995) Single stage repair of aortic arch obstruction and associated intracardiac defects in the neonate. *American Journal of Cardiology*, **75**, 370–375.

Sinden AA, Sutphen J. (1995) Growth and nutrition. In: *Moss and Adams Heart Disease in Children and Adolescents*, Volume 1, (eds G.C. Emmanuelides & H.D. Allen), 5th edn. pp. 366–373. Williams and Williams, Baltimore.

Sreeram N. (1996) Hypoplastic left heart syndrome: current treatment options and outcome. *Current Paediatrics*, **6**, 156–161.

Thorne S, Deanfield J. (1996) Long term outlook in treated congenital heart disease. *Archives of Disease in Childhood*, **75**, 6–8.

Walker C. (1991) Down's syndrome and congenital heart defects. *Intensive Care Nursing*, **7**, 94–104.

Wren C. (1996) Fetal cardiography. *Current Paediatrics*, **6**, 145–149.

7 | Nursing Management of Babies with Genetic Problems

LEARNING OUTCOMES

After reading this chapter and studying the contents the reader will be able to:

O Describe the function of chromosomes and genes.
O List the types of genetic problems.
O List patterns of inheritance.
O Describe current antenatal testing, prediction and counselling.
O List the current ways of genetic testing.
O Identify family emotional problems caring for a genetically disabled baby.
O Describe the team help the baby needs on discharge.
O Discuss the ethical problems encountered with the genome project.
O Describe current genetic treatments and progress.

CAUSES OF GENETIC DISEASES

A genetic disease is one that has been inherited from one or both parents. They have passed on a faulty gene that has resulted in an abnormality of the baby. The gene may have been inherited from their own parents or it may have been changed by some outside factor.

Teratogenic factors

When diagnosing a genetic disease, other causes of abnormalities in the fetus that affect development must be excluded to assess the risk of the parents' next baby inheriting the problem.

Teratogens are factors capable of disrupting fetal growth and producing malformations. The resulting genetic changes in the fetus will not be inherited by other children of the same parents unless the same factors prevail during the pregnancy. Teratogens include some drugs, infections, poisons and radiation. For example:

- Drugs such as thalidomide, phenytoin or tetracyclines taken in the first trimester of pregnancy cause multiple deformities in the baby.

- Diseases such as rubella, cytomegalovirus and toxoplasmosis also adversely affect the fetus, if contracted by the mother in the first trimester, by inducing genetic changes that cause abnormalities.
- Excessive alcohol consumption during pregnancy induces genetic changes in the baby, giving a characteristic appearance with congenital heart disease, growth retardation and learning difficulties.
- Exposure to radiation has been known to cause tumours and mutagenic effects resulting in damage to the germ cells before fertilisation and damage to the developing fetus.

Chromosomes

Chromosomes are structures composed of DNA (deoxyribonucleic acid), a chemical protein that codes and transmits information within the cells in the body. Chromosomes lie within the cell nucleus and divide when the cell divides. Each chromosome carries countless genes which control the functions and workings of the body.

Every human being has 46 chromosomes in each cell of the body. These are seen under the microscope as 23 pairs of rod shaped bodies. Each chromosome is numbered by geneticists in order of size. The biggest two are called the X and Y chromosomes and they determine the sex of the individual. The normal female has two X chromosomes and the male an X and a Y chromosome. The gametes (sperm and ova) contain only 23 single chromosomes. At conception a sperm and an ovum come together to form a fertilised egg which contains 23 pairs of chromosomes.

The chromosomes of an individual are assessed under a microscope and then arranged in pairs in order of size for convenience.

The characteristic chromosome pattern of an individual is called the karyotype.

Genes

Genes are the units of inheritance and there are countless numbers on each chromosome. Each gene consists of a sequence code of the building blocks of DNA. DNA has three functions, it stores and transmits information, it copies itself accurately, it can mutate and the mutation can be inherited. If there is an abnormality in the parent this may be reproduced in the offspring who inherits the faulty gene.

Chromosomal abnormalities

Any irregularity in the number or gross structure of the chromosomes causes great disruption in the functioning of the individual affected. This is because the body is unable to sustain the loss or gain of so much genetic material contained in every part of the chromosome. Many fetuses with chromosome abnormalities are non-viable and miscarry. There are in general four types of chromosomal abnormality:

- Trisomy or addition of a chromosome.
- Monosomy or missing chromosome.
- Deletion or missing part.
- Translocation – where a part has broken off and rejoins another chromosome.

Trisomy

Babies who gain an addition to any of the pairs of chromosomes will have a condition known as a trisomy. The syndrome that results is called by the number of the chromosome that has a triple chromosome.

Trisomy 21

Babies exhibit characteristic facial features, have learning difficulties of differing degrees and often have heart or intestinal defects. This is commonly called Down's syndrome.

Trisomy 13–15

The babies have heart defects, eye and hearing abnormalities, cleft lip and palate and severe mental impairment. The life span is generally 3 months. Trisomy 13 is commonly called Patau's syndrome.

Trisomy 17–18

Infants have many anomalies and skeletal malformations and only about 10% survive the first year. Trisomy 18 is known as Edward's syndrome.

Triple X syndrome

These babies with three female chromosomes remain infantile with some learning difficulties. They are not infertile and produce normal offspring.

Klinefelter syndrome

This is found in boys who have an extra X chromosome. They are sterile, with testicular atrophy and enlarged breast tissue.

Monosomy

Babies who have one of a pair of a chromosome missing have a monosomy. The best known is Turner syndrome.

Turner syndrome

These children have only one X chromosome and are always female. There are no ovaries, often webbing of the neck and skeletal abnormalities. There may be learning difficulties.

Deletions

Deletions occur when a part of a chromosome is missing. All chromosomes have a long and short arm and the position of the deletion can thus be broadly identified. Deletions are responsible for many different syndromes.

Prader–Willi syndrome

This affects boys and is caused by a deletion on the long arm of chromosome 15. The baby has a flat face, hypoplastic genitalia and learning difficulties. In the neonatal period there will be hypotonia and a poor swallowing reflex necessitating treatment. In later childhood this hypotonia improves and overeating with resultant obesity becomes a problem.

Angelman syndrome

This is a deletion also on the long arm of chromosome 15 which affects girls. These children have developmental delay, jerky movements and dysmorphic features (Connor & Fergusson-Smith 1991).

Duchenne muscular dystrophy

This deletion is on the short arm of the X chromosome and only affects males though it is inherited from females. Males appear normal at birth but gradual weakening of the skeletal muscles causes death in late teenage years.

Translocations

These occur when a part of one chromosome breaks off and joins another during fertilisation. As there is no loss of genetic material the offspring is not affected but when their turn comes to reproduce, their offspring may have genetic problems or be miscarried. This is because the translocation affects the gametes and the genetic information given in the translocated chromosomes cannot form a normal baby. Some forms of trisomy 21 are as a result of a translocation.

Abnormalities of the genes

Many genetic abnormalities occur because of a fault in a single gene. As there is a gene for every function and action of the cells in the body a fault in any one gene can be disastrous. If the gene for producing and maintaining a function of the body such as mucus production or muscle or bone tissue is defective this has devastating effect on the individual. It is estimated that this type of defect makes up 10% of all human malformations (Sadler 1990). Some gene abnormalities do not become apparent until later life, for example Huntington's chorea, hypertrophic cardiomyopathy and polycystic kidney disease. As research progresses, more diseases of early and late onset are being found to have a genetic origin which can often be predicted at birth.

GENETIC TESTING

When a genetic disease is found in a family, testing of all members will often reveal more information on the way the gene is inherited. An assessment of the chance of having another affected baby can be made if the way the disease is passed on is known.

Some chromosome and gene faults are carried forward to the next generation even though there is no evidence of disease in the parents. The people with these genetic faults are known as carriers and when their blood is tested their carrier status will be apparent and can have significant predictive value for the next generation. Some carriers of a genetic

problem will have the disease themselves and the way this is passed on to future generations will depend on the inheritance pattern (see Figure 7.1).

Genetic testing of the family is an emotive matter and cannot be carried out without sensitive preparation. Confidentiality is a major concern and families may not want other relatives to know of their genetic problem. Genetic testing could lead to revelations about paternity, which were either unknown or kept secret and the damage that could occur by such disclosures is of paramount concern. Mothers should have an opportunity to see the counsellor alone to discuss such matters.

Late onset disorders or the diagnosis of carrier status raises other issues that can profoundly affect people. The discovery of an intrinsic fault in genetic material has deep and far reaching psychological effects on the individual. A person may decide never to marry or have a partner or children in case of passing on the fault. Their perception of themselves as a whole and adequate person is lost. Anger and bitterness may blight their lives.

Genetic counselling

Genetic counselling is seen as ethically the most important part of genetic medicine especially as research progresses. Genetic counselling should be undertaken before any testing is done. A counsellor will find out how the patient feels about the test and explain common reactions to the results. Arguments for and against testing are examined and options evaluated. Discussions include the options that are available if the test is positive, for example, information on antenatal testing when pregnant and the treatments currently used for the disease. Acceptance of the genetic fault and the feelings this arouses should be explored (Smith & Marteau, 1995).

The aim of antenatal counselling is to inform the parents of the consequences of the disorder, the probability of the baby developing and transmitting it and the ways this may be prevented or helped. The counselling will be non-directive, that is, facts will be given along with the predictions, as far as known, and then parents talk through their fears and worries. Advice and direction are not given as this is considered the concern of the individual and there must be no pressure to make any decisions. This type of counselling is essential, after diagnosis of a genetic disease, so that normal psychological ways of functioning are maintained in individuals and families (Emery & Pollen 1984).

Prediction of inheritance of genetic abnormalities

Genetic diseases are inherited from one or both parents. A baby's genetic inheritance is decided at the moment of fertilisation. The gametes, the ova or sperm, are the only cells in the body to contain a single set of chromosomes, giving the fertilised ovum one set of chromosomes from each parent. There is no certain way, at present, to tell at conception, which genes the baby will inherit. Once the ovum has been fertilised and it is possible to examine the genetic material it contains, abnormalities can be detected. Many faulty fetuses are rejected by the mother's body and it has been estimated that the percentage of genetic abnormalities in natural abortions is 50 times that seen at full term (Connor & Fergusson-Smith 1990).

Each disease has its own pattern of inheritance which cannot be ascertained by blood tests alone. By delving into the family history a pattern may be seen, so that the risks for

future children can be assessed (Fig. 7.1). Blood testing of family members will show if they too carry the gene and could pass it on to their other children.

GENETIC INHERITANCE PATTERNS

Whole chromosomal abnormalities

The addition or subtraction of a whole chromosome such as in Down's syndrome or one of the trisomies does not follow a pattern in a family. There are no carriers but the risk to another child of the same parents is slightly higher than the general population risk.

Deletion pattern of inheritance

Deletions in chromosomes, where there is a part of the genetic material missing, can follow an inheritance pattern but often the abnormality produced is difficult to predict. This is because the deletion may be unstable and smaller or larger pieces of the chromosome may be deleted at each conception altering the severity of disease with each child of the same parents.

If the parents' genes are normal the recurrence risk is not increased above the general population incidence, but their child will pass on the faulty chromosome with the usual unpredictable results.

Translocation pattern of inheritance

If one parent has the translocation there is a one in four risk of passing it on. If they have normal chromosomes and the translocation occurs in the fertilised egg, there is only the usual statistical population risk of the next baby inheriting it.

Single gene disorder inheritance pattern

More than 4300 human single gene disorders are known at the time of writing and this number is increasing as research progresses. The pattern for inheritance can often be worked out from the way the gene passes to the baby from the parents (Fig. 7.1).

Autosomal dominant

The faulty gene can be passed by either male or female partner; only one has to have the affected gene. Those who have the gene have the disease and there is a 50%, or one in two, risk of their offspring inheriting the disease (Fig. 7.1a). Diseases such as achondroplasia, Huntington's chorea, myotonic dystrophy and osteogenesis imperfecta are included in this pattern of inheritance.

Autosomal recessive

The faulty gene has to be carried by both parents and the child has to inherit both copies. Neither parent has to have the disease but there is a 25%, or one in four, risk of the offspring inheriting and two-thirds of the unaffected siblings will be carriers (Fig. 7.1b). Cystic fibrosis, galactosaemia and phenyl-ketonuria come into this pattern of inheritance.

X-linked recessive

The faulty gene is on the sex chromosome X. This means that males are affected but women carry the gene. Of the sons of carrier females 50% will be affected and 50% of the daughters will be carriers. There is no risk to the sons of an affected male but all his daughters will be carriers (Fig. 7.1c). Duchenne muscular

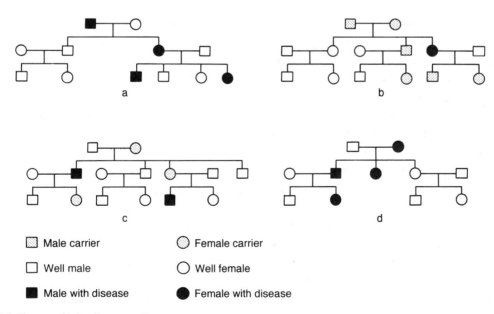

☐ Male carrier   ◯ Female carrier

☐ Well male   ◯ Well female

■ Male with disease   ● Female with disease

Fig. 7.1 Types of inheritance pattern.
(a) Autosomal dominant.
(b) Autosomal recessive.
(c) X-linked recessive.
(d) X-linked dominant.

dystrophy, haemophilia, fragile X syndrome and red–green colour blindness are in this category.

X-linked dominant

This is rare and can be passed on by males and females (Fig. 7.1d) The males are usually so severely affected that often spontaneous abortion occurs so that usually only females present with the disease. Vitamin D resistant rickets and incontinentia pigmenti fall into this category.

A FETUS WITH GENETIC PROBLEMS

Prenatal testing

If there is a known genetic problem in the family, genetic counsellors may have been consulted antenatally. The parents will be advised to seek chorionic villus sampling as the predictive treatment of choice, because the results are obtained a few weeks earlier than other antenatal tests. The parents should be informed of the slight risk of miscarriage after this procedure. It is difficult to obtain figures for the incidence of abortion entirely due to chorionic villus sampling, as a fetus with a chromosomal abnormality has a high chance of spontaneously aborting in the first trimester and a first pregnancy always carries high risks of miscarrying (Harper 1991). Parents need this information and also need to know that the finding of a chromosomal fault may not always mean a lethal abnormality.

Fetal sampling

Chorionic villus sampling (CVS) will take place at 8–11 weeks gestation. The chorion is the outer layer of the fetal sac and the villi are the cells within it. A biopsy is taken under ultrasound guidance by the transabdominal approach as the cervical route carries a higher risk of miscarriage (Connor & Fergusson-Smith 1991). The biopsy will take between 5 and 30 mg of tissue for fetal karyotyping, sexing, biochemical studies and DNA analysis. The results take 2–3 weeks as the cells have to be cultured and grown in the laboratory and examined at the right stage of development.

It is hoped that in the future this procedure can be made safer, so that all at-risk pregnancies can be tested at this gestation. Emery & Pollen (1984) state that there is no proof that the mother is less upset if termination takes place earlier rather than later. Other studies have shown that later termination improves the mother's psychological health because of the 'bonding' process between mother and fetus which allows the mother to grieve for a 'real' baby (Marteau *et al*. 1989).

Amniocentesis

Amniocentesis is carried out at 16–18 weeks of gestation. A sample of the amniotic fluid is taken transabdominally and the cells grown in culture. The results take 2–3 weeks. Amniocentesis is offered to older mothers who are at risk of producing a trisomy 21 baby, to those with higher levels of alpha-fetoprotein in the blood (indicating a fetus with a neural tube defect) and to any mother who has had a previous baby with a genetic abnormality.

When the results are known and there is an abnormality, parents need as much information as is available and the quickest appointment to have a scan. The wait for a scan to have an abnormality confirmed or otherwise will be fraught with anticipatory anxiety for most couples and can lead to marital upset.

The mother may suspend her investment in the pregnancy by, for example, taking up smoking again or not eating healthy foods (Marteau *et al.* 1989).

Ultrasound scanning

Abnormalities are often seen on routine biophysical profile scanning in the 16th to 18th week of pregnancy. If a more definitive diagnosis is needed, to confirm the genetic status of the fetus, an amniocentesis will be done.

Effects of antenatal diagnosis on the family

When a genetic problem is diagnosed parents will be referred to the genetic team, if they wish, to talk to counsellors. The counsellor will ask questions in a controlled and skilled manner to help explore deep seated worries. At this stage the counselling may be similar to bereavement counselling as parents want to talk about their guilt, anxiety, sense of loss and failure. They will want to know if their other children will have this disease and may be helped by predictive counselling involving testing of other family members.

Considering termination

Some parents will have religious or moral grounds for wishing to continue the pregnancy, even in the face of known severe abnormalities. Giving the fetus rights is a contentious issue (Carter 1990). There is a broad spectrum of thinking even among the churches themselves, the Catholic and Evangelical churches believe that the unborn human has from its beginning as much right to life as an adult. The Methodist Church states that 'as the fetus is totally dependent on the mother for at least twenty weeks, she has a total right to decide whether to continue the pregnancy' (Methodist Church 1990). Parents may never even have considered the possibility of a termination and do not even know what they want or should do. If they have religious beliefs these may contain clear guidance and if they wish they can have the help of the hospital chaplain or another religious advisor.

The society SATFA, (Support Around Termination for Abnormality) has trained counsellors who have been through the experience of the diagnosis of a damaged fetus. Parents can be offered their address by the hospital staff for further help and support in making their decision.

Not all families see problems in the same way and for some the decision will be easier than for others. The whole family may be involved in the process but pressure should not be put on parents by any of the parties concerned. They must have time to come to terms with the diagnosis and make a decision that is right for them.

BIRTH OF A BABY WITH A GENETIC DISEASE

The birth of an abnormal baby is a shattering blow to the parents. Any abnormality should be shown to the parents in the labour ward with as much explanation as is possible at the time. Mother and baby should remain together on the postnatal ward unless treatment in the neonatal unit is needed. It is easier then for the parents to accept and begin to love the baby immediately.

If the parents do not notice a problem, the features that give grounds for suspicion should be gently and sensitively pointed out. They must not be 'protected' by silence and must be told if a chromosome sample is to be sent for testing. Sometimes fears are proved wrong and the parents have been worried unnecessarily, but if they are not told until the chromosome results are obtained that their child has a genetic disease, their reactions are doubly compounded by grief at the 'loss' of their beloved child (Harper 1991).

Diagnosis

A sample of the baby's blood is sent for genetic testing. The results can take 24–48 hours for a simple chromosome count for Down's syndrome or one of the other trisomies, but may take up to 10 days or more for a detailed analysis.

Fluorescence in situ *hybridisation (FISH)*

Detailed diagnosis is helped by a new technique developed in the last few years for revealing microscopic deletions of chromosomes. Fluorescence *in situ* hybridisation (FISH), uses a fluorescently marked piece of DNA holding a specific normal chromosome, from a DNA bank. This can be matched with a patient's chromosome to highlight minute abnormalities that were previously difficult to see allowing for more accurate genetic diagnosis.

Restriction fragment length polymorphisms (RFLPS)

Diagnosis of gene abnormalities depends on gene tracking using restriction fragment length polymorphisms. This is complicated procedure but simplified means that radioactively labelled sections of DNA, called DNA probes, are used to measure and compare lengths of DNA in a defective chromosome to ascertain the missing genes.

Positive results

When the results of the genetic testing are known the parents should be interviewed. It is vital that the parents are calmly given all the information available, on their baby's condition. If the baby was not diagnosed antenatally, they will be in a state of bewilderment and confusion over the disaster that has overtaken them. The doctor should allow plenty of time for questions and speak carefully and truthfully. Parents will remember this interview for a long time and some phrases used may be engraved on their minds for ever (Jupp 1992).

The parents will want to know the prognosis and treatment for their baby. If there is a complicating condition needing immediate surgery, parents may not want to go ahead with it, maybe thinking the baby should not live. Parents must be counselled carefully as it is within the powers of medical staff to take out a court Care Order if they think the parents' views are not in the child's best interest (Children's Act 1989, see Department of Health 1991). The neonatal nurse can play a supportive role in these cases, making sure the parents understand all that is going on and acting as their advocate with the medical staff.

Practical help

This is a difficult time of adjustment for the parents. The nurses may have formed a relationship with them before diagnosis and can help them form a bond with and accept their baby. Many parents may feel insecure about handling the baby especially if it is their first. A baby with a genetic disease is a person first, the disease is secondary and this must be communicated to the parents. When the parents see the nurse handle their baby lovingly they will gain confidence and comfort. It is not always necessary to say a great deal, the parents may just want someone to talk to about their feelings.

Parents of babies with genetic problems in neonatal units are always riddled with guilt and this is magnified by the inescapable fact that they did pass a disease on, even though they had no control over it. They will need constant reassurance and information about their baby given simply and repeatedly until they feel calmer and more rational about the situation. Guilt feelings may take days or weeks to resolve and may persist after the baby goes home (Harvey 1987). A support group or unit counsellor can help parents talk through these feelings.

Family adjustment

Mothers and fathers may react differently to the news that their baby has a genetic disease. Fathers focus on instrumental concerns such as financial strains while mothers worry about the emotional strains. It has been found that fathers tend towards a steady adjustment and gradually return to normal but mothers have many different feelings of being burdened, overwhelmed, embarrassed in public, fear of the future and a resentment of people whose children are not handicapped (Cunningham 1988). The mother may feel imperfect because she has given her baby faulty chromosomes and may feel she has let her family down.

Siblings will have to go to school and tell friends that their long awaited new baby is handicapped and may feel resentful at the attention given to the new child. Grandparents may become very important, either offering support to the parents or having difficulty coming to terms with the baby themselves.

The finding of a genetic disease in a healthy family inevitably leads to friction and the altering of family relationships. Sometimes members will cast about looking for a scapegoat and dredge up old grievances and feuds causing distress and hostility in the family.

Discharge

When a baby has a genetic problem, a multi-team approach to treatment is usually needed so that the needs of the baby are identified and met in a co-ordinated fashion. Health professionals who may be involved include physiotherapist, occupational therapist, speech therapist, health visitor, paediatrician, GP, social worker, child psychologist.

The baby's discharge must be carefully planned with community services primed to follow up the family and health visitor supervision to co-ordinate and advise parents. This follow-up must be arranged on the neonatal unit before discharge and carefully explained to the parents before they leave.

Common genetic disorders often have support groups that can help the parents. Some units have a system for supporting parents of a baby with a specific problem. This may consist of parent telephone supporters who can be contacted for mutual support and friendship. Not all parents will wish to make such contacts but can be given relevant addresses for use later (Yeo 1994).

Implications for the future

The toll on family life is great as the parents, usually the mother, has to attend various clinics with the baby. Many hospitals centralise their clinics and give appointments and treatments where possible, in one place on the same day. Treatments that were once only undertaken in hospital can now be done at home with special training for the family (Brennan & Vickers 1990). This prevents the trauma of repeated hospitalisations for routine therapy. The whole family is likely to be disrupted and the siblings may be unwittingly neglected as parents care for the sick baby. There may not be much parents can do about this situation because of their heavy commitments to the baby.

Prolonged counselling may be needed if parents blame themselves for passing this disease on to their baby. They will always be able to contact the genetic counsellors and may need advice if they plan another child.

GENETIC DISORDERS ENCOUNTERED ON THE NEONATAL UNIT

It is interesting to look at the more common genetic defects seen in the neonatal unit to gain some knowledge of the treatment needed and outcome for the baby.

These diseases will be looked at with regard to present and future help the baby and family will need. The outlook for these diseases is considered, as parents often want to know what will happen to their child in the future and whether help and support will be ongoing for them.

DOWN'S SYNDROME

This is the most common chromosomal abnormality and is found in 1 in 650 live births. There is a much higher incidence at conception as more than 50% spontaneously abort and 20% are still born (Roberton 1993). The incidence of the disease is related to the ageing of the ovum so an older woman is more at risk. This condition is also called trisomy 21 because there are three chromosomes at this

position, thus instead of having 46 chromosomes, the baby has 47. The parent's chromosomes are usually normal and the risk to the next child is only slightly higher than the normal population risk.

The translocation anomaly

Five per cent of Down's syndrome babies will have a translocation where a piece of genetic material breaks off one chromosome and attaches itself to another. This causes one chromosome to have too much, usually number 14, and the other, chromosome 21, too little. For estimating the risk factors of this inheritance parental blood has to be tested. If a parent has the abnormal chromosome there is a one in four chance of passing on the abnormality to any other child they have. Other members of the family are offered testing and prenatal diagnosis in these cases.

Diagnosis

Down's syndrome is suspected when alpha-fetoprotein (AFP) levels in maternal blood are measured at 12–15 weeks gestation. The level of this substance, which is produced by all human fetuses, is reduced when a Down's syndrome baby is being carried, especially if the mother is over 35 years of age. A Down's syndrome baby produces less AFP which may be because of impaired fetal kidney function (Brizot *et al.* 1996).

Ultrasound scanning can raise suspicions if the baby has a flat occiput and small head with typical facial features and a thickening at the back of the neck. Heart and intestinal defects may also be seen (Proud 1994). Mothers identified as carrying a Down's syndrome baby will be offered termination.

Common features of the disease

No one baby will have all the physical features of Down's syndrome. The most common are muscle hypotonia, eyes that slant up and out with folds of skin that run vertically between the inner corner of the eye and the bridge of the nose (epicanthic fold). A large tongue that tends to protrude, small ears, nystagmus and a single palmar crease.

Many Down's syndrome babies have serious congenital heart defects, usually an atrial or ventricular septal defect, an atrioventricular canal or Fallot's tetralogy. There is also a higher risk of oesophageal atresia, duodenal atresia and Hirschsprung's disease. As many as 25% of these babies will require surgery in the first year of life (Walker 1991). All have learning difficulties ranging from mild to severe (Table 7.1).

are together. They must be told if a chromosome test is to be done on their baby even though the result may not always be certain. Parental reactions to the diagnosis range from shock, denial, disbelief and anger to adaptation and adjustment. Parents may never have heard of the words used to describe their baby's condition such as trisomy or chromosome, and other medical terms. They may try to explain away the characteristics of the baby by saying someone else in the family looks the same. They may feel that once they accept the baby's condition they will be overcome by anxiety and not be able to cope. Parents who rejected a termination after the diagnosis of Down's syndrome, may also find the reality difficult to cope with.

All parents will be referred to a genetic counsellor who will be able to explain more fully how this has happened and how best to

---

Table 7.1 Common features and defects in Down's syndrome.

Common features	Common defects
Upward slanting eyes	Congenital heart
Prominent epicanthic folds	Duodenal atresia
Low nasal bridge	Oesophageal atresia
Small mouth turned down at corners	Hirschsprung's disease
Protruding tongue	
Hands short and broad	
Wide gap between big toe	
Muscular hypotonia	
Learning difficulties	

At birth

Parents may not notice any problem so it is essential that features in the baby that are giving rise to concern are pointed out sensitively as soon as possible when both parents

help the baby. Some parents do not wish to have this counselling but it can guide them to a healthy adjustment rather than struggling with their confusion and grief.

Many babies will not require treatment at birth but may be admitted to the neonatal unit for assessment of a heart defect. Such defects are often severe and require major surgery in early infancy. Drugs to control heart failure will be started and referral will be made to the cardiac team who will decide the best time for surgery. Babies who require surgery for cardiac or other anomalies in the neonatal period will have the same problems as normal babies undergoing similar treatment.

Learning problems

The process of learning for a Down's syndrome baby is slower than normal and it takes longer for them to learn every function. Parents need help and patience teaching their child and it may be useful for them to see a table of milestones and the approximate times that their child can expect to attain them (Table 7.2).

The portage system introduced in 1986 is a system whereby parents help their child by getting them to repeat various tasks with a set weekly target.

Social aspects

It is not always the case that the family will have enough support as this may depend on their location. They may fall within the catchment area of a Local Authority that offers specialist help to enhance the abilities of the child. Many Down's syndrome children are able to attend a nursery with normal children, others may need a specialist nursery.

When the child is 2 or 3 years old, educational needs will be assessed. The 1981 Education Act recommended that children with Down's syndrome be integrated into normal schools, which is often the best option for parents as the child can then live at home and have local friends. Though some parents will see a place in the protective environment of a special school as best.

Children with Down's syndrome are usually very friendly and if the parents are not embarrassed by them, others will react positively. For the child to achieve the greatest potential, early structured teaching methods and good social integration are the goals.

Table 7.2 Comparing the learning of a Down's syndrome baby with that of a normal baby. (Adapted from Cunningham (1988), Selikowitz (1990).)

Milestone	Average age	
	Down's syndrome	Normal
First smile	3 months	$1\frac{1}{2}$ months
Sits unsupported	9 months	6 months
Finger feeds	10 months	9 months
Crawls	15 months	9 months
Stands unsupported	18 months	11 months
Drinks from cup	20 months	12 months
Uses spoon	22 months	14 months
Walks alone	26 months	12 months
Bowel control	36 months	22 months

Future

Depending on the local education authority's policy, children up to the age of 16 years will be in full-time education. There may then be a place in a sheltered workshop where they can enter the job market, though this will not be suitable for all people with Down's syndrome. Better health care and diet means that many people with Down's syndrome live well into middle age. There are increasing numbers getting married and living happy fulfilled lives often with their parents or in small protected communities (Cunningham 1988).

CYSTIC FIBROSIS

Cystic fibrosis (CF) is a complex inherited disorder. It is the most common life-threatening disease in the United Kingdom affecting 1 in 2500 people. The cause is a faulty gene on chromosome 7. The current theory is that the fault causes too much chloride and too little water secretion in the epithelial tissues. This results in the formation of dehydrated viscus mucus in the lungs and pancreas which prevents their normal function (Hull & Thomson 1994).

It is an autosomal recessive disorder which means both parents must carry the gene. Neither of the parents may be affected but one in four of their children may be and two-thirds of the others will be carriers. In the population as a whole 1 person in 25 people is a carrier of the cystic fibrosis gene. If untreated, 75% of babies will die in their first year (Ferec *et al.* 1995).

Diagnosis

This disease is not usually diagnosed ante-natally unless the mother has had a previous child with cystic fibrosis. If this is the case she will be offered prenatal testing in the form of chorionic villus sampling or amniocentesis. If the result is positive she may be offered a termination.

Common features of the disease

The thick sticky mucus causes repeated chest infections and inflammation of the lungs leading to chronic lung disease. Thick mucus in the pancreas causes obstruction of the pancreatic ducts which prevents secretion of pancreatic enzymes and therefore induces pancreatic insufficiency leading to poor weight gain and failure to thrive. The children do not look different except that they are often frail and small. They have intelligence within the normal range.

At birth

When the baby is born there may be no indication of the condition. Some health authorities adopt a policy of screening for cystic fibrosis using blood from an additional blood spot on the Guthrie testing card. The argument against this is that it does not improve the long term outlook for the baby. But those in favour of screening say that early diagnosis improves short term morbidity and benefits the family by allowing the planning and screening of future pregnancies (Ferec *et al.* 1995).

Babies who do not pass meconium in the first 48 hours may have cystic fibrosis. About 15% of babies with cystic fibrosis present in the neonatal period with meconium ileus caused by abnormally tenacious meconium clogging the small intestine. The baby presents with abdominal distension and bile stained vomiting. X-rays typically show dilated bowel with air/fluid levels and trapped gas in the meconium. The condition usually needs to be resolved by surgery, which involves resecting the obstructed segment and the formation of a double-barrelled ileostomy for postoperative irrigation.

If there is no meconium ileus, a later symptom is steatorrhoea. The stools are fatty, loose and strong smelling as a result of fibrous scarring in the pancreas. The pancreatic ducts become blocked and eventually stop pancreatic juices reaching the intestines. This results in malabsorption, failure to thrive and recurrent chest infections.

Blood will be taken for measurement of immune reactive trypsin (IRT) if there is a possibility of CF. This test is based on the reaction of the body's defences to the pancreatic enzyme trypsin. CF is positively confirmed by a sweat test which is done at 4–6 weeks. There are abnormally high salt levels if the baby has cystic fibrosis.

Nutrition

Nutrition is a very important aspect of the care of a baby or child with CF. Babies and children with CF have chronic respiratory infections which result in increased metabolic needs, but because of the infections appetite is usually poor. All parents are referred to a dietitian – usually one with an increased knowledge of the specialised needs of a child with CF. Pancreatic enzymes should be started immediately following diagnosis to prevent mucus starting to block the pancreatic ducts and preventing essential enzymes reaching the gut. The enzymes come in capsule form and must be given with every milk feed, snack or meal. Over the years there has been modification of the capsules, first the concentration of lipase was increased to reduce the number of capsules required with each meal and second the gelatin surrounding the capsule

was changed so that it is unaffected by stomach acid and passes through to the duodenum before the coating is lost. This ensures that the enzymes are acting at the site where natural pancreatic enzymes would be released. Fat-soluble vitamins are poorly absorbed and need to be supplemented, especially vitamins A, D, E, and K.

Parents can become obsessed with their child's weight and feeding behaviour, little or no weight gain being a reflection of parenting skills. The obsession can be so great that parents may focus on their child's food intake for most of the day. This in turn can lead to food manipulation and bribery by the child for extra treats if food is eaten. The families need to understand the difference between normal and abnormal eating behaviour. Another factor is the increased salt need in a child with CF especially in hot weather. It appears that certain children are prone to acute salt loss and extra salt should be considered in any case where the child shows signs of becoming lethargic. In extreme cases of weakness or dehydration an intravenous infusion of saline may be indicated.

At school the child may encounter problems when taking enzymes with snacks and meals, especially as it now appears customary to lock up drugs as a routine safety procedure. Most teachers are happy to help once the child's needs are understood.

Older children can suffer from a meconium ileus equivalent and a child may present with abdominal pain, distention, vomiting, and constipation from faecal matter mixed with thick mucus collecting in the gut, usually around the caecum. This can almost always be treated medically.

A child with severe nutritional problems may need short periods of hospitalisation for nasogastric or in extreme cases intravenous feeding. Good nutrition may delay a decline in lung function and optimum nutrition leads to improved health and as a consequence a better quality of life.

Physiotherapy

The inevitable lung damage in CF means that physiotherapy plays an important role in the management of the condition. This should begin at the time of diagnosis even if the lungs are clear, and continue at least twice a day for life. Parents will be taught how to do this by physiotherapists and helped to establish a regular routine incorporated into the playtime of the child. It is an essential preventative measure to help minimise long term fibrotic changes in the lungs, which can occur following infective episodes.

Family adjustment

Owing to the chronic nature of CF, the uncertainties of the progress of the disease and long term prognosis, there is a great impact on family life. If the baby needed surgery, parents have to come to terms with looking after a baby with a stoma and this may overshadow the diagnosis of CF at first. The first few days after diagnosis will be a bewildering blur of information, advice and teaching and it is important not to overwhelm the family at this time. Members of the CF support team should be introduced gradually so that the family are not swamped by a number of new people entering their lives at once. The parents will need emotional support from the staff to enable them to cope with the impact of the disease and may benefit from talking to a counsellor.

Social aspects

The child with cystic fibrosis will go to a normal school but may have periods away with chest infections. Physiotherapy and the enzyme regime have to be ruthlessly pursued for the child to have the best chance of a healthy life. Even so some will have such damaged lungs that a lung transplant may be needed in their early teens if they are to survive.

The future

The CF gene has now been isolated and there have been many studies investigating the possibility of gene therapy. At present no treatment for CF actually corrects the gene defect in the specialised epithelium but research is investigating gene therapy for reducing lung damage. The most hopeful trial currently in the UK and USA involves introducing normal copies of the affected gene into the lungs of patients with CF. This therapy is not designed to introduce the gene into the reproductive cells, so that permanent genetic changes will not occur or be passed on. The problem with this kind of therapy is that the treated cells die and the cells that grow to replace them still carry the defective gene. This means that the treatment has to be repeated every 2–4 weeks (Hull & Thomson 1994).

New genetic approaches to CF may drain financial resources from other important areas of research, such as infection control and screening programmes. These have been the means of improving life expectancy and life quality for sufferers of this condition up to the present. Life expectancy 50 years ago was less than 2 years but today reports show an average life expectancy of 20–25 years and longer, with some sufferers having families themselves.

OSTEOGENESIS IMPERFECTA

This is a group of disorders affecting the skeletal structure of the body. Osteogenesis imperfecta manifests in increased fragility of the bones so that they fracture very easily. This is caused by a defect in collagen, the principal constituent of the white fibrous connective tissue which makes bone, tendons and cartilage. The fault lies in two genes, one on chromosome 7 and the other on chromosome 17. These two genes work in co-ordination to produce collagen. In osteogenesis imperfecta (OI) these genes are abnormal or missing resulting in a disease that has varying degrees of severity. The two genes mutate causing different degrees of the same disease and even different inheritance patterns. Some types are autosomal dominant, where there is a one in two chance of the baby having the disease, others are autosomal recessive where there is a one in four chance. Even in a family with a history of the disease it is impossible to predict the way the mutant gene will appear in an individual. Occasionally a family with no history of the disease will produce a baby with osteogenesis imperfecta. The incidence appears to be similar in all races and affects males and females equally with a general population risk of 1 in 20 000 (Connor & Fergusson-Smith 1991).

Common features

The severity of the disease varies from a few fractures in childhood through to multiple fractures *in utero* and death. Osteogenesis imperfecta has many different manifestations but in the main can be classified into four types with different inheritance patterns (Table 7.3).

In all types the fractures occur in the long bones and more frequently in weight bearing limbs. The bones heal leaving deformities of bowing and shortening. There is hyperlaxity of the ligaments and joints because of the defective connective tissue. Even finger joints may be affected and bend back when holding objects. The skull may be abnormal in shape owing to the pressure from the cranial contents on the soft bones and this may lead to tooth loss and hearing problems. The eyes are often very blue as a result the thin sclera and there is usually short stature.

In the most severe cases there is extreme fragility of the bones, macrocephaly, a triangular shaped face, kyphosis and scoliosis and very short stature. These badly affected patients are wheelchair bound by adolescence.

Prenatal diagnosis

For families with a history of osteogenesis imperfecta, chorionic villus sampling can be done at 8–9 weeks or amniocentesis at 16–26 weeks. If osteogenesis imperfecta is diagnosed the parents can opt for termination. There is no way of knowing at this stage how badly the baby will be affected because of the variability of the mutations of the gene but if another family member or sibling is severely affected it is likely that this will be the type inherited.

For families with no history, ultrasound scanning may diagnose the disease. Undermineralisation of skull bones and fractures may show up and cranial bones can be compressed easily by the transducer (Phillips *et al.* 1991). Positional deformities may occur due to the pressure of the abdominal and uterine walls.

At birth

If the baby is born with fractures the disease is

Table 7.3 Common features of osteogenisis imperfecta.

Type	Severity	Symptoms
Type 1 Dominant	Mildest Mild to moderate	Fragility of bones Normal appearance Bruise easily Early hearing loss Short stature
Type 2 Recessive	Prenatally lethal	Multiple fractures *in utero*
Type 3 Recessive	Severest among survivors	Severe fragility of bones Deformity on healing Macrocephaly Triangular face Scoliosis and/or kyphosis Severe osteoporosis Extremely short stature Wheelchair bound in teens
Type 4 Dominant	Less severe	Moderate fragility of bones Osteoporosis Bowing of bones Short stature Lax joints

fairly easy to diagnose. In many cases diagnosis may not occur until the baby has a fractured bone. Before this later diagnosis is made there may be worries that the baby was injured deliberately which adds to parental distress.

If the baby is diagnosed *in utero* or has obvious deformities at birth, management during the neonatal period is based on careful handling. The parents and staff should be made aware of how to lift the baby supporting head, trunk and buttocks. Care must be taken when changing nappies and gentle unhurried handling is needed. Even changing the nappy can cause a femoral fracture if the legs are held up during the procedure. If there is a family history or the diagnosis was made prenatally then these babies should not be tested for congenital dislocation of the hips as the examination itself can cause fractures.

Treatment

These children spend long periods in hospital while fractures are healing or surgical treatment is undertaken. The main goal is to achieve the best possible mobility and keep fractures to a minimum to get maximum independence and allow for easier social integration.

There are currently no drugs available to help prevent fractures. Dietary advice is to avoid fluoride deficiency and obesity. Splints are used in the treatment and prevention of fractures. They are often used on the lower limbs for support. Sometimes an intramedullary rod can be inserted to stabilise the bone. Braces may be needed to prevent the hyperextension of joints in some patients. Hydrotherapy helps improve muscle strength. Occupational therapists will provide practical aids. Patients with rib deformities and scoliosis, which decrease pulmonary capacity, are at risk of repeated respiratory infections.

Social aspects

During the early years there may be a delay in reaching some of the milestones such as sitting and walking but intellectual and emotional development is unaltered. These children have the standard range of intelligence and benefit from normal schooling. They are often absent for long periods so that home or hospital tuition may be necessary.

Parents

The parents of a child with a new mutation of osteogenesis imperfecta or a familial one will need to understand that fractures are inevitable and in no way reflect badly on their care. They will be taught how to use the various aids to make life easier for themselves and their child. It will be difficult not to be over protective as the need to prevent fractures may override the child's need to become independent. Financial help may be needed for hospital visits and special equipment.

Future

The incidence of fractures decreases with the onset of puberty and in many cases stops completely. In women who reach puberty there is an increased risk of osteoporosis.

A baby born with osteogenesis imperfecta today has a better prognosis than a baby born 30 years ago, owing to better medical and orthopaedic care both surgical and non-surgical. Most patients with osteogenesis imperfecta become productive members of society. The better their social adjustment and academic background the greater is their chance to advance in a competitive world.

DIGEORGE SYNDROME

This is caused by a microdeletion on chromosome 22, which involves a variety of problems concerned with the face, heart and neck structures such as the parathyroids and the thymus, which controls immune response. It is an autosomal dominant condition with males and females equally implicated. Sporadic cases and new mutations have been reported in families with no deletion in their chromosomes. The incidence of DiGeorge syndrome is 1 in 66 000 (Davies 1992) and accounts for 1% of congenital heart defects.

In some families, parents may appear normal or may have sub-clinical problems but produce children with a variety of symptoms from simple cleft palate or mild congenital heart problems to the severe DiGeorge type with heart defects and immunodeficiency (Driscoll *et al.* 1991). DiGeorge type abnormalities have been reported to occur partially and fully in many different disorders (Table 7.4). If the mother is a diabetic or abuses alcohol, the baby might have a deformity which includes a deletion on chromosome 22.

Common features

The main problems of this syndrome are major heart defects and primary immunode-

Table 7.4 Syndromes associated with DiGeorge anomaly.

Syndrome	Organs affected
Truncus arteriosus Fallot's tetrology	Midline heart defects
Velocardiofacial syndrome, Shprintzens	Facial and heart disorders
CHARGE	Coloboma Heart defects Atresia of choanae Retardation, mental and somatic Genital hypoplasia Ear anomalies
Familial congenital heart disease	Heart defects
Zellweger syndrome	Cystic kidneys
Kallmann syndrome	Hypotrophic gonadism
Holoprosencephaly	Mid-line facial anomaly
Diaphragmatic defects	Hernia Hypoplasia
Gastrointestinal anomalies	Gastroschisis Exomphalos
Genitourinary anomalies	Bladder exstrophy Cloaca

ficiency owing to absent or hypoplastic thymus and parathyroid glands. The baby will have dysmorphic features, which are not always obvious at birth, mild learning difficulties, hearing problems and sometimes cleft lip and palate.

Severe cardiac anomalies are responsible for many deaths within the first week. Other babies die in the first month from infections owing to immunodeficiency. Those that survive suffer from failure to thrive and repeated infections because of immunodeficiency problems. The severity of immunodeficiency problems will depend on the amount of functioning thymus (Campbell & McIntosh 1992).

Diagnosis

If there is no history in the family, the heart defect may be discovered on the routine biophysical scan at 14–16 weeks. The mother will be informed of the problem and a detailed cardiac scan is performed as soon as possible with her permission.

If the baby has DiGeorge syndrome there will usually be aortic arch problems. There might be an interrupted aortic arch, where a piece of the aorta is missing, or coarctation or narrowing of the aorta. This means the baby will not have a complete circulation and will die of heart failure within the first few days of life unless treated.

The mother may be offered a termination at this stage or can have an amniocentesis to check if the baby has the deletion on chromosome 22 which could indicate that immunodeficiency disease may be present. Even with the diagnosis of a deletion on chromosome 22 it is impossible to predict how badly the baby will be affected by the immune problems (Wadey *et al.* 1993).

At birth

If the mother does not opt for a termination she will be sent to a regional neonatal unit for delivery. Undiagnosed babies are well at birth and the dysmorphic features not always obvious at this stage. Within the first 24 hours the baby will get progressively breathless and exhausted as the ductus arteriosus closes. (The ductus arteriosus is part of the fetal circulation, joining the aorta to the pulmonary artery, which closes off naturally during the first few days of life.) When the duct closes the baby will not have a complete circulation and will die.

All babies who have heart problems concerning the aorta should be treated for DiGeorge syndrome with the immunity disorder. This means strict universal precautions during handling to ensure no infection is caused and the use of irradiated blood in which the antibodies have been destroyed. Major heart surgery, using cardiopulmonary bypass techniques, is necessary in the first few days of life.

The immunodeficiency disease in DiGeorge is caused by the absence of T cells. These are the most important cells in the immune system as they control the regulation of antibody production, the secretion of growth factors and lymphokine production which regulates other non-specific immune effector cells.

Without these cells the slightest infection can develop into an overwhelming disease.

Family adjustment

After the operation the main problem for the parents, when their baby has recovered, is the immunodeficiency disease. At first this might not seem to be such an issue to them, especially after the drama of the heart surgery and the days in the intensive care. Education of the family must begin as soon as it is obvious that the baby is going to survive the heart surgery (Davies 1992).

Immunodeficiency means the baby is susceptible to repeated infections with the constant threat of death from overwhelming infection. Colds turn into pneumonia and a childhood disease such as rubella or varicella could prove fatal. Live vaccines must not be given and parents will have to keep a constant vigil to protect their baby from infection.

To build up an antibody level, intravenous infusions of immunoglobulin need to be given every 3–4 weeks with daily antibiotic cover. The long term treatment of choice now is a bone marrow transplant from a suitably matched donor. This gives long lasting results and holds out a great deal of hope for these children (Davies 1992).

Discharge

The baby's discharge must be carefully planned with community services primed to follow up the family. It is likely that the parents will need the help of a dietician and physiotherapist to promote good nutrition and treat repeated chest infections that damage to the lungs. Parents will be referred to an immunology specialist and have follow-up care from the cardiologist, paediatrician and geneticist.

There are two support groups who can help parents with information and advice: The Primary Immunodeficiency Association and Contact a Family. These organisations send out information and give addresses of the nearest group or family that can help (Appendix 1).

Future

Survival depends on the severity of the heart condition and the amount of functioning thymus. Severe DiGeorge syndrome poses ethical problems as the cost of the specialised treatment necessary is very high. The surgery requires highly skilled surgeons and specialised equipment: nursing care is critical, needing experienced, qualified staff. Often these babies die soon after surgery and if they live their quality of life may be poor as they succumb to repeated infections. The most optimistic outlook lies in advances in surgical cardiology and refining of bone marrow transplants (Davies 1992).

Less severely affected babies survive reasonably well with careful treatment. The fairly minor learning difficulties mean they can have a reasonable quality of life in the community with minimum support.

THE HUMAN GENOME PROJECT

The human genome project is a multi billion pound international project to map human genes and define the chemical structures of their DNA. There are 50 000 to 100 000 genes spaced along the 23 pairs of chromosomes and through this exciting research new genes are being mapped and their structures examined. Knowing the location of a disease-causing gene is the first step in developing a useful diagnostic test. Discovering the abnormal DNA structure of the diseased gene to find the flaw allows potential treatment to correct or eradicate it.

The idea of the project came from a molecular biologist, Walter Sinsheimer, in 1985 in California. The Human Genome Organisation (HUGO) parcels out work to research teams all over the world and the results are collated in the USA, Britain, Germany and Japan. The organisation itself has run into many problems as it is proving prohibitively expensive and is involved in international wrangling about ethical dilemmas.

In Britain an independent project is running. This is a simpler and less expensive project than the American one which will research and record the sequence of the genes. Co-ordination of work done throughout the country is being collated at Northwick Park Hospital, London. Knowledge of the human genome means that human beings born or unborn can potentially be screened for their genetic faults. The abuses this could lead to are enormous and research into ethical implications has been allocated 3% of the project's budget (Hodson 1992).

Mapping the entire genetic blueprint and finding genes for the thousands of inherited disorders could revolutionise medicine. Doctors will one day be able to create a genetic readout of their patients' genes and give them a breakdown of inherited traits that could cause ill health later in life. There may even be a genetic basis for behavioural traits and some studies have suggested genetic links for aggression and homosexuality (Lees & Winter 1996).

If the genetic blueprint is mapped while treatment for genetic diseases is in its infancy, ethical problems lie in the possibility of discrimination because of genetic predictions. This could lead to problems in choosing a partner, gaining employment, health care, mortgage and insurance. Careful legislation will be needed to ensure medical research does not hinder humanity instead of help.

GENE THERAPY

Defining the structure of the genes opens the door to overcoming genetic problems by developing gene therapy. Geneticists are concentrating on developing a gene augmentation therapy whereby a healthy gene replaces a missing or defective gene. Proposals for human gene therapy must clear several issues. The safety of the procedure for the patient and general public, the benefits to the patient as opposed to the risk and the useful information that is to be gained from a clinical trial (Miller 1992).

The essence of gene therapy is gene transfer, which is very much in its infancy. The first approved trial of gene transfer into humans in May 1989 did not involve gene transfer at all but was performed to track a tumour infiltrating lymphocytes in a patient with melanoma (Miller 1992). The cytokine gene transferred into the tumour cells stimulated the host to an immune response against the tumour cells.

Gene therapy involves two possible ways for curing genetic disease. A new gene can be implanted at a very early stage of embryogenesis so that the gene is incorporated into the individual's germ line, either the ova or sperm. This is not considered ethical for humans as the new genes would be passed from generation to generation with unknown results. This method is very exciting and promising but does raise profound ethical concerns about genetic manipulation.

The second method, gene augmentation involves inserting the relevant gene into developed tissue, not into the germ line of the individual. This works by cloning the normal gene of the individual in bone marrow, putting it in a suitable vector (carrier) and introducing it into the body to target specific cells (Strauss 1996).

Research is ongoing into the use of viruses as suitable vectors because of their ability to enter and infect cells of the body. The viral agents are removed from the vector before introduction and a number of types of virus are being investigated. These are currently, the retrovirus associated with tumour cells, adenoviruses and adeno-associated virus which have properties that ensure efficient targeting of the necessary gene. So far no one of these has proved the ideal in clinical trials and the retrovirus risks infecting the germ line cells (Coutelle 1996). It is possible that viruses such as the Herpes virus or Epstein Barr virus, which have different infecting properties, may be of use (Strauss 1996). It is essential that the function of the virus is completely understood to minimise problems such as the spread of cancer, tumour growth and mutations (Karpati *et al.* 1996). There is also the fear that the gene introduced this way may get out of control and escape into the germ line putting the future reproductive health of the human race in jeopardy.

Recent developments in genetic research

A recent development is the genetic screening of very early stage embryos resulting from *in vitro* fertilisation (IVF) techniques. IVF usually results in the production of several embryos. These are genetically examined and only those which will not develop a known genetic disease are implanted. This has been carried out where the parents are carriers of a disease and is specialised, expensive and unlikely to be routinely available.

Previously unknown mechanisms for genetic changes are also being investigated. This concerns how the gene is passed from the parents. For example, in some deletion syndromes such as DiGeorge, not all patients will have the full deletion, and other defects affect only males or are carried through the female line. It is hoped that this research will cast light on inheritance patterns and help in more accurate prediction risks for the family (Korf 1995).

There is at present a clinical trial on cystic fibrosis patients using adenovirus as a vector and the airway route for delivery. The treatment has to be repeated frequently as the healthy CF gene is lost as the viral cells die. Repeated usage may cause interference with the patient's immune system (Williams & Lessick 1996). Other gene therapy treatment has been tried on conditions such as severe combined immune deficiency disease. Although good results were obtained in trials, the intervention is only helpful for the life span of the white blood cell used.

Gene therapy holds exciting potential for the near future. The diseases the scientists are most hopeful about helping are defects caused by a single gene, such as cystic fibrosis. Genetic engineering may offer a solution in the future when genes can be manipulated and altered. For the present, genetic counselling with the offer of termination is the only preventative measure available for genetic abnormalities and their disruptive problems.

REFERENCES

Brennan VM, Vickers P. (1990) *Nurses and Primary Immune Deficiency Disorders*. Baxter Healthcare.

Brizot ML, McKie AT, Von Kaisenberg CS, Farzineh F, Nicolaides KH. (1996) Fetal hepatic alpha-fetoprotein mRNA expression in fetuses with trisomy 21 and 18 at 12–15 weeks gestation. *Early Human Development*, **44**, 155–159.

Campbell AGM, McIntosh N. (1992) *Forfar and Arneil's Textbook of Paediatrics*. 4th edn. Churchill Livingstone, Edinburgh.

Carter B. (1990) Fetal rights – a technologically created dilemma. *Professional Nurse*, **5** (11), 590–594.

Connor JM, Fergusson-Smith MA. (1991) *Essential Medical Genetics*, 3rd edn. Blackwell Scientific Publications, Oxford.

Coutelle C. (1996) Gene therapy for cystic fibrosis. *Annales Nestle*, **54**, 15–24.

Cunningham C. (1988) *Down's Syndrome. An Introduction for Parents*. Souvenir Press, London.

Davies EG. (1992) Immunodeficiency. In: *Forfar and Arneil's Textbook of Paediatrics*, (eds AGM Campbell & N McIntosh) 4th edn. Churchill Livingstone, Edinburgh.

Department of Health. (1991) *The Children's Act 1989: An Introductory Guide for the NHS*. Department of Health, London.

Driscoll DA, Budarf ML, Emanuel BS. (1991) Antenatal diagnosis of DiGeorge syndrome. *Lancet*, **338**, 1390.

Emery AEH, Pollen I. (1984) *Psychological Aspects of Genetic Counselling*. Academic Press, London.

Ferec C, Verlingue C, Parent P, *et al.* (1995) Neonatal screening for cystic fibrosis. *Human Genetics*, **96**, 542–548.

Harper PS. (1991) *Practical Genetic Counselling*, 3rd edn. Butterworth-Heinemann, Oxford.

Harvey D. (1987) *Parent Infant Relationships*, Volume 4. John Wiley, Chichester.

Hodson A. (1992) *Essential Genetics*. Bloomsbury, London.

Hull J, Thomson AH. (1994) Genetics of cystic fibrosis. *Current Opinion in Paediatrics*, **6**, 136–140.

Jupp S. (1992) *Making the Right Start*. Opened Eye Publications, Cheshire.

Karpati G, Lochmuller H, Nalbantglu J, Durham H. (1996) The principles of gene therapy for the nervous system. *Trends in Neuroscience*, **19** (2), 49–54.

Korf BR. (1995) 'New' mechanisms of genetic disease. *Current Opinion in Paediatrics*, **7** (6), 695–697.

Lees MM, Winter RM. (1996) Advances in genetics. *Archives of Disease in Childhood*, **75**, 346–350.

Marteau T, Johnston M, Shaw R, Michie S, Kidd J, New M. (1989) The impact of prenatal screening and diagnostic testing upon the cognitions, emotions and behaviour of pregnant women. *Journal of Psychosomatic Research*, **33** (1), 7–16.

Methodist Church. (1990) *Status of the Unborn Human*. Methodist Publishing House, Peterborough.

Miller AD. (1992) Human gene therapy comes of age. *Nature*, **357** (11), 455–460.

Phillips OP, Shulman LP, Altieri LA, Wilroy RS, Emerson DS, Elias S. (1991) Prenatal counselling and diagnosis in deforming osteogenesis imperfecta. *Prenatal Diagnosis*, **11**, 705–720.

Proud J. (1994) *Understanding Obstetric Ultrasound*. Books for Midwives Press, Cheshire.

Roberton NRC. (1993) *Textbook of Neonatology*, 3rd edn. Churchill Livingstone, New York.

Sadler TW. (1990) *Langmans Medical Embryology*, 6th edn. Williams and Wilkins, Baltimore.

Selikowitz M. (1990) *Down's Syndrome the Facts*. Oxford University Press, Oxford.

Smith DK, Marteau TM. (1995) Parental reaction and adaptability to the prenatal diagnosis of fetal defect or genetic disease leading to pregnancy interruption. *Prenatal Diagnosis*, **15** (3), 249–259.

Strauss M. (1996) Strategies in gene therapy. *Annales Nestlé*, **54**, 1–14.

Wadey R, Daw S, Wickremasinghe A, *et al.* (1993) Isolation of a new marker and conserved sequences close to the DiGeorge marker HP500 (DS1340). *Journal of Medical Genetics*, **30**, 818–821.

Walker C. (1991) Downs syndrome and congenital heart defects. *Intensive Care Nursing*, **7**, 94–104.

Williams JK, Lessick M. (1996) Genome research: Implications for children. *Pediatric Nursing*, **22** (1), 40–46.

Yeo H. (1994) Support from people who know. *Child Health*, **2** (1), 32–35.

8 Nursing the Critically Ill Baby

LEARNING OUTCOMES

After reading and studying this chapter the reader will be able to:

○ List the conditions that could lead to a critical illness in a new-born baby.

○ Demonstrate an understanding of the care of a baby in respiratory failure and cardiac failure.

○ Describe medical and nursing management of a baby with renal failure and undergoing peritoneal dialysis.

○ Identify the clinical manifestations of disseminated intravascular coagulation (DIC).

○ Discuss management of the neurologically damaged baby.

○ Discuss the support needed by the parents of a very ill baby.

THE CRITICAL BABY

Neonatal intensive care has been described as the most successful of all medical technologies (Neonatal Association Working Party 1994). New therapies and improved techniques mean that the intensive care unit is successfully treating babies with ever more serious conditions. Nurses who look after these very ill babies give a high standard of experienced and skilled care often under difficult and stressful circumstances.

An illness can be defined as critical where there is a risk of failure of one or more systems of the body. The baby will have a primary illness which may overwhelm and involve other organs separately or together. Often the course of the baby's illness is acute and critical, lasting only a few days before the baby improves or succumbs. Sometimes the illness is prolonged, lasting many weeks with numerous acute episodes involving different systems of the body. Eventually the baby may die and the nurse has to face the emotional conflict and distress of the family as well as personal feelings.

Predisposing causes of critical illness

All new-born babies whether preterm or term

have the potential for a critical illness. There are many factors which make birth and the neonatal period fraught with danger for the baby:

- There are forces that may have adversely influenced fetal development such as smoking, substance abuse or intrauterine malnourishment.
- The physical changes necessary to enable the baby to progress from intrauterine to extrauterine life do not always occur properly.
- There is a low resistance to infection.
- There may be trauma involved in the birth process.

As a result of these factors the baby may be ill at birth or develop an illness during the neonatal period. A baby can become seriously ill very quickly from apparently minor symptoms so the aim of the neonatal intensive care unit is to recognise the significance of early symptoms and initiate treatment to prevent a critical illness.

Babies who are ill at birth are treated aggressively to prevent worsening of the condition and those with minor problems such as raised respirations, poor feeding, unstable temperature or blood sugars are carefully monitored for any escalation of symptoms.

The precipitating factors to critical illness are varied but conditions that predispose to it are:

- Birth asphyxia
- Meconium aspiration
- Intrauterine infection
- Extreme prematurity
- Respiratory distress
- Twin to twin transfusion, polycythaemia in one, anaemia in the other

- Congenital malformations, diaphragmatic hernia, hypoplastic lungs
- Genetic problems such as Patau's or Edward's syndrome

RESPIRATORY FAILURE

The system needing primary support most often in acute neonatal disease is the respiratory system. Respiratory distress syndrome is the most common illness affecting preterm babies, owing to lack of surfactant in the lungs. Difficulties, at birth or afterwards, also affect the production of surfactant causing worse respiratory distress. In term babies the mature pulmonary vasculature is affected by hypoxia and acidaemia causing a serious respiratory illness.

Acute disease

Preterm babies

Respiratory distress often results in an acute illness caused by immaturity of the respiratory system and lack of surfactant (Chapter 4). Respiratory distress syndrome is self-limiting, lasting about 7 days, and the aim of treatment is to support the baby through the course of the disease.

Term babies

The most common respiratory disease to affect term babies is persistent pulmonary hypertension of the newborn (PPHN) or persistent fetal circulation. During intrauterine life the pulmonary vasculature is hypertensive ensuring resistance that enables blood to bypass the lungs through the fetal circulation. When the baby is born and takes the first few breaths, oxygen acts on the vasculature caus-ing resistance to fall (Table 6.1). This lowers the pressure on the right side of the heart closing the foramen ovale and starting the closure of the ductus arteriosus.

If the baby is hypoxic the pulmonary vessels constrict causing increased vascular pressure against which the right side of the heart cannot force blood towards the lungs. The fetal circulation then persists and causes blood to flow away from the lungs, preventing the normal fall in pulmonary vascular pressure. This results in severe systemic hypoxic condition that is difficult to treat (Mitchell 1996).

Chronic disease

Respiratory distress syndrome can cause acute illness in the preterm baby (see Chapter 4) and may leave residual lung damage which can cause ventilator dependence. Babies who have conditions involving malformations of respiratory organs, heart, intestinal tract or kidneys may also develop chronic ventilator dependence.

In these conditions the baby remains venti-lated for days or weeks in a sub-critical state, not improving or deteriorating but needing many supportive interventions and drugs. There may be frequent respiratory collapses with deterioration in vital signs, plummeting oxygen levels and rises in carbon dioxide due to lung damage.

Respiratory collapse

A respiratory collapse may occur at any time during an acute or chronic illness and may be a frequent occurrence during the treatment of any ventilator dependent baby. There are a number of causes for a respiratory collapse which may occur together or singly:

- Blocked endotracheal tube
- Pneumothorax
- Pulmonary interstitial emphysema
- Consolidation of areas of the lungs
- Infection
- Inhalation of fluids
- Cerebral haemorrhage

Symptoms

There will be a sudden drop in oxygen saturations usually accompanied by brady-cardia. There may be little or no movement of the chest wall signifying a blocked or dis-placed endotracheal tube. The endotracheal tube may be difficult to hand bag, needing more pressure than expected to produce chest movement because of consolidation of one or both lungs. The chest may be asymmetrical owing to a massive pneumothorax. If there is a raised temperature, the collapse may be due to pneumonia caused by bacteria or inhalation of fluids.

Emergency treatment

The patency of the airway is paramount to keep the baby oxygenated. Emergency mea-sures must begin immediately to prevent prolonged hypoxia while the exact cause of the collapse is being sought.

The first action must be to detach the baby's endotracheal tube from the ventilator and hand bag the tube until the oxygen saturations are above 90%. A stethoscope should be used to listen to the chest for air entry during this procedure. Mechanical ventilation can recommence if all appears well, as the drop in saturations may have been due to exhaustion on the part of the baby in response to hand-ling. Pain, instability of the nervous system or fragility of the infant can be causative factors for this and there is often an improvement when the baby is left to rest and given extra oxygen for a short time.

If the oxygen saturations do not improve after 30 seconds of bagging or if they fall again when the baby is returned to the ventilator, the ventilator rate should be increased and a chest X-ray ordered.

Further investigations

A chest X-ray will reveal the presence of pneumothoraces, air leaks or consolidation due to lobar pneumonia (Fig. 8.1). Blood gases will be measured to assess respiratory status. Blood cultures should be made in cases of suspected infection. If cerebral haemorrhage is suspected an ultrasound scan of the head may be arranged to check the extent of the bleed.

Treatment

The result of the blood gases and chest X-ray will often ascertain the state of the lungs and suggest the course of treatment needed. Respiratory status may be improved by changes in the rate or pressures of the ventilator. Consolidation of the lungs in pneumonia is treated by physiotherapy and frequent changes of position for postural drainage.

Paralysis is often necessary when babies need high ventilatory rates and pressures. This will ensure maximum compliance with the ventilator and prevent breathing against the pressures, which can cause pneumothorax. Continuous pain relief must be given to these babies as owing to the paralysis, they will not be able to respond in a recognisable way to pain (Sparshot 1996).

Antibiotics will be commenced immediately after blood cultures are taken to prevent worsening illness from infection. They will be continued, changed or stopped according to the results obtained after 24 hours' growth in the laboratory. If a pneumothorax is revealed on X-ray, a chest drain will be inserted to drain the air away until the lung has healed (Flores 1993).

Treatment of pneumothorax

A pneumothorax occurs when some of the alveoli in the lungs collapse allowing a pocket of air to collect (Fig. 8.1). If not treated the pocket of air grows as more air is trapped with every breath. This prevents efficient ventilation and oxygenation until treated.

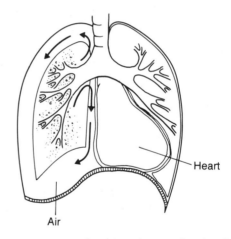

Fig. 8.1 Diagram of pneumothorax, showing the pathway of air from the lung tissue into the pleural space. The heart is pushed to the left because of the pressure in the right side of the chest.

When a pneumothorax is suspected in respiratory collapse, a strong light is shone through the chest, which shows the position of a translucent expanse in the lungs, filled with air. A sterile butterfly needle is inserted into the area thus revealed, with the tube end in a bottle of sterile water so that air does not enter the lungs. Bubbling in the water will show that the correct part has been treated and there is usually a noticeable improvement in the baby's condition.

Chest drain insertion

A permanent chest drain is inserted for continuous draining of air until the alveoli reinflate. This is a very painful procedure for the baby, necessitating cutting through a thickness of skin to insert the chest drain between the ribs. Lignocaine skin anaesthesia must be used, even in an emergency, to prevent stress and shock to the baby. Lignocaine should be given even when the baby is on maintenance pain relief to ensure sufficient anaesthesia.

The procedure is done using aseptic technique. The drain will usually be inserted through the second or third intercostal spaces anteriorly. Lateral drains use the third or fifth intercostal spaces. The site of entry should be chosen carefully because of permanent scarring and in a girl it may interfere with breast development (Fig. 8.2).

The drain enters the chest for about 2–3 cm. It is then attached to tubing which ends in an underwater seal. Bubbling and oscillation of the water with respiratory efforts will signify the success of the procedure. The tube is

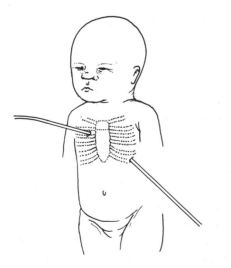

Fig. 8.2 Diagram showing sites for insertions of pleural drains, only one is usually necessary.

secured with tape or clear plastic dressing to make an airtight seal. Then the chest is X-rayed to check it is in the most effective position.

Nursing care of a baby with a chest drain

After the insertion of a chest drain the baby will be shocked and exhausted. Adequate warmth and a period of rest must follow for the baby to recover.

The drain should be checked hourly and a record kept of bubbling, oscillation and drainage. If movement ceases in the drain the baby should be watched closely for signs of deterioration. The drain may be blocked or out of position causing another accumulation of air in the lungs and a further X-ray will be needed.

The dressing around the drain should be inspected frequently to ensure there is an airtight seal. Any serous fluid seeping through should be reported and the dressing renewed, using aseptic techniques to prevent infection. Bottles and tubing must be changed using aseptic precautions every 24 hours and any drainage recorded. The drain must be clamped before tubing is changed to prevent air getting into the chest.

Care should be taken that the drain does not become dislodged when removing the bottles and tubing. There should always be two clamps at the cotside to clamp off the drain when carrying out any activity involving moving the baby or tubing. The weight of the tubing may drag the drain out of the chest but this can be prevented by placing a piece of strapping around the tube and pinning it to the undersheet. It should be unpinned before moving the baby or changing the sheets. The chest drain will cause pain and discomfort on moving, so handling should be done with care. Pain relief should be given to every baby with a chest drain.

The water in the bottle must cover the end of the tubing and care must be taken not to tip the bottle as this will let air enter the chest. The bottle must be lower than the site of entry of the drain otherwise water will enter the chest from the bottle. The bottles should be secured to a stand or the incubator to prevent accidental spilling.

Removal of chest drain

When the drain has stopped oscillating and the baby remains stable, the collapsed area of the lung has probably reinflated. The drain will be clamped for 24 hours and the chest X-rayed before removal to check that there is no re-accumulation of air. The drain is removed using aseptic precautions taking care to ensure that no air enters the chest. The skin can be closed with skin closures, a purse-string suture should not be used as it causes disfiguring scarring (Bernbaum & Hoffman-Williamson 1991). After the drain has been removed the site should be checked for a day or two to ensure that the skin closures are intact and that the wound is healing well.

Physiotherapy

Consolidation of the lungs is often caused by a pneumonia. This infection may give rise to a thick exudate which will clog up areas of the lung making it necessary to raise pressures and rates of the ventilation for adequate oxygenation. To improve the baby's condition and reduce ventilatory requirements this exudate needs to be removed. Physiotherapy is usually prescribed to loosen secretions and allow them to be removed through the endotracheal tube. Many units will have an accessible physiotherapist but nurses looking after babies with respiratory problems need to be taught to perform physiotherapy for the times when the physiotherapist is not available.

To perform physiotherapy, gentle percussion of the chest or vibrations using the fingertips is necessary. This is applied on every third or fourth breath and can be very effective at loosening and removing secretions. Endotracheal suctioning should always follow physiotherapy and the amount and colour of secretions recorded. Treatment every 4–6 hours may be necessary in the early stages with changes of position at least once a shift and possibly more often to prevent lung stasis. Physiotherapy will continue until the consolidation has improved as seen on X-ray or the secretions are being easily removed from the endotracheal tube.

Other nursing treatments

When the cause of the respiratory collapse has been found and treated, the baby often appears pale and exhausted. A long rest period should follow to assist recovery. The baby may be hypothermic after chest drain insertion or re-intubation and require a higher ambient incubator temperature or a blanket for warmth. After the collapse, there may be hypotension due to pain and shock, which can be improved by an infusion of fresh frozen plasma. Blood sugar may be unstable after a traumatic event because of the stress, pain and possible drop in temperature. Regular checks with glucose test strips should be carried out and if the blood sugar is low a more concentrated solution of dextrose maintenance fluids can be given or intravenous fluids can be increased as prescribed until the blood sugar is within normal limits.

Sequelae

Babies may suffer many respiratory collapses during their stay on the neonatal unit and most will eventually make a good recovery. Others may develop chronic lung disease from the initial disease and become ventilator dependent. If the baby is suffering from a congenital progressive atrophic disease or one of the trisomy syndromes such as Edward's or Patau's syndrome they might never be able to breathe on their own and decisions may have to be taken about the continuation of aggressive treatment. A baby who is ventilator dependent may become weakened by repeated episodes of collapse and infection and may go on to suffer the failure of other bodily systems.

CIRCULATORY FAILURE

Sick babies who have suffered episodes of hypoglycaemia, hypotension and hypoxia during episodes of respiratory collapse often incur coronary damage. This may cause the myocardium, or muscle layer, of the heart to become weakened, resulting in inefficient pumping of blood and poor oxygenation of vital organs such as kidneys, gut and brain. If there is an underlying congenital heart defect or patent ductus arteriosus, this may cause an escalation of heart failure.

A hypoxic episode from a blocked endotracheal tube, or any problem such as infection, electrolyte imbalance, deep suction causing vagal stimulation or neurological complications, may cause a cardiac arrest in these compromised babies.

Chronic heart failure

Symptoms

In chronic failure the onset may be gradual, over a few hours or days. The baby will be increasingly sweaty, restless and grey looking. There will be tachypnoea, tachycardia, enlarged liver, weak peripheral pulses and peripheral oedema (Paul 1995).

Diagnosis

There may be an underlying known cardiac defect which is already being treated and an ultrasound scan carried out on the unit can verify previous findings or diagnose new problems. A chest X-ray will demonstrate worsening cardiomegaly or pulmonary oedema.

Blood will be sent for culture in cases of suspected infection. Blood gases and serum electrolytes will be taken for assessment with a view to altering management of the condition.

Treatment

Treatment of chronic heart failure will be tailored to suit the underlying problem but, in general, comprises treatment to support and strengthen the failing heart. Ventilatory support will be given if necessary, to ensure adequate exchange of gases and good oxygenation of the blood. Maintenance fluid may be restricted in an effort to reduce pulmonary oedema caused by the inefficient circulation.

Drug therapy will include diuretics to prevent reabsorption of sodium in the kidneys, allowing more fluid to be excreted. This controls oedema in the lungs and tissues, easing the load on the heart. Diuretics can cause electrolyte imbalance so serum electrolytes need daily assessment.

Dopamine, a vasodilator, decreases vascular resistance and increases blood flow to the organs. It is given by continuous infusion to raise the blood pressure and a low dose improves renal function.

Digoxin improves the strength of the heart beat and controls arrhythmias. Dobutamine can be given as a continuous infusion to increase cardiac output and blood pressure, thus improving tissue perfusion and stabilising arrhythmias.

Acute failure

Sudden cardiac arrest can occur in a baby who has no history of heart problems. It may happen in response to a hypoxic episode, a reaction to suctioning, handling, or infection. There may be sudden bradycardia or extreme tachycardia (supraventricular tachycardia) accompanied by a fall in blood pressure which will not improve in spite of hand bagging the endotracheal tube, sometimes the heart will stop completely.

When the heart stops pumping, the brain is starved of oxygen and if this persists for more than a few minutes, permanent brain damage may result from the effects of hypoxia. Resuscitation to restart the heart must, therefore, be swift and efficient.

Cardiopulmonary resuscitation

The teaching of current resuscitation skills is mandatory in hospitals and nurses looking after small babies need to know how to adapt adult measures to suit their patients.

When the heart rate fails to return to normal after a few minutes of bagging, medical help should be summoned for further interven-

tional measures. For cardiopulmonary resuscitation at least two staff will be needed for hand bagging, cardiac massage and drug administration. It is helpful to have someone who can act as a runner, drawing up drugs and infusions of colloid. An intensive care unit should always have a trolley laid with items for re-intubation and drugs for emergency resuscitation.

Procedure

If the endotracheal tube is thought to be blocked it should be replaced or suctioned swiftly. The baby will be placed supine with the chin supported with one person to bag the airway while the other performs chest compressions.

There are two methods of doing chest compressions, the thumb method and the two-finger method. The method used may depend on preference, operator's skills or ease of access. The thumb method involves placing both thumbs side by side over the mid sternum, with the hands encircling the chest. The fingers should be supporting the baby's back. If the baby is very small, one thumb can be placed over the other (Fig. 8.3). For the two-finger method, the tips of the index finger and the middle finger are placed over the middle of the sternum while supporting the baby's back with the other hand.

For either method the sternum is depressed 1–2.5 cm ($\frac{1}{2}$ to 1 inch) then released, allowing the heart to refill, the thumbs or fingertips should be kept in contact with the sternum. This counts as one compression. A new-born baby's heart will beat at 120–180 depending on size so compressions should begin at 120 a minute or more if the baby is very small. The chest should not be squeezed or the xiphoid sternum pressed, as this may compromise the lungs (Kenner 1992). If the pressure is applied too low down or too heavily on the sternum

Thumb placement

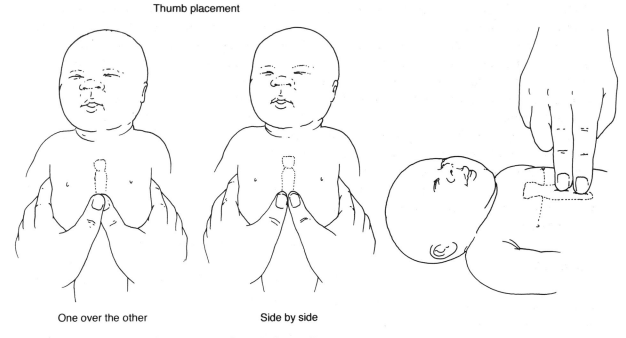

One over the other   Side by side

Fig. 8.3 Diagram showing position of hands for cardiac massage.

there is a risk of rupture of the liver causing fatal haemorrhage.

After 30 seconds the pulse should be checked. The compressions must be stopped briefly to listen with a stethoscope. Once the heart rate reaches 80, the compressions can cease but bag and mask ventilation should be continued until the heart rate is above 100 and the oxygen saturations are above 90%. First line drugs used for cardiopulmonary resuscitation are adrenaline and sodium bicarbonate.

Adrenaline
Adrenaline is a vasoconstrictor which raises the blood pressure and increases the heart rate in asystole or bradycardia. This should be given through a major vein, but can be given in a dire emergency into the endotracheal tube.

Sodium bicarbonate
This is used to correct the metabolic acidosis that develops as a result of hypoxia. It should

be given slowly and with great care to prevent tissue necrosis. Fast administration has been implicated in the development of intraventricular haemorrhage (Crawford & Morris 1994).

Other drugs such as calcium gluconate, calcium chloride and atropine can be given as necessary, to strengthen and support the heart.

When assisting at a resuscitation the person drawing up the drugs must keep a note of the drugs given and their effect. These details will be required later when an assessment of the emergency takes place.

Stores of glycogen in the brain, liver and heart muscle, which can produce energy by anaerobic glycolysis, enable neonates to survive 20 minutes of complete oxygen deprivation (Roberton 1993). If the heart has not restarted after 15 to 20 minutes in spite of vigorous efforts, a decision will have to be made as to whether to continue, as after this time permanent neurological impairment will be incurred.

Psychological effects on parents and staff

A cardiac arrest resuscitation, whether a success or failure, is an emotive and stressful event for all concerned. The people involved may need to go over the events with their colleagues for reassurance and maybe to regain their confidence, if they feel they did not act quickly or observantly enough. It often helps to have an informal meeting of staff involved to discuss events and feelings in a supportive atmosphere. Some may wish for retraining in cardiopulmonary techniques. Parents too will be very frightened and disturbed by this event and will need to know the causes of the problem and whether it will happen again.

Sequelae

The hypoxia that ensues during a cardiac arrest requiring lengthy resuscitation will have profound effects on other systems of the body. The brain, liver, intestine, kidneys and the heart muscle itself will all have been depleted of glycogen and oxygen. This will exacerbate the baby's underlying condition. There may be irreversible neurological damage, acute tubular necrosis or renal cortical necrosis causing kidney failure.

ACUTE RENAL FAILURE

Renal failure in the neonate can be prompted by a number of factors. This is because there is a high vascular resistance in the arterioles of the normal new-born baby's kidneys which makes them vulnerable to decreased renal blood flow. Renal blood flow is decreased in conditions causing hypoxia, hypotension, heart failure or severe infection and could result in renal damage and failure.

If the blood flow to the kidneys is impaired there is an abrupt reduction in glomerular filtration rate (GFR) of the kidney. GFR is the rate of filtration of blood through the nephrons of the kidneys which produce urine. Urine output falls and toxins and waste products cannot be excreted (Seaman 1995). Added to this, the immaturity of the kidneys at birth predisposes them to intolerance to fluid overload and salt excretion.

Symptoms

Renal failure will be suspected when urine output falls and blood tests reveal acidosis and abnormal electrolytes. The potassium will be high, the creatinine rising, urea levels high and there may be low blood sugar (McHugh 1997). Seizures or cardiac arrhythmias may occur as a result of the abnormal electrolytes.

There will be a fluid imbalance, with more fluid retained than excreted, and there will be oedema from the retained fluid. Urine output will fall to under 1 ml per kg per hour and there may be blood in the urine.

Treatment

There are two types of renal failure in the neonate. Prerenal failure and acute renal failure (ARF). Prerenal failure may be present due to essential fluid restriction in problems such as cerebral oedema or cardiac defects. Urine output in these cases will improve when the baby is given fluid, such as fresh frozen plasma, albumin or blood to expand the circulating blood volume, and diuretics. This treatment is used with caution in fluid restricted babies.

Treatment aims to improve the urine output to above 1 ml per kg per hour. If it does not increase urine output then the baby is most likely to have ARF. Dialysis will then be needed to prevent a build-up of toxins, remove fluid from the body and to restart renal function.

To improve recovery rates peritoneal dialysis should be undertaken before serious fluid imbalance has developed. The criteria for dialysing the baby will depend on:

- Continuing oliguria.
- Rapidly rising plasma potassium, urea and creatinine.
- The need for nutritional maintenance and drug treatment.
- Failure to improve by conservative management.

Peritoneal dialysis

Dialysis is carried out to remove fluid and toxins from the baby. Abdominal peritoneal dialysis is the dialysis of choice for neonates because it is safer than haemodialysis in sick small babies. The peritoneum is a highly vascular semi-permeable membrane with a large surface area which makes it ideally suited for the exchange of fluids that occurs during peritoneal dialysis.

Setting up the dialysis

The procedure is carried out on the neonatal unit using full aseptic techniques. The baby will usually be ventilated, paralysed and sedated because of other aspects of the illness. The baby's bladder should be catheterised so that an accurate fluid output can be recorded.

Lignocaine as a local anaesthetic should be injected into the area of the abdomen to be used, even if the baby is on continuous pain relief. The area used is the midline following the linea alba between the umbilicus and the pubic symphysis where major organs are less likely to be involved. A small cut is made in the skin with a scalpel and the cannula inserted into the peritoneum. The cannula is secured either with a suture or tape.

The cannula is attached to a tubing set with two branches. One end enters a bag of dialysate fluid, the other enters a bag to receive the drainage. The system is a closed one to prevent air entering the peritoneal cavity and to prevent infection. The cycles should start with drainage, to release any fluid put in during insertion. A system of taps on the tubing allows each part of the cycle to be controlled (Fig. 8.4).

One cycle consists of letting about 30 ml of dialysate run into the peritoneum by gravity, allowing it to dwell while dialysis takes place across the peritoneal membrane, then draining by gravity (Haycock 1993). Some neonates do not tolerate 30 ml at a time as it further compromises respiration. A smaller amount may be used though this may not be as efficient.

It is important to record the time the fluid takes to enter the abdomen and to drain. Usually cycles are organised by taking 20 minutes to run in, 20 minutes resting in the abdomen and 20 minutes out. This can be varied according to the tolerance of the baby and the success of the dialysis.

Cross-flow dialysis

Cross-flow dialysis uses two catheters, one for fluid in, the other for fluid out. Fluid is introduced and released at the same time irrigating the peritoneum continuously and does not

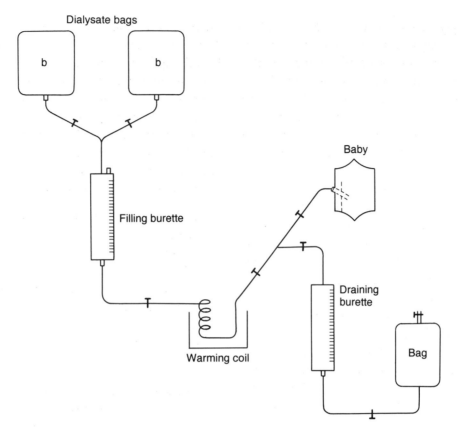

Fig. 8.4 Diagram showing closed system for performing peritoneal dialysis. (Adapted from Fleming *et al.* (1989).)

cause the abdominal distension that occurs when the fluid is given as a bolus.

Fluids used

Fluids used are intended to remove excessive fluid and consist of dextrose and saline solutions to which sodium, bicarbonate and potassium can be added to control the electrolytes. The higher the glucose concentration the more fluid is removed.

The fluids will be heparinised so that the catheter does not block, and warmed before being given to prevent cooling of the baby. Serum electrolytes should be taken frequently, at least 6-hourly to ensure the correct dialysate concentration is given.

Peritoneal dialysis is continued until the fluid balance is satisfactory and the potassium is below 6 mmol/l (Roberton 1993). When this has been achieved conservative measures will be reinstated until renal function returns to normal.

Complications with dialysis

There may be problems with the catheter – blocking, leaking and inefficient drainage are common. Fluid run in before most of the last cycle has drained could cause fluid overload. Dehydration can occur if the baby responds well to the dialysis so meticulous fluid balance and electrolyte assessment is needed.

Hyperglycaemia may be the result of absorbing sugar into the blood from the dialysate solution, especially if the infant is dehydrated. This can exacerbate acidosis and cause electrolyte disturbances. It can also cause more rapid osmotic diuresis so that the dialysis fluids may have to be given more slowly. Blood sugar levels need to be monitored 4–6 hourly.

Hypotension may result, if there is hypovolaemia because too much fluid is removed, and can be avoided by attention to fluid balance.

Peritonitis may be a problem if the catheter has had to be reinserted a number of times. Infection also may occur as a result of fluid leakage into the dressing around the catheter entrance, as the dialysate is a good medium for bacteria. If leaking persists the catheter should be removed and reinserted at another site. If peritonitis occurs the fluid returned may be cloudy and the baby will be pyrexial and irritable with abdominal distension.

Haemodialysis

Dialysis of the blood is technically difficult in preterm babies. The need for high-flow vascular access, systemic coagulation by the use of heparin and the development of hypotension causes problems in preterm babies (Hutchison & Gokal 1995).

Alternative developments to traditional techniques for haemodialysis are being explored. Continuous arteriovenous haemofiltration (CAVH) is a relatively inexpensive extracorporeal renal replacement therapy using a vacuum suction pump to overcome the problem of needing a high blood flow. Prediluting the blood with an electrolyte solution before it reaches the machine means that minimum heparin is needed (Stapleton & Wright 1992).

Two catheters are inserted, one arterial the other venous into major vessels (Table 8.1). The two vessels are cannulated and attached by tubing to the CAVH machine. All tubing and the filter is heparinised and the fluid is removed and replaced, slowly and continuously (Fig. 8.5). It is a well tolerated method which uses only a small amount of blood and avoids the need for fluid restriction. Adequate parenteral nutrition can be given concurrently. The disadvantages include:

- Haemorrhage if there is disconnection at the tubes.
- A high risk of sepsis.
- It is not suitable for premature babies because of the risk of IVH (Stapleton & Wright 1992).
- Impaired circulation of the limb if femoral access is used.

Table 8.1 Access for continuous arteriovenous haemofiltration.

Arterial access	Venous access
Umbilical	Umbilical
Femoral	Jugular
Radial	Subclavian
Tibial	Brachial
Brachial	Femoral

Care of a baby with acute renal failure

Fluid balance

Maintenance fluid requirements may be restricted to insensible loss replacement which may be estimated at 20–30 ml per kg daily (Roberton 1993). Urine output should be calculated hourly and the volume added to the fluids allowed. Intravenous or arterial lines should be flushed using the smallest

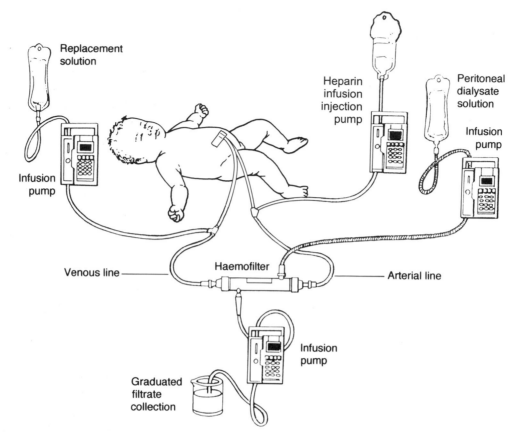

Fig. 8.5 Continuous arteriovenous haemofiltration. Access is through the umbilical artery and vein. The baby's blood pressure forces blood through the filter. Blood is heparinised through the arterial line. Replacement fluid can be added to arterial or venous line. Fluid removal is regulated at the infusion pump filter outflow and filtered through dialysate in the haemofilter. (Adapted from Merenstein and Gardner (1993).)

possible volume of fluid and this should be added to the fluid balance.

Accurate measurement of urine output is essential (Fox 1992). A catheter may be passed into the baby's bladder and left to drain into a closed system to ensure volume accuracy. If the baby has an indwelling catheter the urethral area should be inspected frequently for redness, infection and correct placement. If the catheter comes out and has to be reinserted it is important to use full aseptic precautions to prevent bladder infection. When emptying the closed system, gloves should be worn, as usual when handling body fluids, to prevent the spread of hepatitis B which may be in the urine.

A urine sample should be sent at least daily for measurement of electrolytes. This sample does not need to be sterile, just clean. Urine should be ward tested 6–8 hourly and the results recorded.

Blood tests

Blood will be sent for assessment of electrolytes, gases, glucose at least once a day and blood glucose estimated on the ward with glucose test strips 6–12 hourly. If the baby is hypoglycaemic a stronger intravenous dextrose solution can be given instead of increasing the amount of fluid.

Drug therapy

Metabolic acidaemia may sometimes be corrected by sodium bicarbonate infusion. Dopamine in low 'renal' doses may be given as a continuous infusion to improve renal blood flow.

Nutrition

If acute renal failure persists for more than a day or two, providing adequate nutrition will become a problem. It will be impossible to ensure the energy needed while fluid restrictions prevail and this in itself can be an indication for dialysis (Haycock 1993).

Good nutrition is important for all critically ill babies but those in renal failure require extra energy because of the catabolic reaction in the blood, to the toxic constituents from the ailing kidneys. The aim is to increase the anabolic reaction of the body, by extra nutrition, to prevent a build-up of these toxins. Babies in acute renal failure need at least 20% more energy than for normal growth (Haycock 1993). Enteral fluids can be given if the baby's condition allows – breast milk or formula with added energy.

If the baby is to be fed intravenously, a central venous line will be inserted so that energy-rich parenteral fluids such as 20% dextrose with lipids and proteins can be given.

Oedema

The baby with renal failure often has gross oedema. The skin is fragile and liable to break down leaving weeping areas at intravenous cannulation sites etc. Sore areas need to be kept dry and clean to prevent infection and swabs should be sent for bacteriological assessment if the area looks infected.

There may be pressure sores as a result of the oedema. Changes of position help prevent sore areas but are difficult to achieve with a baby on dialysis as this may move the peritoneal catheter causing leakage or blockage. Bean bags can be used to support limbs or relieve pressure on other parts of the body and an inflated mattress or soft sheepskin can be used.

The site of the intravenous cannula may be oedematous, making assessment of the site difficult. To prevent extravasation into the tissues, infusion pump pressures must be carefully monitored and the cannula resited when pressures rise.

If the condition allows, the baby should be weighed daily. This poses a challenge as moving these critical babies and manipulating life-sustaining equipment often results in physiological instability. Weighing is essential to gauge the extent of fluid retention. Electronic mattresses which fit under the mattress of the incubator have been found to be reasonably accurate (Engstrom *et al.* 1995, Torrance *et al.* 1995) though accuracy does depend on the incubator tray contents like linen, nappies, and attachments such as chest tubes and splints for intravenous lines weighing the same each time.

Parents

Renal failure in the baby is distressing for the parents as there is often massive oedema making their baby unrecognisable. The parents at this stage will be living from hour to hour in a state of anxiety and anguish. The aim of the treatment and its expected results should be discussed with them before it is undertaken.

The baby's nurse will offer support and detailed information on the progress of the dialysis and the baby's comfort and well being. Parents may wish to know about the equipment used and will often cling to fluid balance results or the voluntary passage of urine from the baby as a sign that their baby is improving or worsening.

They need to know the possibility of a poor outlook at this stage, though to tell them there is no hope when treatment is being carried out makes the treatment and the suffering of their child seem futile.

Sequelae

Acute renal failure in the new-born is a potentially reversible problem if uncomplicated by other severe illness. However, many of those affected are ill in other ways so that the overall mortality rate of babies needing peritoneal dialysis is at least 50% (Haycock 1993). Many babies who are very sick may incur, at this stage, complications with the clotting mechanisms of the blood such as disseminated intravascular coagulation.

DISSEMINATED INTRAVASCULAR COAGULATION (DIC)

This is a syndrome in which the clotting mechanism of the blood becomes abnormal. There is a reduction in platelets, prothrombin, fibrinogen and clotting factors resulting in haemorrhage and the formation of thrombi. There may be multiple thrombus sites which can cause tissue necrosis and ischaemia in areas of the brain, lungs, renal system, liver, gastrointestinal tract. There can be severe

uncontrolled haemorrhaging in the same organs. The disease is devastating in a sick baby and potentially life threatening.

DIC is usually secondary to and triggered by another serious disease. The baby will be ventilated and paralysed, there may have been respiratory problems, cardiac failure and acute renal failure.

Causes

DIC is a confusing disease because of the paradox of clotting and haemorrhage problems taking place at the same time (Emery 1992). The common mechanisms that trigger DIC include birth trauma, sepsis, shock, and hypoxia, all frequent problems in sick new-borns. These factors can lead to inappropriate systemic activation of the haemostatic mechanism (Table 8.2).

Table 8.2 Mechanism of disseminated intravascular coagulation.

Activation of homeostasis by birth trauma, sepsis, hypoxia etc.
↓
Clots in the circulation and fibrinogen degradation
↓
Inhibition of platelets and impaired clotting
↓
Ischaemic tissue damage and haemorrhage

Symptoms

The clinical manifestations of DIC will be extremely variable. Bleeding is the most common symptom and may occur at multiple sites from venipuncture, umbilical catheter sites, heel pricks, chest drain and dialysis entry scars. Gastrointestinal, pulmonary, renal or intraventricular haemorrhaging may occur. There may be haematuria, haematemesis or blood in the stools. Pulmonary or intraventricular haemorrhage can also take place. There may be petechiae and purpura of the skin.

The thrombotic signs will include skin necrosis such as digital gangrene, renal failure from renal thrombosis, paralytic ileus or abdominal distension, pulmonary embolism, central nervous system involvement, lethargy and seizures.

Diagnosis

This is made on the clinical signs and a combination of laboratory blood tests. These tests will include clotting factor studies and pro-thrombin time, which assesses fibrinogen and fibrinogen degradation products (Roberton 1993). The results will show abnormal clotting studies, low platelets and raised fibrin degradation products and abnormal red blood cells.

Management

This is a very difficult disease to treat successfully but in general the goals are early diagnosis, control of haemorrhage and elimination of the fibrin degradation products that cause the thrombi.

Clotting factors will be replaced by transfusions of fresh frozen plasma. Vitamin K is given to help prevent bleeding. Severely affected infants or those not responding to fresh frozen plasma may be given an exchange transfusion of blood not less than 48 hours old to replace the clotting factors and wash out toxins that are perpetuating the disease (Roberton 1993). Blood that has been stored in citrate phosphate dextrose has a low pH and high $PaCO_2$, which may cause metabolic stress to the baby, and should not be used. The use of intravenous heparin therapy is controversial as it increases the risk of bleeding

(Roberton 1993). It is normally reserved for babies with thrombotic complications in a large vessel (Emery 1992).

Nursing care of a baby with DIC

Babies with this disease bleed easily so that drugs must be given either intravenously or orally to prevent bleeding from an intramuscular injection. Intravenous resitings of cannulas and heel prick punctures should be kept to a minimum. It is fortunate if the baby already has a central venous line for intravenous feeding and drugs, and an arterial catheter for blood sampling. Invasive procedures should be forestalled where possible to prevent bleeding and trauma. Any bleeding, orally, rectally, intercranially or from the lungs could develop into a major haemorrhage.

The baby will already be seriously ill, requiring all the skills of an experienced neonatal nurse. The baby will be on many different infusions for other system failures, and possibly on renal dialysis. The charting of infusion rates and changes, ventilator and airway management, drug regimes, fluid balance, observations of chest drains, catheter and intravenous sites, wound sites, clinical changes in the baby and support for the family will challenge nursing and medical skills.

Parents

Sensitive, supportive care of the parents of a baby who reaches this critical state is essential. Every stage of the disease and treatment will be discussed and the expectations of the outcome realistically given. Ideally parents should be staying in hospital accommodation or living nearby so that they can arrive quickly if there is a major change. Some parents wish to stay at the incubator continuously, realising the short time they may have with their baby. They will get tired and stressed and need to be encouraged to leave for a break, if only for a few hours to have a meal and a bath. This often refreshes them to a small degree and enables them to cope more adequately. Sometimes mothers will ask if they should give up expressing milk for their baby at this stage when there is the likelihood of dying. Psychologically it is probably beneficial for the mother to continue expressing. There may be some hostility at this stage if the parents think their baby has suffered enough or that too many interventions are being made when the baby is so ill.

There will also be parents who will visit infrequently and not appear to realise how sick their baby is. They may have shut off their emotions to protect themselves or be afraid to commit themselves to the baby in case of a poor outcome. The nurse can do little except make sure they know everything about the baby's illness and the likely outcome.

Parents can be asked if they wish to have an appropriate religious ceremony at this stage. This often upsets parents as they think they are being told their baby is going to die. For those parents who appear to have shut off their emotions, this request sometimes provokes an emotional crisis as realisation occurs to them. This may have a devastating effect as they now have faced the reality of their situation and the services of a counsellor may be needed to help them cope. A short appropriate ceremony can be arranged at the cotside if wished, with the family religious advisor or hospital chaplain and members of the baby's family in attendance.

Many parents at this stage may be sinking into a quicksand of emotion. Relationships within the family are put under great pressure. Normal difficulties in the extended family can become magnified. Parents may

loose their ability to solve simple problems or carry on normally with their daily lives (Orford 1996). Parents of a critically ill baby often need the help of a trained counsellor who will support them and allow them to talk through their feelings and grief. Some units have such a counsellor but all will be able to refer parents on if they wish. Nurses will continue to offer supportive help, encouraging parents to help make the baby comfortable, encouraging them to write down how they feel in a daily diary if this appeals to them.

Sequelae

Disseminated intravascular coagulation needs to be recognised early in babies who are likely candidates, as survival rates improve with early diagnosis and aggressive treatment. There is a high mortality rate of 50–80% in sick babies (Emery 1992). Some babies have an intercranial haemorrhage or thrombosis in the brain vessels which leads to convulsions and an adverse neurological outcome.

ADVERSE NEUROLOGICAL OUTCOME

Sometimes in spite of all the care and technology a baby will sustain a severe cerebral catastrophe that will either cause death or serious neurological impairment. If a major cerebral event occurs it is possible that death will ensue shortly whatever measures are taken. If the baby has a cerebral haemorrhage or thrombus, the neurological damage is assessed by neurologists and paediatricians. If the outcome is judged to be so poor as to encompass no reasonable quality of life for the baby, then treatment will be discontinued.

Causes

Clots from disseminating intravascular coagulation may block a major vessel in the brain causing irreversible damage such as brain necrosis. There may have been a periventricular haemorrhage soon after birth which has recurred or worsened. Cerebral oedema and hypoxia from severe birth asphyxia may have caused irreversible damage. Meningitis, hypoglycaemia or severe metabolic disease can also cause a baby to have severe neurological damage.

Symptoms

The baby may have fits involving twitching of some or all limbs, cycling movements, yawning, sneezing. There may be arching of the body, apnoea and cyanosis during the seizures. The fontanelle may be bulging if there has been a haemorrhage or swelling of the brain.

Diagnosis

Blood will be taken for bacterial culture, electrolyte assessment and white cell count. Ultrasound scanning may show blood in the ventricles if there has been a periventricular haemorrhage. Cystic changes may be seen owing to the re-absorption of blood into the brain matter causing periventricular leucomalacia. Necrotic areas may be shown on the scan.

A lumbar puncture may be done if meningitis is suspected as the cause of the symptoms. There may be frank blood in the cerebrospinal fluid if there has been an intercranial haemorrhage.

Treatment

Underlying causes such as hypoglycaemia and metabolic imbalance will be corrected. Intravenous phenobarbitone will be commenced and if this does not control the fits, intravenous paraldehyde is the next choice; then clonazepam, diazepam or phenytoin. It is possible that a baby may need two or more of these drugs to control the seizures. Once under control, they can cautiously be withdrawn. Usually phenobarbitone is continued for several days longer than the others as maintenance anticonvulsant therapy (Roberton 1993).

Nursing care of a baby with convulsions

The nurse is usually the first to observe 'odd' movements in the baby. Exact recording of events and their duration are helpful in diagnosing and treating the cause. During the convulsion, care should be taken that the baby does not choke or block the airway, if ventilated. Ideally oral feeds should be discontinued until the fitting is under control to prevent vomiting and inhalation. Hand bagging may be necessary during the seizures if there is a profound bradycardia or drop in oxygen saturations.

When anticonvulsant therapy is started, records of convulsions will continue to be kept to assess the efficacy of the drugs. Intravenous phenobarbitone should be given slowly to prevent cardiac or respiratory arrest. Paraldehyde can be given in a plastic giving set if the solution is very dilute otherwise it dissolves the tubing. It degrades with exposure to light so tubing and syringe must be covered with foil or opaque plastic and the solution changed every 6–8 hours. Severe burns result if it infiltrates the tissues and ideally it should not be given with other infusions so that the site can be closely observed.

Parents

They will be able to do very little for their baby at this stage as any touch may produce a fit. As the anticonvulsant therapy begins to work their baby will appear deeply uncon- scious and may have distortion of facial muscles. The likelihood of having a brain damaged child is a nightmare for parents and many fear they will not cope. They will go through many agonising emotions and may even ask for treatment to be discontinued. Ideally an experienced nurse who under- stands the emotions that these parents are going through should look after the baby. Parents at this stage may be frightened if there is an unfamiliar nurse looking after their baby in case the complicated treatment needed is misunderstood. There may be hos- tility if the parents feel that the unit was in some way to blame and they may vent their anger on staff.

DISCONTINUING TREATMENT

Issues about the continuation of treatment arise when the benefit of continuing life- prolonging measures becomes open to doubt. The criteria normally used for judging this are:

- If the condition is judged to be terminal so that death is inevitable.
- If there is so much neurological damage that the baby has no potential for future development (Doyal & Wisher 1994).

The neonatologist looking after the baby may decide that it is in the baby's best interest to discontinue treatment at this stage. The normal high standard of intensive care will be maintained until this decision is reached (Campbell & McHaffle1995).

Parents

Parents will be interviewed by the neonatol- ogist and the position carefully explained. They may be shocked at the finality of the situation even though they know how ill their baby is. The baby's nurse should be present at this talk to enable information to be relayed back later as parents are often so distressed that they may forget or misunderstand what has been said.

After explaining the situation a short time should be given for them to come to terms with their baby's death. This should not be too long once the decision that further treatment is futile has been made. It is immoral to continue to treat a severely impaired and suffering baby even in the interests of the parents' feelings (Doyal & Wisher 1994). No court will compel a doctor to give a neonate life-saving treatment against clinical judgement.

Parents may have expected this to happen or they may have clung to hope until the last minute. They will want to know what the next step is and will be told that all drugs and interventions such as mechanical ventilation will stop but pain relieving drugs will con- tinue. They can if they wish hold the baby, stay at the incubator during this time or take the baby into a private room. Requests for a short delay in discontinuing treatment, until an important family member or friend has been contacted, will be respected. The parents will have formed emotional relationships with the nurses who have looked after their baby during the struggle for survival and they will need their support during their baby's last moments. Parents and nurses will go through the sad process of death together so that both can say their farewells. (This subject is dealt with fully in Chapter 9.)

REFERENCES

Bernbaum J, Hoffman-Williamson M. (1991) *Primary Care of the Preterm Infant*. Mosby, St Louis.

Campbell AGM, McHaffle HE. (1995) Prolonging life and allowing death: infants. *Journal of Medical Ethics*, **21**, 339–344.

Crawford D, Morris M. (1994) *Neonatal Nursing*. Chapman and Hall, London.

Doyal L, Wisher D (1994). Towards guidelines for withholding and withdrawal of life prolonging treatment in neonatal medicine. *Archives of Disease in Childhood, Fetal and Neonatal Edition*, **70**, 66–70.

Engstrom JL, Kavanagh K, Meier PP, Boles E, *et al*. (1995) Reliability of in-bed weighing procedures for critically ill infants. *Neonatal Network*, **14** (5), 27–33.

Emery ML. (1992) Disseminated intravascular coagulation in the neonate. *Neonatal Network*, **11** (8), 5–13.

Fleming PJ, Speidel BD, Marlow N, Dunn PM. (1989) *A Neonatal Vade Mecum*, 2nd edn. Edward Arnold, London.

Flores MT. (1993) Understanding neonatal chest X-rays. *Neonatal Network*, **12** (8), 9–15.

Fox MD. (1992) Measurement of urine output volume. *Neonatal Network*, **11** (2), 11–18.

Haycock GB. (1993) Acute renal failure in the newborn infant. *Care of the Critically Ill*, **9** (6), 250–254.

Hutchison AJ, Gokal R, (1995) Peritoneal dialysis in the ICU. What is its role. *Care of the Critically Ill*, **11** (3), 111–113.

Kenner CA. (1992) Neonatal care. In: *Nurse's Clinical Guide*. pp. 265–297. Springhouse Corporation, Pennsylvania.

McHugh MI (1997) Acute Renal Failure. *Care of the Critically Ill*, **13** (2), 55–7.

Merenstein GB, Gardner SL. (1993) *Handbook of Neonatal Intensive Care*, 3rd edn., Mosby Year Book, St Louis.

Mitchell A. (1996) Persistent pulmonary hypertension of the newborn. *Journal of Neonatal Network*, **2** (3), 5–10.

Neonatal Association Working Party. (1994) Long stay neonatal care; a national survey. *Journal of Neonatal Nursing*, **1** (1), 19–22.

Orford T, (1996) Crisis and crisis intervention. Psychological support for parents whose children require neonatal intensive care. *Journal of Neonatal Nursing*, **2** (1), 11–13.

Paul KE. (1995) Recognition, stabilisation and early management of infants with critical heart disease. *Neonatal Network*, **14** (5), 13–20.

Roberton NRC, (1993) *A Manual of Neonatal Intensive Care*, 3rd edn. Edward Arnold, London.

Seaman SL. (1995) Renal physiology. *Neonatal Network*, **14** (5), 5–11.

Sparshot MM. (1996) The development of a clinical distress scale for ventilated newborn infants. *Journal of Neonatal Nursing*, **2** (2), 5–10.

Stapleton S, Wright J. (1992) Continuous arteriovenous hemofiltration. *Neonatal Network*, **11** (4), 12–25.

Torrance CR, Horns KM, East C. (1995) Accuracy and precision of neonatal electronic incubator scales. *Neonatal Network*, **14** (5), 35–39.

9

Nursing Management of a Dying Baby

LEARNING OUTCOMES

After reading and studying this chapter the reader will be able to:

○ Discuss the decision process leading to withdrawal of treatment.
○ List the babies that are likely to die.
○ Describe the care of the dying baby.
○ Identify practical steps to be undertaken after death.
○ Demonstrate an understanding of the grief process.
○ Discuss the support the family and staff need during and after the death.

THE DECISION TO WITHDRAW TREATMENT

A few decades ago in Western societies, severely malformed and very preterm babies frequently died as there was not the technology to keep them alive. Today neonatal intensive care units are able to help such babies but as the technology improves so ethical questions arise about the poor outcomes of some babies saved by the use of aggressive medical treatment. The medical profession has tried to set up criteria for the selection of those who will benefit from high-tech support. Decisions on the life or death of a baby are emotive, as well as being a sensitive legal matter and any such proposals must meet with ethical and legal requirements before being universally acceptable (Doyal & Wisher 1994).

There have been attempts to deal with this situation. Lorber, in 1972, proposed criteria for the treatment of infants born with spina bifida and hydrocephalus (Kuhse & Singer 1985). Nelligan, in 1979 (as cited in Whitelaw 1986), suggested guidelines for discontinuing treatment of severely asphyxiated babies. None of these suggestions were legally accepted.

In 1981 Dr Leonard Arthur was tried on a charge of attempted murder. He acted on the belief that non-treatment of a baby with Down's syndrome who had been rejected by his parents was justified (Raphael 1988). Since 1989 there have been a series of court cases that have substantially clarified the situation. Now there are a range of situations in which selective non-treatment can be said to be lawful.

Doyal & Wilsher (1994) offered proposals that they hope will lead to written guidelines for withholding and withdrawing treatment. These are based on a duty of care which states that aggressive technological treatment must be in the patient's best interest as judged by a competent body of medical opinion. These proposals when expertly and carefully thought out are within today's legal remit.

Considerations

When the decision about aggressive treatment is considered, the question is complicated and may be seen from different angles. Will the life saved be full of suffering, an intolerable life with frequent hospitalisations and surgery; or a life of a severely handicapped person which may seem to many as without meaning?

There may be great costs and hardships for the family which has to care for a handicapped baby. The burden on the family will be considered but is not the main issue, as it is the baby alone who must be considered.

The cost of saving any baby should not be considered as, ethically, this has no place in the decision to end a life. It may be argued that the treatment of extremely small babies is justified to increase scientific knowledge (Stewart 1990; Campbell & McHaffle 1995). In this case should the cost to society and the community in terms of institutional care then be considered (Schlomann 1992)?

Issues about the continuation of treatment arise when the benefit of continuing life-prolonging measures becomes open to doubt. The criteria normally used for this are when the baby's condition is judged to be terminal so that death is inevitable or if there is so much neurological damage that the baby has no potential for future development (Doyal & Wisher 1994).

The decision makers

Medical staff

The decision will finally be made after considering all the facts and what the best outcome can be. This will be done principally by the neonatologist looking after the baby, as he or she is the one answerable in law. The decision will usually be made in conjunction with other senior doctors of different specialities, who are concerned with the treatment of the baby.

Nursing staff

Neonatal nurses have the most contact with the babies and they get to know them in a way no other health care professional does. They put into practice decisions about treatments. They may even be asked to implement decisions with which they do not agree (Elizondo 1991). Clause 8 of the UKCC Code of Conduct (1992) states that in the exercise of professional accountability the nurse must report to an appropriate person at the earliest opportunity any conscientious objection relevant to professional practice. In law, however, there are only two areas in which nurses are allowed to refuse to take part; that of abortion and that of artificial procedures to achieve conception and pregnancy (UKCC 1992). In practice the general consensus of feeling among nursing staff is considered during the decision-making process.

Parents and family

Parents must be involved in the decision making. They need to be kept fully informed at every stage of their baby's illness and of the possibility of death. When the time comes they should not feel that they alone carry the whole burden of decision. They should be consulted and informed but not led in a patronising way to agree with a decision made by the medical staff without questions or discussion. Reasonable time, possibly a day or two, should be allowed for them to come to terms with their baby's death and there should be no unseemly rush to discontinue treatment until they are ready.

BABIES THAT DIE

When it is evident, before or shortly after birth, that a baby's condition is incompatible with life the parents will be told and they will have to face the miracle of birth and the tragedy of death in a short time (Orford 1996).

Often a baby may be resuscitated first and later found to have a lethal malformation. A baby born at the very early gestational age of 23 weeks may live for some days but often in spite of high-tech intervention cannot survive. Some babies will improve at first and later develop serious complications and die after a number of weeks or the decision may have to be made to discontinue treatment (La Pine *et al.* 1995).

A baby may have been in the unit for many weeks with a serious congenital problem. Despite aggressive intensive care, possibly frequent surgery and many interventions there is no progress and the baby continues to deteriorate. Often the suffering of such a baby is very difficult for staff and the family to bear.

The dying baby

When the baby is very sick the possibility of death must be explained to the parents. The nurse looking after the baby will get to know them well and help them to accept that the baby might die. If there is a unit counsellor they may wish for further help.

Parents may want a religious service for the baby, according to their faith. This can be carried out at the baby's cotside with the family present. Even if they have no particular wish an appropriate religious adviser or the hospital chaplain can be supportive. A ceremony can be a meaningful ritual, with nurses and relatives present and there will be a baptismal certificate or other symbol to add to mementoes of the baby's life. Parents may wish to bring in family and friends to see the baby at this stage so that they can say their farewells.

Family reactions

Even when parents are kept fully informed, they may be unable to take in and accept that their baby is dying. Denial and anger are common reactions. The anger is often directed at the medical and nursing staff for poor management or wrong treatment. A great deal of time and patience is required from staff to enable parents to air their feelings while maintaining honesty and support.

When the baby is very ill parents may withdraw from the infant to try to make the separation easier. This may never be expressed but is indicated by fewer visits and less contact with the baby (Orford 1996).

If it has been a twin pregnancy, where one twin dies, the parents are faced with a confusion of thoughts and feelings. The mother's nurturing commitment is needed for the surviving baby, delaying grief reactions for the other. It is important that parents have a tangible memory of both babies including photographs of them together. The surviving twin should be told when growing up, about the dead sibling. Even so survivor guilt and confusion of identity, which may affect personality development, is common (Lewis & Bryan 1988).

Grandparents experience grief and disappointment because their expectations of a full term, healthy grandchild have not been fulfilled. In addition they have the pain of seeing their own child suffer, and they feel helpless without being able to prevent the hurt. They may experience survivor guilt in wishing that they, not the baby might die. For the grandmother specially, uncompleted grief from an earlier bereavement such as stillbirth or neonatal death of a child of her own, for example, may surface (Borg & Lasker 1982).

Withdrawing treatment

Intensive care treatment will be maintained until the decision is made to discontinue treatment. When death is inevitable and the parents have discussed the discontinuation of their baby's treatment with medical staff, family and friends, a time may be decided to start withdrawing treatment.

Parents may wish to wait for a particular relative or friend to see the baby or may need more time before the actual death. This time should not be prolonged and is unethical if the baby is suffering. Parents may need this explained to them if there are too many delays. The nurse who is looking after the baby at this time should be one who knows the family, supporting the parents as much as they need.

Death

When the family is ready, invasive procedures are discontinued and the siting of cannulas and taking of blood specimens stopped. Unneeded equipment and tubing should be removed and the baby kept pain free with analgesic drugs as appropriate. If ventilation is discontinued the parents should be told of possible changes in appearance, for example the baby may appear cyanosed or pale.

The parents may wish to take the baby into a quiet room. It may be the first time they have held the baby and they may want family and friends around them. If they wish photographs to be taken this is usually arranged. The nurse will stay with the parents as appropriate to offer practical help, psychological support and answer questions, sharing the grief with the family (Henley & Kohner 1991). Other members of staff may wish to say goodbye and this helps the family and staff in the mourning process.

When death comes the parents may wish to wash or bath the baby and dress him or her in their own clothes. A Moses basket may be provided that they can put the baby in afterwards. They may wish to have hand and foot prints made and to collect a lock of hair. These mementoes will be treasured for many years and validate the memory of their baby as a person (Thomas 1996).

Staff should be aware of the needs of parents from different cultures, though it is best not to assume generalisations. The family should be asked what they wish to do. They may wish for prayers to be said before and after death and there may be rituals for washing and laying out, which are important to them. Others may require non-believers to wear gloves when touching the baby after death. The nurse looking after the family should be aware of whether some unit practices are offensive to those of another culture. When needed a mature adult interpreter should be used. The family may need extra help with the procedures after death (Firth 1993).

After the death

The parents must be allowed as much time as they wish with the baby, before and after the death. The doctor will confirm the death when advised by the nurse. When the parents leave, the baby will be labelled in accordance with hospital regulations and taken to the mortuary. If the parents express a wish to see the baby during the next few days this can usually be arranged with the pathologist. There may be a room, specially designated, in the mortuary where they can sit with their baby. Alternatively arrangements can be made for a room on the unit or the chapel to be used.

The procedures of registering the death will be explained and this should be backed up with written information. For some parents the making of funeral arrangements will be helpful as it assists them to accept their loss and start to deal with their grief. Others may be too distraught and need help from a hospital staff member, a social worker or a chaplain. It may be necessary to call in a grandparent of the baby to help. It must, however, be remembered that parents should not be deprived of tasks which can help them in their grief (Kenner 1992).

If the parents are to arrange the funeral they will need the baby's death certificate for the undertaker. Parents of babies who die in the late evening or night may not be able to obtain a death certificate until the next day. They may not wish to come back to the unit where their baby died and if this is the case arrangements should be made to see them elsewhere.

A follow-up appointment should be made for them to see the neonatologist or unit counsellor in a few weeks. Then they can discuss any aspects of their baby's death that they wish. If they have consented to a post-mortem they will be told the results at this meeting. The neonatologist will see how the family are progressing and assess their need for further counselling. Davies (1983) maintained that an unhurried interview with the doctor at this stage was therapeutic in itself.

The funeral

All major religions teach that there is some kind of continuity after death. Religions and their rituals help mourners to make sense of the loss and provide a framework for a process of mourning; allowing time to pass and time to let go. The ritual of the funeral has an important function (Jolly 1987; Dyregrov 1992). It helps to make the unreal real and gives the opportunity to say goodbye. It also offers others the chance to show support.

It is advisable that a funeral ceremony is held in which both parents can plan and participate if they wish, and if culturally acceptable. In the past, the funeral was often arranged in haste by the father, and the mother and siblings were left out and had no concrete memories. The plans for the funeral should be in accordance with the family's beliefs and customs and include concepts that hold a special meaning. This ritual also creates a closure, the baby's life completed, symbolised by the filling in of the grave or the completion of the ceremony (Firth 1993).

UNDERSTANDING THE GRIEVING PROCESS

Grief in adults

There are five stages of grief (Kubler-Ross 1969) which the bereaved person passes through: denial and isolation, anger, bargaining, depression and acceptance.

These stages manifest themselves in the initial numbness when death is acknowledged intellectually in an absence of appropriate feeling, the person may be as if in a dream. This is followed by a sense of disbelief, and often the pain of acute grief expresses itself in crying or shouting. There may be a searching for the dead person and anger at them for leaving. There may be anger with God, the professionals and themselves, in the form of guilt. Bargaining may occur at the same time as denial and shock, as an attempt to delay or prevent the loss. It usually takes place with 'whoever the parents think the supreme being to be' (Merenstein *et al.* 1993). The coming of depression marks a level of acceptance and an acknowledgment of the need to be sad. Eventually after weeks or months, adjustments to the loss usually leads to acceptance.

The stages may not necessarily be in the above order and the duration varies. Many parents experience disorganisation and physical ailments. There may be an inability to sleep or make decisions even to the point of being unable to meet their own or their children's needs (Orford 1996).

In the neonatal setting some grief expressions will already have occurred because of the loss of the healthy baby the family were expecting.

Grief in children

It is important that children are included in the preparation for death as well as birth. They should be told the facts, as even young children sense that something is wrong. If possible they should be taken to hospital to visit their baby and explanations should be given about the illness and possibility of death, in a manner appropriate to their age.

Dyregrov 1992 showed that grief affects children of different ages in relation to their cognitive development. Below the age of 5 years they do not understand that death is final and have concerns about the physical well being of the dead baby, worrying if the baby will be kept warm and fed. They do not understand that death happens to everyone. Euphemisms such as 'gone to sleep' should not be used, as the child may fear sleeping in case they might die too. It should be remembered that their thinking is magical and they may believe that their wishing caused the baby's death.

From the age of 5 to 10 years children gradually understand death as irreversible, though the thinking may still be magical, such as the dead person may see or hear. At this age they feel compassion for others and even try to console a grieving parent. They may understand that death is caused by outer or inner events such as an accident or illness. If they are given detailed and truthful explanations about the events around death they will be able to cope with the event. At this age too they may keep their grief to themselves and suppress their feelings.

From 10 years onwards through to adolescence, the concept of death becomes more abstract. There is an understanding of the long term consequences of death and that it could happen to them.

The most common immediate reactions of children of all ages are shock, disbelief, dismay and protest, apathy or resuming usual activities for a while. Further responses are anxiety, flashbacks, sleep problems, anger, guilt, regression, social isolation, fantasies and personality changes.

When a sibling dies the other children may lose parental attention, while guilt on behalf of the parents may reduce the usual discipline boundaries. The parents may be paralysed by their own distress leaving the children to cope alone or be over protective trying to make the children or child take the place of the dead sibling. The child may have felt jealous of the new baby and wished to get rid of it and will feel guilty for having caused the death. When a baby dies the other children are at the centre of tension in the family and are always affected.

Support for the bereaved

After the death of a baby, the mother's body continues to remind her of the pregnancy. She experiences the continuation of lactation and maybe painful perineal or abdominal stitches. Analgesics can be given but sedatives are not recommended as they only delay the pain of grief. The couple are often so distressed in their sorrow that communication is impaired (Alderson 1992) and fathers often cope by plunging themselves into their work (Forrest 1982). Western cultural conditioning often makes it difficult for men to talk about their grief, giving their partners and children the impression that they do not grieve.

The neonatal nurse who has worked with the family is in a unique position to help parents. She can inform them of the grief process and how it is expressed; encourage them to talk openly to each other and the children; let them know that it will take time to work through the feelings. Written material from support groups helps to reinforce this information. A referral to a support group may be appropriate (Appendix 1).

Community support staff such as mid-wives, health visitors and general practitioners should be informed as soon as possible so that they can offer help to the family.

The best form of support seems to be that offered by a parent support nurse, who has been trained in counselling. This nurse, who is ideally based on the neonatal unit, will keep in touch with the family by phone calls, letters and home visits over an extended period of time according to need (Orford 1996).

It is recognised that a new pregnancy is not advisable until the grieving process has been completed. It is better to wait at least 6 months before conceiving again (Forrest 1982). A new pregnancy deprives the mother of time and space for mourning and unresolved grief may carry on into the next generation (Bourne 1984).

Staff support

The death of a baby creates a heavy emotional burden on the nurses who care for the baby and family. It is important that staff members have their individual ways of relieving tension, such as relaxation techniques, hobbies, sports and holidays. Even more crucial is a general atmosphere of mutual support on the unit. Staff need to care for each other and to develop skills to listen empathetically and non-judgementally to colleagues.

A regular organised staff support group may meet on the unit regularly. Praise for work well done is often appropriate as well as an acknowledgement that the work is stressful. There should be an opportunity to air difficulties and to share feelings. Hopefully staff will feel safe enough to be open about their vulnerability and humanity and will give support as well as receive it. Teaching about how to cope more easily with the work may be included at these meetings (Marshall 1982).

A different kind of support group may meet

after certain incidents to share facts, air feelings and discuss the impact of the event on individual staff members. On some units interdisciplinary support groups have been set up, meeting regularly away from the unit. There is a trained counsellor in attendance and members relate on an equal basis (Wright 1991).

Conclusion

Nurses should reflect on the ethical issues involved in neonatal intensive care and keep themselves informed about the current ethical and legal debate so that they can be knowledgeably involved in decision making on the unit.

The utmost is done to ensure that the death of a baby is dealt with appropriately according to present knowledge of ideal care. The practice should be audited regularly and improvements implemented where necessary to ensure that the care given is suitable to individual needs.

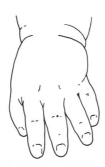

REFERENCES AND FURTHER READING

Adams M, Prince J. (1990) Care of the grieving parent with special reference to stillbirth. In: *Midwifery Practice. Postnatal Care*, (eds J. Alexander *et al.*). Macmillan Education, Basingstoke.

Alderson P. (1992) *Saying Goodbye to Your Baby*. SANDS (Stillbirth and Neonatal Death Society), London.

Bourne S, Lewis E. (1984) Pregnancy after stillbirth or neonatal death. *Lancet*, July 7, 31–33.

Borg S, Lasker J. (1982) *When Pregnancy Fails*. Routledge and Kegan Paul, London.

Campbell AGM, McHaffle HE. (1995) Prolonging life and allowing death: infants. *Journal of Medical Ethics*, **21**, 339–344.

Davies DP. (1983) Support after perinatal death: a study of support and counselling after perinatal bereavement. *British Medical Journal*, **286**, 286–287.

Doyal L, Wisher D. (1994). Towards guidelines for withholding and withdrawal of life prolonging treatment in neonatal medicine. *Archives of Disease in Childhood, Fetal and Neonatal Edition*, **70**, 66–70.

Dyregrov A. (1992) *Grief in Children, A Handbook for Adults*. Jessica Publications, London.

Elizondo AP. (1991) Nurse participation in ethical decision making in the neonatal intensive care unit. *Neonatal Network*, **10** (2), 55–58.

Firth S. (1993) Cross cultural perspectives on bereavement. In: *Death, Dying and Bereavement*. (eds D. Dickenson & M. Johnson), pp. 262–268.

Forrest GC. (1982) Support after perinatal death, a study of support and counselling after perinatal bereavement. *British Medical Journal*, **285**, 1475–1479.

Henley A, Kohner N. (1991) *Miscarriage, Stillbirth and Neonatal Death. Guidelines for Professionals*. SANDS (Stillbirth and Neonatal Death Society), London.

Jolly J. (1987) *Missed Beginnings*. Lisa Sainsbury Foundation and Austen Cornish Publishers, Great Britain.

Kenner CA. (1992) Neonatal care. In: *Nurse's Clinical Guide*, pp. 265–297. Springhouse Corporation, Pennsylvania.

Kubler-Ross E. (1969) *On Death and Dying*. Tavistock/Routledge, London.

Kuhse H, Singer P. (1985) *Should the Baby Live?* Oxford University Press, Oxford.

Lewis E, Bryan EM. (1988) Management of perinatal loss of a twin. *British Medical Journal*, **297**, 1321–1323.

Marshall K. (1982) *Coping with Caring for the Sick Newborns*. pp. 5–13, 31–43, 103–143. W.B. Saunders, London.

Merenstein GB, Gardner SL, Costello AJ. (1993) Grief and perinatal loss. In: *Handbook of Neonatal Care*. (eds G.B. Merenstein & S.L. Gardner) 3rd edn. pp. 531–562. Mosby Year Book, St Louis.

Murray L, Cooper PJ. (1991) Postnatal depression and infant development. *British Medical Journal*, **302**, 978–979.

Orford T. (1996) Psychological support for parents whose children require neonatal intensive care. *Journal of Neonatal Nursing*, **2** (1), 11–13.

La Pine TR, Jackson C, Bennett FC. (1995) Outcomes of infants of less than 800 gms at birth. *Paediatrics*, **95**, 479–483.

Raphael DD. (1988) Handicapped infants; medical ethics and the law. *Journal of Medical Ethics*, **14** (1), 5–10.

Schlomann P. (1992) Ethical considerations of aggressive care of very low birthweight infants. *Neonatal Network*, **11** (4), 31–35.

Stewart AJ. (1990) Dilemmas in neonatal units. *Professional Nurse*, **5** (6), 318–322.

Thomas J. (1996) When a baby dies. *Journal of Neonatal Nursing*, **2** (4), centre insert.

UKCC. (1992) *Code of Professional Conduct*. United Kingdom Central Council for Nursing, Midwifery and Health Visiting, London.

Whitelaw J. (1986) Death as an option in neonatal intensive care. *Lancet*, **i**, 328–331.

Wright B. (1991) *Sudden Death; Intervention Skills for the Caring Professions*. Churchill Livingstone, Edinburgh.

Nutrition in the Neonatal Unit

10

LEARNING OUTCOMES

After reading this chapter and studying the contents the reader will be able to:

○ Discuss the importance of adequate nutrition for small babies.
○ List the nutrients essential for complete intravenous feeding.
○ Describe the methods of giving intravenous fluid, the complications and care of a patient receiving it.
○ Demonstrate the ability to calculate daily fluid requirements.
○ Identify different methods of giving enteral feeds.
○ Discuss support for baby's family to establish breast or bottle feeding.

IMPORTANCE OF NUTRITION

The provision of adequate nutrition plays an important part in the successful management of sick and low birth weight infants. Early attention to meeting the needs of basal energy and growth requirements has been shown to maximise potential for development for babies in neonatal units (Van Beek *et al.* 1995). The maturation of all the organs is improved by the optimum intake of energy.

In the third trimester of pregnancy the fetus triples its body weight so that babies born before this time will have depleted nutritional reserves (Morgan 1992). It is thus obvious that low birth weight infants have more nutritional requirements than full term infants, because they have less body fat and need more energy for growth (Davies *et al.* 1996).

Adequate growth

Energy is essential for basic functional requirements and maturation of the brain and other organs as well as for growth (Morley 1994; Van Beek *et al.* 1995). The principle of good nutrition is to provide energy and other nutrients to match the growth rate of the age-matched unborn fetus. This growth rate in the last trimester of pregnancy is 14–17 g a day

(Crawford & Morris 1994) and to maintain this it is estimated that the preterm baby will need 420–500 kJ (100–120 kcal) per kilogram a day (Dear 1992).

Method of feeding

Wherever possible the new baby is enterally fed with breast milk from the mother. Breast milk contains immunoglobulins which help mature the baby's immune response, it is easily digested and contains 270–300 kJ (65–70 kcal) per 100 ml which can be supplemented with extra energy in the form of glucose if weight gain is poor.

If the baby is sick and/or very small enteral feeds may not be tolerated because of immaturity of the gastrointestinal tract or the illness. Development of parenteral (intravenous) nutrition solutions has meant that such babies can survive and grow adequately on a carefully worked out regime. The improved survival rate of the very low birth weight babies owes much to the provision of appropriate intravenous nutrition.

INTRAVENOUS NUTRITION

Total parenteral nutrition is the provision of all nutritional requirements by the intravenous route. In 1944 Helfrick and Abelson first reported the possibility of using intravenous nutrition for infants but because of the lack of technology and expertise the idea was not developed. In 1960 total parenteral nutrition was reported as being solely responsible for the growth and development of a sick infant in America (Krollman *et al.* 1994). Since that time research has produced a regimen of carbohydrates, fats and vital elements which

can now be tailored to suit the requirements of each baby.

The fluid cannot be purchased in the complete form needed on the neonatal unit and has to be made to order by the pharmacy. It is made up in aseptic conditions in laminar flow cabinets or isolators by trained pharmacy staff. Great care is taken in the preparation and accuracy of the prescription. The provision of total parenteral fluid is expensive and time consuming and not available in every hospital.

Indications for parenteral nutrition

Parenteral nutrition is given for a variety of reasons in the neonatal unit:

- Babies of extreme prematurity and/or very low birth weight have immature gut function leading to intolerance of milk feeds and poor weight gain.
- Sick babies who are ventilated, receiving paralysing agents and sedation will have poor gut motility from the drugs and illness.
- Babies whose gut is being rested to treat necrotising enterocolitis.
- Babies with intestinal defects such as malrotation, midgut volvulus, intestinal atresias, complicated meconium ileus, gastroschisis and omphalocele.
- Babies with conditions requiring neonatal surgery such as tracheo-oesophageal fistula or diaphragmatic hernia before surgery.
- Babies who have had large amounts of bowel removed because of intestinal disease may need parenteral nutrition for many months maybe years, until their gut is able to digest enteral feeds (Wise 1992).

Calculating parenteral nutritional requirements

Requirements are calculated on the baby's weight and age in days. The maximum energy level for growth is reached gradually over a number of days as glucose, fat and protein content is increased and the baby's system tolerates it. The aim is to achieve the optimum energy intake at day eight of the baby's life.

Energy requirements

The baby will need 420–500 kJ (100–120 kcal) a day in order to grow. This energy initially comes from glucose; for example, 12.5% glucose will give 210 kJ (50 kcal) per 100 ml, and 20% glucose will give 340 kJ (80 kcal) per 100 ml.

Fat requirements

Fats are an important source of energy and an essential component of all tissue. Loss of dietary fats causes fatty acid deficiency which results in calcium and vitamin malabsorption and lack of synthesis of long chain polyunsaturated fatty acids (LCPs), which influence the growth stimulating factor and retinal function in preterm babies (Koletzko *et al.* 1989). LCPs are normally deposited in the fetus in the last trimester of pregnancy so preterm babies are often born before building up any stores.

The fats are given in an emulsion, as lipids and come in 10% and 20% solutions. Lipid 20% has 80 kJ (20 kcal) in 10 ml and can contribute up to 50% of energy intake. Fats are poorly metabolised in preterm babies and can cause lipaemia or high cholesterol levels in the blood. They must be introduced gradually building up the amount over a few days as tolerated (Table 10.1)

There has been some controversy over the giving of fats to small babies. It has been claimed that fat might be the cause of some babies developing pulmonary problems (Van Beek *et al.* 1995). There is thought to be a link with bronchopulmonary dysplasia and babies who are given fat emulsions when they have respiratory distress (Cooke 1991). At the time of writing there has been no conclusive proof of adverse effects and intravenous fats are commonly given to babies in neonatal units.

Fat metabolism is affected in the presence of sepsis, jaundice or respiratory distress, so is discontinued when these conditions prevail. For this reason the lipid infusion is often given as a separate solution so that if it has to be discontinued, the rest of the fluid prescribed is still usable.

Protein requirements

Protein is needed to achieve normal growth and the best growth results are obtained with a protein intake of 2.5–3.5 g per kilogram per day (Fleming *et al.* 1991). This is given in the form of nitrogen which is given as a solution. This solution mimics the pattern of amino acids found in cord blood and breast milk. Protein is introduced gradually from day three and increased reaching the maximum at day eight to reduce the risk of aminoaciduria and hyperaminoacidaemia (Table 10.1).

Electrolytes and trace elements

Daily blood assessment of sodium, potassium, nitrogen and urea levels is needed for all babies receiving total parenteral nutrition. Trace elements will include phosphorus, iron, magnesium, zinc, manganese, copper, iodine. These help to keep body electrolytes stable and encourage the absorption of nutrients for optimum bone and skin growth.

Vitamin supplements

Babies need fat-soluble and water-soluble vitamins in equal amounts to prevent deficiencies. Vitamins A, D, E, K, B_1, B_6 and C are given as standard practice in parenteral nutrition.

Fluid balance

To maintain normal body fluid composition a number of factors need to be taken into account:

- Insensible losses from sweating, overhead heaters and phototherapy.
- Ongoing losses, i.e. from large aspirates or diarrhoea or from exudating lesions such as open spina bifida, gastroschisis or exomphalos.
- Urinary output.
- Necessary fluid restrictions such as in renal

failure, heart failure, birth asphyxia or patent ductus arteriosus.

Calculating fluid requirements

The amount of fluid given will be calculated on weight, number of days of age and any fluid restrictions required (Table 10.1).

The age of the baby
Most units will have a fluid protocol for the TPN regime (Table 10.1).

Intravenous feeding commences with 90 ml per kilogram per day of 10% dextrose with added electrolytes, for babies under 1.5 kg, within the first hour after birth. Fluids are increased on a daily basis until preterm infants after day 8 receive 180–200 ml per kilogram. This is the maximum amount to which the fluid is increased. Further increases are made as the baby gains weight.

Medical status of the baby
In the presence of such conditions as patent ductus arteriosus, pulmonary oedema,

Table 10.1 Intravenous feeding guidelines for the neonatal unit. (Printed with kind permission of Dr Mark Drayton, Neonatologist, University Hospital of Wales.)

	Total daily fluid intake ml/kg per 24 h		Nitrogen (g)	Intralipid 20% (ml)
Day	Weight < 1.5 kg	Weight > 1.5 kg		
1	90	60		
2	110	90		
3	130	110	0.06	
4	150	140	0.12	2.5
5	170	150	0.18	5.0
6	180	160	0.24	7.5
7	190	170	0.30	10.0
8	200	180	0.30	12.5
9	200	180	0.30	15.0

congestive cardiac failure or renal failure, fluids may have to be restricted to prevent lung damage from fluid stasis. If the baby is asphyxiated at birth or at risk of cerebral oedema, fluid is restricted.

During the use of phototherapy lamps for the treatment of jaundice, many units increase the amount of fluid given. There is no documented evidence that this fluid loss needs replacing but there is a need for additional energy requirements to achieve and maintain enzyme activity for the degeneration of the bilirubin (Edwards 1995). Fleming 1991 advocates 1 ml per kilogram per hour increase in fluid, other authors advise an increase of 25% to 30% of daily fluids (Blackburn 1995; Edwards 1995).

Untreated hypoglycaemia may lead to convulsions and neurological damage so that any baby with blood glucose levels of 2 mmol/l or below is at risk (Roberton 1993). If hypoglycaemia is a problem, intravenous fluid volume can be increased or the dextrose solutions strengthened if fluid restrictions are essential.

Administration of total parenteral nutrition

Total parenteral nutrition is administered intravenously. It can be given by peripheral venous line, central venous line or umbilical venous catheter.

Peripheral line

A peripheral line is not the most suitable way to give parenteral nutrition, as solutions have to be less concentrated and there is risk of chemical burns if tissue infiltration occurs. It is usually impossible to give enough energy for adequate growth using this method. Peripheral lines are used only where there is diffi-culty in siting a long line or if intravenous feeding is to be used for a relatively short time.

Administration

The line must be continuously monitored on a pressure pump as the fat and vitamin content in the fluid may cause deep 'burns' around the site if the fluid extravasates into the tissues. The strapping of the needle and the splinting of the limb should allow clear observation of the cannula site. These lines need frequent replacing as small veins cannot take the volume of fluid needed for long.

Whether the line is peripheral, central or arterial, the bag of parenteral solution and the lipid, if used, is changed daily. The bag label is checked with the doctor's prescription on the baby's chart. If there is extra sodium, potassium or any other additive in the solution, this should be re-affirmed with the doctor with the day's urea and electrolyte results.

The baby's armband is checked with the prescription to ensure the correct fluid is being given to the right baby. Two nurses should do this and both sign the chart when they have connected the fluid and checked that the infusion pump is set to deliver the prescribed amount.

Central venous line

The advantage of a central venous line is that the solution is delivered into the superior vena cava where it is rapidly diluted by the volume of blood, making the risk of damage to blood vessels minimal. Concentrated solutions can be given to ensure optimum growth and weight gain.

A limb does not have to be splinted as the silastic catheters used for cannulation are flexible and move with the patient without fear of being dislodged.

Complications of a central venous line

In spite of the advantages gained by the use of a central venous line, there are a number of major complications that can occur.

Infection
This could come from contamination at the time of insertion or when changing lines or solutions. Current infection rates vary from 6% to 20% and cause raised temperature, glycosuria, high white cell count (Reid & Frey 1992). As sites are so precious in babies on long term parenteral nutrition, infections in these cases are often treated with antibiotics given through the line.

Mechanical complications
These may occur from catheter malpositioning and may include, thromboembolism, pneumothorax, thrombophlebitis, hydrothorax.

Catheter occlusion
The catheter may become blocked with a blood clot, this can be treated by an injection of urokinase to dissolve the clot. Occlusion may also occur because of crystallisation in the line, possibly due to drugs given. In this case the line is removed.

Administration

The fluid should be given through a pressure pump and monitored carefully as for a peripheral infusion. The entry site should be inspected frequently to ensure it has stayed in position and that there is no reddening or swelling indicating thrombophlebitis. The baby should be monitored and observed for

any changes which may herald the onset of the complications listed.

Checks should be made when starting an infusion or changing the bags as for a peripheral line. When changing the fluid bags, syringes and giving sets, strict aseptic techniques should be used. Fluid bags are renewed each day. A bacterial filter may be used to protect the line from infection. In these cases the complete giving set only has to be changed every 3–4 days, the decreased infection risks being cost effective.

Umbilical catheter

The umbilical venous route is not the most common way of giving parenteral nutrition because of the risk of necrotising enterocolitis. It is, however, another route that can be used if necessary (Morgan 1992).

Complications
If the catheter falls out there is a risk of copious bleeding in a very short time. The baby should not be nursed prone as this prevents observation of the catheter entry site and could lead to unseen bleeding. There may be reddening and swelling of the abdomen around the site.

Administration

Umbilical venous fluids are administered in the same way as peripheral and central line fluids. Aseptic technique should be used when changing sets and bags.

Drug compatibility with parenteral fluid

When the baby is acutely ill there will be infusions of drugs running concurrently with the parenteral nutrition. Ideally the baby should have a second line for the administration of drugs but in practice this is not always possible.

Some drugs will react with the parenteral fluid and cause crystallisation and precipitate in the line causing blockage or emboli in the vein. Chemical instability or inactivation of the given drug can also be caused with drugs that do not mix well (Maguire 1994). Drug manufacturers' instructions usually contain advice on fluid compatibility and should always be read carefully. If there is any doubt, the hospital pharmacy must be consulted. Maintaining venous access is often critical and an understanding of fluid and drug incompatibilities is essential.

Complications of parenteral feeding

In spite of the advances made and the proven success with parenteral feeding there are complications which can occur from long term use.

Cholestatic jaundice

This is a heralded by a rise in the serum conjugated bilirubin concentration. It occurs as a result of intestinal stasis in babies who have had a prolonged period of parenteral feeding. A small volume of enteral feed should be given, wherever possible, to stimulate the production of gastrointestinal hormones which play a major role in gut development and improve the excretion of bile.

In this condition, the baby's skin turns slowly to a deep khaki colour which may take many months to clear. The long term outlook seems to be good though there is insufficient follow-up evidence to be certain (Dear 1992).

Catheter-related sepsis

Ideally the central line should be used only to supply parenteral nutrition to reduce the risk of sepsis caused by repeated infusion changes. Meticulous attention to asepsis when dealing with lines and bag changes helps prolong the life of the line. If infection is suspected in a precious line antibiotics, such as vancomycin, can be given through the line in an attempt to eradicate the infection.

Monitoring parenteral feeding

Clinical observations

Temperature, respiratory rate and heart rate should be recorded 4–6 hourly for the early detection of infection. Blood glucose should be assessed by glucose test strips 6–8 hourly to ensure there are no drastic rises or falls in blood sugar levels. Fluid intake and output must be recorded accurately.

Blood tests

Routine blood tests for making adjustments to the fluid content should include:

- Plasma electrolytes urea, glucose, creatinine, daily.
- Plasma calcium, magnesium, phosphate, bilirubin weekly.
- Full blood count and platelets weekly.

If lipid infusions are being used they should be stopped for 4 hours before blood tests to ensure the results are not adulterated by the fat in the blood (Kelnar *et al.* 1995).

Weight gain

The baby should be weighed twice weekly. A weight gain of 12 g per kilogram per day can be expected on parenteral nutrition, and there will be a greater gain as the baby recovers from any illness. Weight gain alone is not always a sign of good nutrition. Head circumference and length should be monitored to ensure that both are developing at the same rate, ensuring optimum bone growth. Many units use charts on which weight and head circumference are plotted on a graph. These are centile charts with lines showing average measurements for age and sex. The number of the centile predicts the percentage of children who are below a particular measurement at a given age. For example, the 10th centile means that 10% of the population are smaller and 90% bigger at that age. Children who are below the 3rd centile or above the 90th centile should be investigated for abnormal growth (McFerran 1996).

Calcium and phosphorus levels need to be assessed to prevent the development of rickets from poor calcium uptake. This is a common complication for very low birth weight babies because of poor solubility of calcium and phosphorus in parenteral fluids.

Transition from parenteral to enteral nutrition

Starting enteral feeding

Breast milk is the milk of first choice for any baby and babies in the neonatal unit are no exception. When the baby is first admitted the mother is asked to consider expressing her milk, which can be kept frozen if not needed immediately.

A small amount of breast milk is given to the baby as soon as possible to stimulate gut hormones that encourage gut maturity. This helps prevent gut stasis and necrotising enterocolitis (Morgan 1992). The milk is given as an hourly bolus or by continuous syringe pump depending on the amount the mother produces. If there is only a small amount of breast milk there will not be sufficient to prime the tubing and syringe set needed for continuous feeding. This amount will be increased 1 ml every 4–6 hours depending on tolerance as judged by stable respiratory rate, small aspirates, bowel action, lack of abdominal distension and stable blood sugars.

It may take many days, sometimes weeks if the baby has an intestinal problem, for the transition to be complete. There may be many stops and starts as the baby learns to digest the milk. The transition process is the same whether the baby is low birth weight, has had surgery or any other problem requiring neonatal intensive care. As oral fluids are increased, parenteral nutrition is reduced. Once the baby is receiving half enteral requirements, lipids are stopped as there is enough fat in the milk. Blood glucose must be monitored during the transition, as there may be a hypoglycaemic reaction if the parenteral fluid was rich in glucose.

ENTERAL FEEDING

Preterm babies 1000 g and over, who are well and have normal glucose levels, are usually given a milk feed within the first 2 hours of birth. The method of delivering milk feeds will depend on the size of the baby. If the baby is below 34 weeks gestation, nasogastric tube feeds are given initially, as the sucking reflex will not have fully developed. The mother will decide whether to express breast milk for this or use formula milk. If the baby is mature enough breast or bottle feeds can be commenced. Fluid requirements are worked out in the same way as for enteral feeds (Table 10.1).

Orogastric/naso gastric tube feeding

Babies born before 34 weeks gestation will have poorly developed sucking reflexes and so will need to be fed nasogastrically. Measurements are taken from the tip of the sternum to the bridge of the nose and across to the top of the ear. When the tube is passed through the nose to this length it will be in the stomach. It is imperative that the tube is proved to be in the stomach not in the lungs or curled in the throat, before any fluid is introduced.

A small amount of gastric fluid is withdrawn from the tube and tested with blue litmus paper for an acid reaction. If a sample is impossible to obtain and the baby's colour and breathing are satisfactory, making it obvious that the tube is not in the lungs, about 5 ml of air can be pushed into the tube while a stethoscope is held over the stomach to hear the crackle of air. The tube is then secured to the baby's cheek with transparent plastic dressing or hypoallergenic surgical tape.

The choice of orogastric or nasogastric tube will depend on the baby's clinical status. If there are respiratory problems or low flow oxygen is being given through nasal cannulae, the tube is generally passed through the mouth as babies are nose breathers and the airway is easily compromised. The orogastric tube is not as easy to secure as the nasal one and the baby can chew and suck on it displacing it from the stomach. The placement of the tube must be checked with litmus paper before each feed; the tube must be well secured and the baby should be asleep or quiet before the feed is given. The baby should not be left alone during a tube feed as milk inhalation or asphyxia could occur if the tube becomes displaced.

Transpyloric tube feeding

Some units pass a weighted tube into the jejunum so that a stage of digestion is bypassed. It is a method of introducing early milk feeds to low birth weight babies and in units familiar with the practice, complications are rare and weight gain is satisfactory (Uttley 1995). This type of feeding may mean that milk is not properly digested because the enzymes secreted by the stomach are not used and raised gut motility and diarrhoea may result. Gastric bleeding is a common complication. Tubes are difficult and time consuming to pass and require an X-ray to show the final position, so the baby is exposed to radiation.

Syringe pump feeding

Small babies do well on continuous feeds given with a syringe pump through a nasogastric or orogastric tube. They manage the slow delivery of the pumped feeds and do not have a stomach full of milk to cope with as when a bolus feed is given. The drawback with this method of feeding is bacterial contamination of the tubes and syringes used (Doolittle & Mills 1992). Scrupulous hygiene should be used when changing the syringes, which should be done at least 4-hourly. Research has shown that fats in the milk adhere to the sides of the tubing so that the baby is not getting the energy expected (Brennan-Behm *et al*. 1994). Minibore tubing has less total surface area for the fats to cling to but there is still high loss. Syringe pump feeding should be replaced by bolus feeds as soon as possible to counteract this loss of nutrients.

Position of baby

The position of the baby receiving continuous feeding can be important, for example, raising the head end of the incubator tray improves gastric emptying and thus prevents vomiting and reflux (Dellagrammaticas *et al.* 1991). Nursing the baby prone encourages gastric emptying (Ewer *et al.* 1994) but the baby should be returned to a lateral position an hour after the feed as the prone position has been implicated in cot death.

Three-hourly feeds

As the baby grows, hourly bolus tube feeds can be started. If there is an increase in oxygen requirements or vomiting, then syringe pump feeds are restarted. When the baby has coped with hourly feeds for a few days an increase to 2-hourly and later 3-hourly feeds can be made. Blood sugar levels must be monitored during all the transition stages to prevent hypoglycaemia.

Non-nutritive sucking

Research has shown that premature babies allowed non-nutritive sucking (a dummy) gained more weight than those who were not. This may be due to release of hormones and enzymes necessary for digestion (Pickler & Terrell 1994). Giving a dummy during a tube feed will help the baby to associate the action of sucking with the feeling of getting a full stomach, which may help to encourage sucking at a breast or bottle later. Non-nutritive sucking has also been shown to accelerate the maturation of the sucking reflex. This allows the earlier introduction of sucking feeds.

Establishing breast feeding

Expressing breast milk

Breast milk significantly reduces the risk of infection in low birth weight babies and reduces the incidence of necrotising enterocolitis (Lucas *et al.* 1994), possibly because of the immunoglobulins in the milk. Mothers of babies in the unit will be encouraged to express their milk, even if they do not intend to breast feed.

For successful expression a mother needs patient help and guidance, equipment will be available on the neonatal unit and ideally there will be a comfortable private room. Breast milk can be expressed by hand or by using a pump. There are several types available and the mother will be given a choice of the unit's methods of expressing so she can decide which suits her needs.

Expressing will ensure that lactation is established and maintained, until the baby is able to feed at the breast, as well as ensuring a supply for present use. Initially breast milk needs to be expressed six to eight times a day to establish lactation (Lang 1997). Once the baby is receiving the milk it may need to be done more frequently to keep up with the demand.

Mothers are usually encouraged to commence expressing as early as possible. There is, however, no evidence to suggest that this is vital. If no sucking occurs, prolactin levels will remain high enough during the first week for a substantial number of women to start expressing (Niefert & Seacot 1985). Some Asian women do not consider it appropriate to put their babies to the breast before the milk comes in on the third or fourth day after delivery but this appears to have little effect on their ability to breast feed if the feeding is then unrestricted (Inan & Garform 1989).

When the mother has been discharged home, if she wishes to carry on expressing, a breast pump and bottles will be supplied from the unit. Breast milk can be stored in a fridge at home for 24 hours or frozen for up to 3 months.

Starting sucking feeds

When the baby starts waking up for feeds, a breast or bottle feed can be offered. Before the baby is 34 weeks gestation the sucking reflexes have not properly developed and this should be explained to the mother to prevent inevitable disappointment. The baby may not be able to complete a feed at this stage but breast or bottle feeds should be offered once or twice a day to promote and strengthen sucking and to help mother–baby interaction. The unfinished feed will be given by nasogastric tube.

Breast feeding

The emotional and physical advantages conferred upon a baby who is breast fed have been well documented and are especially important when the baby is sick or preterm.

Breast milk has been shown to influence and improve later neurodevelopment. Breast fed children scored higher at psychomotor and mental development skills at 18 months than bottle fed babies (Lucas 1994). Many studies have shown the link between improved intelligence and breast feeding due to long chain polyunsaturated fatty acids (LCPs) found in breast milk which give improved vision, brain growth and cognitive development (Morley 1994; Van Beek *et al.* 1995).

Breast milk is more easily digested than the available artificial milks. Carbohydrate is in the form of lactose which promotes the growth of lactobacilli in the gut and helps to prevent gut infections.

Necrotising enterocolitis is a gut infection of unknown aetiology which occurs most commonly in the sick and preterm baby. This serious infection carries a high morbidity and is less common in breast fed babies. Breast milk contains antibodies which protect the baby from other infections, and allergies are less frequent.

Breast milk empties faster from the stomach than formula milk proving beneficial for preterm infants with vomiting problems due to delayed gastric emptying (Ewer *et al.* 1994).

Problems with breast feeding in the neonatal unit

Psychological problems

There are recognised difficulties in the neonatal unit concerning breast feeding (Nyqvist *et al.* 1994). Mothers who have watched helplessly during the acute stage of the baby's illness often find difficulty taking up the role of parent (Nyqvist *et al.* 1994). In many units most of the staff are not, these days, midwives but are often technically orientated people who may have no experience of breast feeding. In many units the nursery nurses support and advise breast feeding mothers and this works well; or the unit may have a family support sister who will help. Opportunities should be made for the baby to be put to the breast for skin-to-skin contact to improve the mother's morale and often her lactation.

Lack of privacy

Privacy and comfort are essential in establishing breast feeding, as noted in a 24 unit survey of breast feeding in neonatal units by Ingram *et al.* in 1994. Women who had been given enough privacy were three times more likely to be breast feeding their babies on discharge. Ideally there should be a room for mothers to breast feed their babies on or close to the unit so that they can be given help and support when needed but still retain their privacy.

Insufficient milk

Expressing over a long period can result in the

gradual suppression of milk (Inan & Garform 1989). This is often due to an unresponsive milk ejection reflex rather than milk production. The mother can be taught to gently massage her breasts to achieve milk ejection. Changing the way the milk is expressed may help, i.e. using a hand pump instead of an electric one for a short while.

Another factor inhibiting the milk ejection reflex is the prolonged anxiety and fatigue of having a baby in the neonatal unit (Jones 1995). At this stage careful counselling may reveal and alleviate such anxieties and will often determine success or failure of breast feeding. Putting the baby to the breast, even if the response is weak and nutritive sucking does not occur, will enhance the milk ejection response and improve the supply.

Weight gain

The baby should be weighed every 3 days, weighing more frequently than this is unnecessary unless there are medical reasons. A gain should be seen at each weighing.

Breast milk can be mixed with formula milk, if the mother cannot supply all her baby's needs, and given by tube or cup. If a small preterm baby does not gain adequate weight on the mother's milk, an energy additive such as eoprotin, a breast milk fortifier, can be added to expressed milk. This is usually added to 100 ml of milk giving an extra 47 kJ (11 kcal) in three scoops.

Giving breast feeds

The mother needs privacy for this and a helper who has plenty of time. If the breasts are full and hard they should be partially expressed before starting, to help the baby take the nipple more easily.

Before giving the feed the mother needs to be comfortable so that she can give full attention to feeding her baby. When feeding sitting up the mother should have her back straight and her lap almost flat. She may need a pillow or two on her lap to raise the baby to just below her breast level. The baby may be wrapped up at first with arms to the side so that he can be brought nearer the breast. The mother can then support the head with the opposite hand and guide the baby on to her nipple (Fisher 1995) (Fig. 10.1).

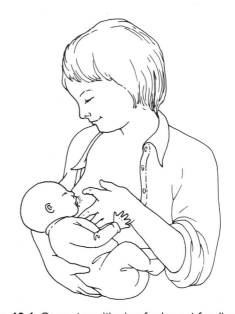

Fig. 10.1 Correct positioning for breast feeding.

Bottle fed babies take the teat and suck continuously. The breast feeding baby's pattern of feeding differs in that there are bursts of sucking followed by pauses then bouts of long deep sucking. The pauses get longer as the feed progresses especially for a preterm baby. Mothers will get to know this pattern and not worry if their baby does not suck at the breast the whole time.

As the baby becomes stronger and is taking all feeds by breast the mother needs help to see the baby as a normal neonate rather than one who needs nursing care. This is more easily achieved if there is a room the mother can stay in with her baby before going home. There she can begin the transition from regulated volume-controlled feeds to the unregulated feeding that is characteristic of the breast feeding baby.

Some mothers get disheartened when they see bottle fed babies going home earlier as they have put on more weight. Even after persevering this far some women may want to give up so that the baby can be discharged earlier. Pointing out the emotional and developmental advantages of a breast fed baby, as well as the financial advantages and convenience may help overcome these doubts.

When discharged home, mothers who are expressing milk or breastfeeding will need support from a range of people. The community midwife or health visitor can introduce her to the National Childbirth Trust or the La Leche League who will have breast feeding counsellors in her area. These support organisations can be contacted by the mother herself if she wishes. (See Appendix 1.)

The Department of Health in 1992 formed the National Breast Feeding Working Group to co-ordinate a programme of action to promote breast feeding. This group hopes to set up regional co-ordinators to 'stimulate initiatives at a local level' (Department of Health 1995a).

Bottle feeding

Bottle feeding is introduced in the same manner as breast feeds, initially one or two feeds a day being offered. The number of feeds is increased as the sucking reflex improves until all the feeds can be taken by bottle.

Small preterm babies who have needed parenteral nutrition or tube feeds are often difficult to bottle feed. They have poorly developed sucking reflexes, are sleepy and sometimes intolerant to handling. Mothers who have looked forward to feeding their small baby with the bottle are often disappointed and feel their skills are inadequate.

Preterm babies do not usually feed eagerly or wake up ready for their feeds. They are often sleepy and need to be kept awake during feeds. This is more easily achieved when bottle feeding starts if the baby is held on the mother's lap facing her. She can then hold the head and control the bottle with her other hand. The baby should not be rushed and if there is breathlessness or cyanosis a rest period must be allowed. It is often the poor feeding ability of the baby that prevents early discharge. Sometimes where it is apparent that the feeding problem will be long term the parents will learn to tube feed the baby ready for discharge.

Cup feeding

This is mainly used as an alternative method of feeding for preterm babies who are breast feeding. It is also useful for babies with cleft lip and palate and for those babies where sucking feeds are unsuccessful because of neurological conditions.

Cup feeding provides a positive oral experience for the baby and avoids the confusion of sucking techniques that may arise from breast feeding, bottle feeding and the use of dummies. This method does away with the need for oral and nasogastric tubes (Lang 1995).

Cup feeding is advantageous in that it stimulates the suck and swallow response and requires little energy expenditure on the part of the baby. There is no fat loss from the milk as there is from gastric tubes and the baby can be held close with eye contact. The stimulation of saliva aids the digestive process.

Method of giving cup feed

A 60 ml measure is ideal for cup feeding as long as the rim is not sharp. The baby should be wrapped to prevent knocking over the cup and sat upright. The measure should be half full and tipped so the milk is just reaching the mouth but not poured in. The rim of the cup is directed towards the corners of the upper lip and gums and rests gently on the lower lip. The cup should be left in position during the feed and not removed when the baby stops drinking. It is important to let the baby pace the intake (Lang 1995).

Formula milks

Low birth weight baby milks have made progress in the last 15 years and are now the formulae of choice for babies under 1800 g (4 lb) whose mothers are not going to breast feed. These feeds have an energy content in the region of 340 kJ (80 kcal) per 100 ml as opposed to ordinary formulae which have about 270 kJ (65 cals) per 100 ml. If the weight gain is poor on formula feeds, whether a premature baby milk or normal milk, energy can be added. Duocal or Maxijul add about 67 kJ (16 kcal) to each 100 ml of milk.

There is much interest in the development of milks with long chain polyunsaturated acids that are thought to promote brain and vision development (Koletzko *et al.* 1989) and many units are now using such formulae.

Advertising of formula milks in hospitals can be seen as endorsing them over breast milk so companies are careful to state that breast feeding is the best method. Recent legislation on advertising in the United Kingdom has overruled the World Health Organisation recommendations (WHO 1981) so as to comply with European Union Regulations. Such advertising is now regulated by 'The Infant Formula and Follow-on Formula Regulations.' (Department of Health 1995b). This recommends that information in advertising formula milks must be written in such a way as not to discourage breast feeding. Milk companies are allowed to promote their milks in hospitals for research and testing purposes and are thus able to give free samples and 'bounty packs' to mothers (Manders 1995). When deciding which milk is best for their baby, mothers may use one that is endorsed by bounty packs or milk used in the hospital. Research projects and equipment are often sponsored by milk companies in return for advertising concessions. The ethical considerations of accepting funding for research or equipment in return for advertising these milks is a difficult issue.

Choice of formula

Preterm formulas are stopped when the baby is 1800 g (4 lb) and normal baby milk is given. Most units will have their favourite formula milk and some give parents the choice. There is minimal difference between formula milks' constituents in spite of the bewildering variety of milks on the market. Most babies will thrive on the milk they are given.

Special dietary milks

Babies who have had bowel surgery, repair of gastroschisis or exomphalos may not tolerate breast or formula milk. In these cases a feed can be given which is free from lactose, galactose, sucrose and fructose such as Pregestimil and Prejomin. These formulas are well absorbed and are especially useful for malabsorption and short-bowel syndromes.

Vitamins and supplements

It is common practice to give all babies, whether breast or bottle fed, 0.3–0.6 ml of a multivitamin preparation a day from 1 month to 2 years of age. Most preparations contain vitamins A, C and D and some, such as Abidec, have vitamin B. Folic acid, which can promote growth and prevent megablastic anaemia, is given in powder form once a day for the first few months.

Poor mineralisation of bone, causing osteopenia and rickets of prematurity, is a common complication of low birth weight whether the baby is breast or bottle fed. This is because it is very difficult to duplicate the *in utero* levels of bone mineralisation in preterm infants. Calcium and phosphorus needed for bone formation are poorly soluble in milk and parenteral solutions so babies of less than 1500 g should have their plasma alkaline phosphatase monitored. Low levels of these minerals should be treated with alfacalcidol and calcium phosphate.

Iron

Full term babies have sufficient iron stores acquired *in utero* to last 4–6 months but babies born before term have low stores. The erythropoietin in the bone marrow of a full term baby is stimulated to produce red blood cells when the haemoglobin drops to about 11 g/dl but a preterm baby's bone marrow is often slow to respond even when the haemoglobin level falls. The rapid growth spurt of preterm babies also means a larger quantity of circulating blood and unless these babies are given iron supplements they develop anaemia during their second month. There is some evidence that iron deficiency anaemia may delay neurological development (Kelnar *et al.* 1995).

There is very little iron in breast milk and though it is added to formula milks there is insufficient to meet the needs of small babies. Iron in the form of drops, such as Niferex, is usually given twice daily from one month of age until the baby is weaned.

REFERENCES

Blackburn S. (1995) Hyperbilirubinaemia and neonatal jaundice. *Neonatal Network*, **14** (7), 15–25.

Brennan-Behm M, Carlson EG, Meier P, Engstrom J. (1994) Caloric loss from EBM during continuous gavage infusion. *Neonatal Network*, **13** (2), 27–32.

Cooke RWI. (1991) Factors associated with chronic lung diseases in preterm infants. *Archives of Disease in Childhood*, **66**, 776–779.

Crawford D, Morris M. (1994) *Neonatal Nursing*. Chapman and Hall, Bury St Edmunds.

Davies PSW, Clough H, Bishop NJ, *et al.* (1996) Total energy expenditure in small for gestational age infants. *Archives of Disease in Childhood, Fetal and Neonatal Edition*, **75**, 46–48.

Dear P. (1992) Total parenteral nutrition of the newborn. *Care of the Critically Ill*, **8** (6), 252–258.

Dellagrammaticas MD, Kapetanakis J, Papadimitreiou M, Kourakis G. (1991) Effect of body tilting on physiological functions in stable very low birthweight neonates. *Archives of Disease in Childhood*, **66**, 429–432.

Department of Health. (1995a) Minister announces establishment of regional breast feeding coordinators. *Department of Health Press Release 95/257*, May 1995. Department of Health, London.

Department of Health. (1995b) The infant Formula and Follow on regulations. *Statutory Instrument 1995 No 77*. HMSO, London.

Doolittle G, Mills M. (1992) Continuous drip feedings in the very low birth weight infant. *Neonatal Network*, **11** (3), 31–35.

Edwards S. (1995) Phototherapy and the neonate. *Journal of Neonatal Nursing*, **1** (5), 9–12.

Ewer AK, Durbin GM, Morgan MEI. (1994). Gastric emptying in preterm infants. *Archives of Diseases in Childhood, Fetal and Neonatal Edition*, **71** (1), 24–27.

Fisher C. (1995) Translating normal breastfeeding management into the neonatal unit. In: *Neonatal Nurses Year Book*, (ed. Neonatal Nurses Association), pp. 2.2–2.6. CMA Medical Data, Cambridge.

Fleming PJ, Speidel BD, Marlow N, Dunn PD. (1991) *A Neonatal Vade Mecum*, 2nd edn. Edward Arnold, London.

Inan S, Garform S. (1989) Establishing and maintaining breast feeding. In: *Effective Care in Pregnancy and Childhood*, (eds M. Enkin, M. Keirze, I. Chalmers), pp. 1359–1374. Oxford University Press, Oxford.

Ingram J, Redshaw M, Harris A. (1994) Breast-feeding in neonatal care. *British Journal of Midwifery*, **2** (6), 412–418.

Jones E. (1995) Strategies to promote preterm breastfeeding. *Modern Midwife* **5** (3), 8–11.

Kelnar CJH, Harvey D, Simpson C. (1995) *The Sick Newborn Baby*, 3rd edn. Baillière Tindall, London.

Koletzko B, Schmidt E, Bremer H, *et al.* (1989) Effects of dietary long chain polyunsaturated fatty acids on the essential fatty acid status of premature infants. *European Journal of Pediatrics*, **148**, 669–675.

Krollman B, Brock DA, Nader PM, *et al.* (1994) Neonatal transformation; thirty years. *Neonatal Network* **13** (6), 17–20.

Lang S. (1995) Alternative and supplementary methods of feeding. *Neonatal Nurses Year Book*, (ed. Neonatal Nurses Association), pp. 2.40–2.48. CMA Medical Data, Cambridge.

Lang S. (1997) *Breast Feeding Special Care Babies*. Baillière Tindall, London, 42–73.

Lucas A, Morley R, Cole TJ. (1994) A randomised multicentre study of human milk versus formula and later development in preterm infants. *Archives of Disease in Childhood*, Fetal and Neonatal Edition, **70** (2), 141–146.

Maguire D. (1994) Drug incompatibilities and infusion sites. *Neonatal Network*, **13** (4), 79–80.

McFerran TA. (1996) *A Dictionary of Nursing*, 2nd edn. Oxford University Press, Oxford.

Manders R. (1995) Advertising infant formula in the maternity area. *MIDIRS Midwifery Digest* **5** (3), 338–341.

Morgan JB. (1992) Nutrition of the very low birth-weight infant. *Care of the Critically Ill*, **8** (3), 122–124.

Morley R. (1994) Influence of early diet on outcome in preterm infants. *Acta Paediatrica Supplement*, **405**, 123–126.

Michie B. (1988) Total parenteral nutrition. *Nursing Times*, **84**, 35.

Niefert MR, Seacot JM. (1985) Contemporary breastfeeding management. *Clinical Perinatology*, **12**, 319–342.

Nyqvist KH, Sjoden PO, Ewaid U. (1994) Mothers' advice about facilitating breast feeding on a neonatal intensive care unit. *Journal of Human Lactation*, **10** (4), 237–243.

Pickler RH, Terrell BV. (1994) Non-nutritive sucking and necrotising enterocolitis. *Neonatal Network*, **13** (8), 15–18.

Reid S, Frey A. (1992) Techniques for administration of IV medications/parenteral fluids in NICU. *Neonatal Network*, **11** (6), 13–19.

Roberton NRC. (1993) *A Manual of Neonatal Intensive Care*, 3rd edn. Edward Arnold, London.

Uttley D. (1995) Transpyloric feeding. *Journal of Neonatal Nursing* **1** (3), 23–25.

Van Beek RHT, Carnelli VP, Sauer PJJ. (1995) Nutrition in the neonate. *Current Opinion in Paediatrics*, **7**, 146–151.

Wise BV. (1992) Neonatal short bowel syndrome. *Neonatal Network* **11** (7), 9–15.

World Health Organisation (1981) *International Code of Marketing Breast-milk Substitutes*. Article 3. WHO, Geneva.

11 | Infection in the New-born Baby

NEW-BORN BABIES' DEFENCE AGAINST INFECTION

New-born babies are particularly susceptible to infection because of the immaturity of their immune system and their vulnerability to infections acquired *in utero*. Admission to a neonatal unit adds to this increased risk by exposing the baby to nosocomial infections that abound in the unit from staff and the environment.

The body's normal defence against bacteria are the skin and the production of lymphocytes which give cellular and humoral immunity.

The skin

The full term baby's skin is made up of an outer layer, the epidermis, and an inner layer the dermis. The epidermis consists of up to five layers with the outermost being the stratum corneum. This is the major barrier of the skin and consists of flat dead cells filled with keratin, a protein, to form a waterproof layer.

During the second trimester of pregnancy the epidermis consists of peridermal cells providing a weak barrier. By 18 weeks gestation keratinisation begins and by 24 weeks gestation a thin poorly functioning stratum corneum has developed. It is not until 34 weeks gestation that the stratum corneum is well developed. If a baby is born before this time the skin will be very thin making it prone to damage and penetration by bacteria.

A baby's skin is colonised at birth by maternal non-pathogenic organisms and will remain so while being handled and cared for by the mother. Babies who are admitted to the neonatal unit will be colonised by the organisms there, which are often pathogenic and possibly harmful.

Lymphocyte production

Lymphocytes are white blood cells which contain immunoglobulins and antibodies to combat infection. The fetus is protected from infection by the maternal immune system and the barrier of the placenta and membranes while lymphocytes develop.

All babies at birth are susceptible to infection until their own immune systems have been matured by exposure to antigen-producing stimuli. Antigens are substances in the plasma which stimulate the production of antibodies in response to infection.

There are two types of immunity produced by the lymphocytes, cellular immunity and humoral immunity.

Cellular immunity

Cellular immunity comes from specialised lymphocyte cells which develop in the liver and bone marrow. B cell lymphocyte development commences at about 6–8 weeks in the fetal liver and cells are mature by 15 weeks. T cells develop from the thymus and are present in the blood at 14 weeks. After 28 weeks there is sufficient cellular immunity to enable the baby to produce some antigens in response to an infection. Immune reaction ability increases *in utero* with gestational age, so earlier preterm babies have a greater likelihood of postnatal infection.

Humoral immunity

This is the immunity gained from immunoglobulins (proteins produced by B cell lymphocytes) which give protection against bacteria and viruses. There are a number of immunoglobulins in plasma each giving protection against different types of bacteria.

Immunoglobulins

These are groups of structurally related proteins that act as antibodies. There are three immunoglobulins of importance to the newborn baby. They are:

- Immunoglobulin G – IgG
- Immunoglobulin M – IgM
- Immunoglobulin A – IgA

Immunoglobulin G
The only immunoglobulin a baby has at birth is immunoglobulin G which has been transported across the placenta. This immunoglobulin will carry specific antigens to diseases the mother has already encountered.

IgG crosses the placenta from the third month of pregnancy onwards so that the baby is able to make its own antibodies from the antigens it contains. When the baby is preterm there will have been less time to gain these passively acquired antibodies allowing vulnerability to postnatal infection. IgG gives protection from diseases such as tetanus, diphtheria, measles, rubella and mumps as well as common strains of streptococci, pneumococci and meningococci. This protection lasts for the first 3 months of life, after that the baby produces its own IgG.

Immunoglobulin M

Production starts slowly in the fetus at about 20 weeks but even by term the levels are low. IgM gives protection against Gram-negative bacterial infections but does not cross the placenta from the mother owing to its large molecular size. This leaves the baby at risk of Gram-negative infections such as *Escherichia coli* (*E. coli*). *E. coli* is a common pathogen which lives in the gut and normally does not cause problems but in the new-born it can give rise to serious infections.

Immunoglobulin A

Immunoglobulin A does not cross the placenta. It is, however, present in breast milk together with a protein called lactoferrin. These two substances act together to prevent gastroenteritis caused by *E. coli*. This makes breast milk intake important, especially for preterm babies, to help combat infection.

INFECTION RISKS AND PREVENTATIVE MEASURES

Prenatally

Though the fetus is protected by the amniotic membranes and the mother's immune system, the low level of natural immunity allows susceptibility to infections that can cross the placental barrier.

Viruses such as rubella, toxoplasmosis, herpes, cytomegalovirus are known to cause fetal abnormalities (Eltringham 1996). Other infections that may adversely affect the baby during pregnancy or at birth include tuberculosis, hepatitis, syphilis and human immunodeficiency virus. Infection of the mother

with varicella-zoster virus a few days before or after delivery can be associated with serious neonatal illness. Listeriosis transmitted from the mother can cause serious systemic infection in the baby.

Preventative measures

Once the mother contracts an infection, such as rubella, toxoplasmosis, cytomegalovirus or herpes, that affects the baby nothing can be done to avoid the damage to the fetus. Preventative measures concentrate on helping the mother to avoid contracting the disease. In the UK there is a programme to immunise young girls at puberty against rubella to reduce the risk of contracting the disease in pregnancy.

Prenatal education on infection risks should include any suspect foodstuffs to avoid (such as soft cheeses which have recently been thought to cause listeriosis, meningitis or septicaemia in the baby). Undercooked meat is implicated in toxoplasmosis infections.

Mothers need to know that toxoplasmosis can be transmitted by domestic pets especially cats (Eltringham 1996). Pregnant women should be advised to wear gloves when dealing with cat litter or gardening. Infection with toxoplasmosis sometimes causes severe intrauterine infection and where identified in pregnancy a termination can be offered. Screening for toxoplasmosis is impractical and expensive needing monthly blood samples to be effective, so is not recommended at present (Kelnar *et al.* 1995).

At delivery

If the mother has an infection in the uterus or vaginal area the baby may contract it (Lamont 1996). Premature rupture of membranes predisposes the fetus to infection from bacteria ascending through the vagina. This can result in septicaemia or congenital pneumonia and one of the causes of preterm labour is thought to be intrauterine infection (Lewis & Mercer 1995).

Maternal genital herpes can cause an infection in the baby which may develop into a fulminating and fatal disease (Kelnar *et al.* 1995). Gonococcal and chlamydial infections of the baby's eyes may occur if the mother is infected with this bacteria. Untreated this condition could cause impaired vision. Candidiasis can be acquired by the baby from the mother's vaginal infection resulting in a candida septicaemia or meningitis. Group B streptococcus acquired *in utero* or at delivery is now the most common cause of neonatal septicaemia and meningitis.

If instruments were used in the delivery there may be abrasions or bruising which could allow the entry of bacteria. Fetal distress before or at delivery is a risk factor for infection (Blumberg & Feldman 1996).

Preventive measures

Women in preterm labour are often given antibiotics, especially if there has been early rupture of the membranes, to prevent maternal and neonatal infection (Lewis & Mercer 1995). A multicentre trial is evaluating the effects of giving antibiotics to all women with premature rupture of membranes or in idiopathic preterm labour. ORACLE (The Overview of the Role of Antibiotics in Curtailing Labour and Early Delivery) is just ending a 3-year trial (Kenyon 1995). The results are not known at the time of writing.

If there is a known vaginal infection, such as herpes, it may be safer to deliver the baby by Caesarian section. The decision will depend on the obstetrician.

After birth

When the baby is admitted to the neonatal unit there is the risk of succumbing to nosocomial (hospital acquired) infections. The Department of Health's revised document on hospital infection control in March 1995 states that one in ten patients acquire this type of infection. It is estimated that 30% of these infections can be prevented with adherence to basic hygiene and aseptic techniques (MacQueen 1996).

A year-long study in one neonatal unit (Drews *et al.* 1995) indicated a rate of 44.4% rate of nosocomial infections in neonates under 1000 g and 10.1% infection rates among babies weighing more than 2500 g.

Nosocomial infections

Nosocomial infection rate could be said to be an indicator of neonatal unit performance as many cases can be avoided by preventative measures (Fowlie *et al.* 1996). Nosocomial infection must be reduced as it causes suffering to the patients, increased length of stay and the need for potentially toxic drugs for treatment. Potentials for nosocomial infection are:

The baby
The baby is a focus for colonisation of bacteria from the environment such as equipment, the hands of staff, or invasive procedures. Because of the low level of immunity at birth, especially if preterm, these bacteria will invade any vulnerable areas, such as abrasions, mucous membranes or the umbilical stump, especially if the vessels are cannulated, causing infections.

The practice of taking relatively large samples of blood for testing and then using packed cells rather than whole blood if the haemoglobin falls, reduces the antibodies in the baby's blood (MacQueen 1996).

Neonatal unit

The environment of the neonatal unit will contain many pathogenic organisms from the staff, equipment, the different diseases that have been treated there, residue from body fluids such as, blood plasma, wound exudate, urine, faeces, sputum, chest and wound drainage.

Inefficient hand washing by doctors' nurses and parents is the most common way infection is transferred from baby to baby. Infections from *Staphylococcus aureus*, Gram-negative and Gram-positive organisms can be traced to this source (MacQueen 1996).

In the unit there will be communal equipment which may be a source of infection. The incubator in which the baby is nursed is artificially warm, and may have humidity added, making a good breeding ground for infection. Shared equipment will include cardio-respiratory monitors, blood pressure machines, washing bowls and baths.

Liberal use of antibiotics in the treatment of infections may produce super bacteria which cause diseases resistant to the usual treatment. Lack of space may lead to crowding of cots in the unit.

Many neonatal units have multidisciplinary involvements, which means there are always large numbers of staff in and out of the unit. Open visiting too encourages many people to visit. They all bring in bacteria and other organisms to add to the soup.

Preventing nosocomial infection

Hospital infection control is an important part of the care of any patient. Prevention begins with educating staff and implementing policies to ensure infection risks are minimised.

Patients and their families are increasingly likely to take legal action if they think the hospital has been negligent.

The Royal College of Nursing has issued universal precautions for health care workers which should be used against all infection. These precautions cover general areas of risk such as the wearing of gloves, covering of broken skin, treatment of needlestick injury, hand washing, spillages of body fluids and safe removal of waste and safe handling of body fluids. These precautions, if followed adequately, will help reduce nosocomial infection.

Hand washing

Everyone is colonised with their own non-pathogenic bacteria so that there is an exchange of bacteria during any handling. The single most effective procedure for reducing this type of bacteria is hand washing. Hand washing must be efficient to be effective. Bacteria lurking in 'missed' areas around the base of the thumb and between the fingers are still dangerous even after the hands are washed. Units should be equipped with elbow taps and paper towels for careful drying as wet hands even when clean carry bacteria that multiply rapidly in damp skin. Chlorhexidine or an iodine based disinfectant can be used after washing to ensure greater cleanliness.

Gloves and aprons

Gloves reduce the transmission of organisms by up to two-thirds in some cases (Madge *et al*. 1992). Plastic aprons are now accepted as cost effective and efficient barriers to prevent contamination of uniforms as cotton gowns allow organisms through especially when wet (MacQueen 1996).

Decontamination of shared equipment

Careful decontamination of used equipment

helps control hospital acquired infection. Disinfectants and antiseptics normally used to clean contaminated equipment, cots and incubators should not be used in nurseries as the danger of inhalation and skin absorption has been found to cause hyperbilirubinaemia in neonates (MacQueen 1996). Washing with hot water and detergent and careful drying will help prevent cross infection. Some manufacturers have their own recommendations about cleaning their equipment and these should be followed.

Equipment such as stethoscopes are known to be a source of transmission of *Staphylococcus* (Wright *et al.* 1995). Methicillin-resistant *Staphylococcus aureus* (MRSA) can be disseminated by the use of shared equipment so that items such as stethoscopes should be provided for each baby and decontaminated when the baby is discharged.

Laryngoscopes must be carefully cleaned to prevent dried secretions on the blade and in the groove being a source of contamination. Decontamination with an alcohol swab after examination of each baby has been shown to be an efficient cleanser.

Unit size

If the unit is small and overcrowded there is little that can be done other than excluding all those who do not need to be there. Visitors and staff should not be allowed in the unit if they have a respiratory infection or gastroenteritis.

Education of staff

Infection causes a high rate of neonatal morbidity and mortality so all measures should be taken to decrease the incidence of hospital acquired infection. Many hospitals have set up infection control teams. The aim is to have a link person with each ward who has up-to-date information on hospital bacteria and ways to control them. The link person can then educate staff on the implications and risk factors of nosocomial infections and how best to combat them.

NURSING CARE OF A BABY WITH AN INFECTION

Babies admitted to the neonatal unit who are at risk from any of the factors identified in Table 11.1 will be screened for infection, and intravenous antibiotics will be started as soon as blood for culture has been taken.

Table 11.1 Increased risk factors for early and late onset infections.

Early onset infection First 48 hours	Late onset infection From 48 to 72 hours
Preterm labour	Preterm delivery
Prolonged rupture of membranes	Meconium aspiration
Prolonged labour	Congenital malformations
Instrumental delivery	Intravenous lines
Fetal distress	Endotracheal tubes
Maternal infection	Cross infection
Foul smelling liquor	Respiratory distress

An infection in a baby in the first few hours of life may be very different from that in a premature baby who has spent several weeks in the intensive care unit.

Early onset infection

A baby who contracts an infection within the first 48 hours after birth will most likely have acquired this *in utero*. The baby may or may not be symptomatic at birth.

Late onset infection

All babies should be examined every day for signs of infection so that treatment can commence before serious deterioration occurs. Many of the signs of infection in babies mimic other neonatal problems such as respiratory distress.

Babies produce a wide range of symptoms in response to an infective illness (Table 11.2). These may begin with minor changes in vital signs and behaviour. There may be localised inflammations such as reddening or swelling, over a lesion or surgical wound. Babies with internal infections may have temperature instability, or subtle changes in colour, tone and activity. Feeds may be refused or not completed and there may be vomiting.

Respiratory symptoms include apnoea or increasing oxygen requirements. There may be gastrointestinal problems with distension, vomiting, diarrhoea or reduced bowel sounds. There may be rashes, jaundice petechiae, pustules or omphalitis. If untreated, any infection may become systemic with neurological involvement. A deterioration in general condition, which cannot be accounted for, needs to investigated for infection.

When to screen for infection

There is argument in some units over which babies to screen for infection at birth (Yoxall *et al.* 1996) because of use of resources and the overuse of antibiotics. The controversy arises if the baby is term, has had a difficult delivery or the mother has had prolonged rupture of membranes. Some units take blood cultures from babies whose mothers have shown signs of infection or who have had rupture of membranes for more than 24 hours.

Table 11.2 Signs of infection.

Early signs	Late signs
Temperature instability	Enlarged spleen
Pallor	Convulsions
Lethargy	Changes in consciousness
Irritability	Respiratory distress
Skin rashes	Abdominal distension
Jaundice	Bile stained, faecal vomiting
Absent bowel sounds	Apnoea, respiratory distress
Poor tolerance to handling	Bulging fontanelle
Tachypnoea	
Poor perfusion	

Antibiotics are then commenced, but will be stopped after 24 hours if the blood cultures are negative. The rationale for this is that though the risk of the baby being infected is small, in the region of 2%, the mortality rate is high for those who do get infected (Yoxall *et al.* 1996). The alternative is to identify early features of infection in these babies and treat appropriately.

Preterm and sick babies admitted to the neonatal unit with a history of being at risk from early onset factors identified in Table 11.1 will have blood cultures taken and antibiotics started. This is because of their lower immunity status and increased susceptibility to infection.

Infection screening

Infection screening is carried out to identify the illness, the bacteria causing it and the effective antibiotic for treatment. In order to do this specimens of the baby's blood, cerebrospinal fluid, sputum, urine and faeces are needed (Table 11.3). A chest X-ray and a full medical examination of the baby should be undertaken so that local signs of inflammation or bulging fontanelle are not missed.

Chest X-ray

A chest X-ray will reveal any pneumonic changes in the lungs, indicating infection.

Blood culture

This is standard procedure before starting antibiotics. Blood is taken from a vein and sent to the bacteriologist for culturing and assessment of organisms present. Normally the result will be known in 24 hours (Table 11.3).

It is important that the blood is taken in an aseptic manner to prevent contamination from the skin organisms of the taker. Gloves should always be worn when handling babies to help prevent contamination. Blood is taken from a freshly cannulated vein and immediately placed into culture bottles. Capillary heel stab samples are easily contaminated so are deemed unsuitable for culture. Blood can be taken from indwelling catheters but the results obtained may show colonisation contamination from the catheter.

Blood should also be sent for blood gas analysis and biochemical studies so that these can be acted on if abnormal.

Table 11.3 Pathology results showing infection.

Sample	Test	Result
Blood	Culture and virology	Growth of bacteria
	Full blood count	White cell count raised, platelets low and haemoglobin low
CSF	Microscopy	Bacteria and white cells seen
	Protein	Raised protein level
Urine	Microscopy	Bacteria and white cells seen
	Culture	Growth of bacteria

White blood cell count and differential blood count

The differential count measures the relative proportions of different leucocytes in the blood and assesses T cell numbers. White blood cell count is raised in infection and thrombocytopenia, a reduction in platelets, will also be found. C-reactive protein (CRP) is produced by the liver and is increased when bacteria set off a chain of inflammatory reactions. Raised levels of CRP have also been found in babies with tissue damage such as in necrotising enterocolitis and intestinal perforation (Yoxall *et al.* 1996).

Lumbar puncture

Babies who start antibiotics should first have had a cerebrospinal fluid (CSF) specimen taken in case of meningitis. Exceptions can be made for those at risk who commence antibiotics at birth and ventilated babies who develop a lung infection. Lumbar puncture should otherwise be carried out on all babies who have a raised temperature, with abnormal neurological symptoms or who are suspected of having meningitis (Hristeva *et al.* 1993). This is an invasive procedure that must be done with full aseptic precautions to avoid injuring the baby and introducing infection.

A lumbar puncture is usually done with the baby in the lateral position but can be done with the baby sitting upright. This position though better tolerated by the baby (Roberton 1993) is not easily carried out when the baby is ventilated or very sick because of the risk of extubation or compromising the airway.

For the procedure using the lateral position, the baby should be held firmly but carefully in the flexed position by the shoulders and buttocks. It is important to keep the neck straight so as not to obstruct the airway. The spine should be horizontal to cot or incubator.

The baby will be draped with sterile towels and the area swabbed. A spinal needle with stilette (22 G) is used and when the needle is in the correct position the stilette is removed and the needle gently rotated to check for the flow of CSF.

It is important to hold the baby still to avoid injury to the spinal cord. It is easier if a third person is ready with the specimen containers. These are usually three universal containers and a small container for CSF glucose assessment as this is often raised in meningitis. About 0.5–1 ml needs to be collected in each bottle. The flow may be bloody at first from needle entry but should clear after a few drops. If it does not clear it could mean that the needle is not in the correct space and needs to be withdrawn and another attempt made. It could also mean that the baby has had a haemorrhage into the cerebrospinal fluid from the brain.

No more than two tries should be made as overzealous attempts may cause damage to the spinal cord. A swab coated with collodion or spray plastic dressing can be put over the area when finished to prevent seepage of CSF. The baby should be nursed flat for 24 hours to prevent seepage of CSF.

Urine

A sterile urine specimen is sent for culture and microscopy. To ensure an uncontaminated specimen, the genital area should be cleaned carefully and dried thoroughly before the specimen bag is put on and urine should be emptied from the bag as soon as possible after voiding. If a specimen cannot be obtained this way a suprapubic tap may be necessary.

Suprapubic bladder tap

This procedure is done to obtain a sterile specimen of urine for culture in the laboratory. It should be done at least an hour after the last wet nappy to ensure that there is urine in the bladder.

The baby should be held firmly to immobilise legs and pelvis. The area is swabbed with an aqueous antiseptic solution, not a spirit based one as this penetrates and damages the skin. A 23 G needle and a 5 ml syringe are used. The needle should be put in just above the pubic symphysis at right angles to the skin and only advanced 2 cm ($\frac{3}{4}$ inch). After withdrawing the needle the puncture site should be covered with a small dressing. Babies find this procedure uncomfortable and will need comforting measures afterwards.

Chest aspirate

The invading bacteria in a chest infection can be diagnosed from endotracheal tube aspirate, which can be collected in a container attached to the suction tubing.

Swabs

Swabs can be taken of ear and throat for bacteriological investigation. Ear swabs have been found to give the most information on pathogens colonising the baby (Eastick *et al.* 1996). Swabs should be sent to the laboratory within 4 hours or kept in the refrigerator overnight if not urgent or if the laboratory is closed (Crawford & Morris 1994).

Treatment

This is often a matter of urgency when the baby is symptomatic. As soon as the infection screen is complete, antibiotics should be started. A combination of these is used from the start to give a broad cover.

When the results of the screening are obtained antibiotics may need to be changed if they do not affect the infecting organism. If the screen is negative, antibiotics will be stopped after 48 hours.

Some units give immunoglobulin therapy to low birth weight babies, or very sick babies to encourage their immune response. This is an expensive product and there have been reports of hepatitis C associated with commercially prepared immunoglobulin infusions (Fasano 1995).

Exchange transfusion is sometimes given for severe toxic shock, using fresh blood which contains immunoglobulins and coagulation factors. This procedure also washes out toxic metabolites (Fleming *et al.* 1991).

Management

A seriously ill infected baby will need full intensive care support with attention given to:

- Blood gas stabilisation
- Fluid and electrolyte balance
- Blood pressure stability
- Correction of anaemia

Parental reactions

Parents are always mystified as to how their baby contracted the infection in such a clean place as a hospital. Explanations about their baby's lack of immunity and vulnerability to organisms that would not harm others help them to understand this more fully. When the baby has been infected *in utero*, tactful information must be given to ensure the mother does not feel guilty or is blamed by the family for the baby's illness.

A diagnosis of pneumonia or meningitis

will have sinister connotations for parents and they will worry that there may be residual brain damage or that the baby will die. There is no reason why they cannot continue with nappy changes and mouth care, though the baby might not be well enough for cuddles or handling.

If the baby has a serious infection after being in the unit for some time the parents will naturally be devastated by the setback. Often the baby has improved after birth and the parents are beginning to relax, when infection strikes. The baby's illness, treatment and prognosis are discussed with them, and worries and questions are answered.

COMMON NEONATAL INFECTIONS

This chapter has looked in general at the reasons, risk factors and causes of neonatal infection. It is interesting to look specifically at the more common diseases that occur in neonatal units.

CONGENITAL INFECTIONS

These are teratogenic infections which cause mild symptoms in the pregnant woman but have a drastic effect on the unborn baby. A teratogen is anything capable of disrupting fetal growth and can include drugs, poisons, radiation, viral agents such as rubella and cytomegalovirus, and organisms such as toxoplasma.

Rubella

This is now rare in the UK as public awareness, through vaccination campaigns, has risen. Babies of mothers infected during the first few months of pregnancy have over 50% risk of heart defects, cataracts and sometimes mental retardation. Other common manifestations include bone lesions, diabetes mellitus and microcephaly. The earlier in pregnancy the mother has the infection, the greater the fetal damage will be. However, infection after 3–4 months gestation carries only a 2% risk of abnormalities, though deafness is sometimes found on follow-up. The rubella immunity status of all mothers is checked and immunisation offered after the baby is born if necessary.

The defects may not have been seen on routine scanning and the mother may not even remember or know if she had rubella when pregnant so the birth of a baby with the typical defects is devastating.

Diagnosis

Even though the mother may have had the infection many months ago the virus remains active and can be recovered from the throat and urine of the baby for many months. The baby may have pneumonia, myocarditis, anaemia, petechial haemorrhage or osteitis at birth. Diagnosis is made by blood and urine laboratory examination on suspected babies.

Treatment

As the virus is still active during the neonatal period, known or suspected cases must be barrier nursed and pregnant staff kept away. Ideally only those staff who are known to have rubella antibodies should care for the baby. When discharged home, parents should be advised of the possibility that the baby could be infectious for up to 3 months and in rare cases up to a year. They should warn any women of childbearing age who are in contact with the family of the risk.

There is no treatment for the disease but symptoms and defects will be treated and corrected as necessary.

Toxoplasmosis

This disease is caused by a parasite that normally lives in cats. Infestation occurs from cat faeces, contaminated foods or unwashed vegetables. Clinical manifestations in the baby include hydrocephalus or microcephaly, cerebral calcification, hepatitis, myocarditis, microphthalmia. The earlier the mother is infected during pregnancy the worse affected the baby will be at birth. Less than 5% of babies affected in the third trimester will have clinical signs at birth. The mother will usually not know that she has been infected by toxoplasmosis.

Diagnosis

This is made from finding the organism in blood and stool specimens in suspected cases.

Treatment

Babies who are suspected of having toxoplasmosis should be barrier nursed and pregnant staff kept away. Treatment consists of a combination of antiparasitic drugs normally taken for up to 12 months.

Cytomegalovirus (CMV)

This is the most common cause of congenital infection resulting in 120–180 symptomatic cases a year in England and Wales (Crawford & Morris 1994).

It is one of the herpes viruses and may be the result of a previous reactivated infection or a new infection. The mother will have had a mild flu-like illness or may not even have felt unwell. The baby will present with a severe generalised disease which includes haemolytic anaemia, thrombocytopenia, microcephaly, pneumonitis, cerebral calcification, chorioretinitis. Infection can occur any time during pregnancy and the baby can be infected during delivery if active maternal infection is present. In these cases the baby is likely to get CMV from the mother during close contact and breast feeding. The virus can also be transmitted through blood transfusions.

Diagnosis

This is made from blood or urine cultures as the disease is still active at birth.

Treatment

The baby may be very ill and need intensive care support. There is no specific drug for this infection but the symptoms and defects are treated. The virus is excreted in the urine and is potentially infective to health care staff, especially if pregnant. The baby should be barrier nursed.

Herpes

There are two strains of this virus. The herpes simplex virus HSV-1 which causes cold sores usually around the nose and mouth, and HSV-2 which causes genital sores. Both occur as a primary infection in adults in which the lesions heal but the virus lies dormant in the cells of the central nervous system. They can be reactivated later to produce lesions.

Congenital herpes infection causes microcephaly or hydrocephaly, chorioretinitis of the eye and vesicular skin lesions. The baby can also be infected if the mother has genital herpes or contracts a primary infection just before labour. This infection has a later onset than other congenital infections the average time being 5 days and has three general patterns of disease. Localised mucosal infection with lesions which appear after 9–11 days usually resolves without adverse sequelae. Localised neurological infection presents later at 15–17 days with a meningitis type of illness and is more serious with a higher mortality and morbidity rate.

The disseminated type of infection causes a serious illness. Clinical manifestations include lethargy, irritability, poor feeding and vomiting which may appear 2–11 days after birth and escalate into a severe multisystem disease. There is a high mortality rate of 50–60% for the disseminated type and of those who survive one-third will have severe neurological defects (Jones 1996).

Diagnosis

The usual infection screening tests should be done. In addition it may be helpful to know the mother's history. If she did not have labial lesions at the time of the birth there may have been an influenza-like illness just before or during labour when a primary infection of herpes took place. The majority of cases of neonatal herpes occur in babies whose mothers were asymptomatic during pregnancy and who have never knowingly had herpes.

Treatment

If a woman has active labial lesions at the time of birth Caesarian section may be done to prevent infection. Aciclovir, an antiviral drug, is given to any baby at risk of a herpes infection. It should be continued for 14 days or until the possibility of infection can be excluded. The baby should be isolated until the antiviral treatment is complete.

Herpes simplex virus-1 causes cold sores

and is very common in adults. If standard infection control procedures are carried out there is no need to exclude staff with active oral lesions from work.

Hepatitis B

Congenital infection is rare. The risk of transmission to the baby occurs during the delivery of a mother who has been infected during pregnancy. The baby will rarely be ill at birth but will develop antibodies to the disease at about 2–3 months then proceed to chronic carrier status (Crawford & Morris 1994). There is a risk that the baby may later succumb to cirrhosis and/or carcinoma of the liver.

Diagnosis

This is made on the mother's history or if the baby becomes deeply jaundiced. Blood cultures will show the organism responsible.

Treatment

Babies whose mothers have the disease are treated at birth by active and passive immunisation, with boosters at 1 month and 6

Table 11.4 Common infective organisms found in the neonatal unit.

Group B streptococci
Escherichia coli
Haemophilus
Listeria
Streptococcus faecalis
Staphylococcus aureus
Pseudomonas
Klebsiella
Methicillin-resistant *Staphylococcus aureus* (MRSA)
Hepatitis B, C

months. Infection control measures to protect health care staff should prevail and specimens for pathology from these babies should be clearly marked on request forms.

SUPERFICIAL NEONATAL INFECTIONS

These are bacterial infections that occur where there is any point of entry for bacteria. If untreated these infections can escalate into systemic diseases.

Umbilical

Umbilical cord infections cause reddening of the area around the umbilicus which could lead to serious skin infection and generalised infection. When an infection occurs a swab should be taken and antibiotics given to prevent fulminating infection.

Skin

There may be infections of the skin over intravenous sites, catheter entry sites, chest drain sites, surgical wounds. The baby's skin should be inspected every few hours, at nappy change time, especially the areas likely to be infected, and red or swollen areas should be swabbed. If there are symptoms of infection, such as an unstable temperature, infection screening should be carried out.

Thrush

This could be acquired from the mother's vagina during birth and reinfection can occur from her during handling. It can also occur in bottle fed babies or as an opportunist infection in babies who are on broad-spectrum antibiotics.

Thrush presents as white plaques on the tongue or inside of the cheek which bleed when rubbed off. Candidal nappy rash of the perianal, vulval or scrotal area is common in these babies and may be distinguished from common nappy rash by the fact that it extends into the skin creases and has satellite areas around the rash. Nystatin or miconazole antifungal preparations are used. Oral preparations are given after feeds and topical cream applied after nappy changing and washing. The mother's nipples should also be treated if the baby is breast fed. Babies on antibiotic treatment should be given oral nystatin routinely to prevent this infection.

Candida septicaemia causes serious illness and is difficult to eradicate. Antifungal treatment with intravenous amphotericin infusions may need to be continued for weeks until the blood cultures are negative.

Eye infections

These cause a purulent discharge from the eye with swelling of the eyelid. Eye infections acquired during birth will present on the first or second day with both eyes usually affected. A swab will be sent and chloramphenicol or neomycin drops used to treat the eye. When treating the eye strict hygiene is necessary. To clean the eye before insertion of drops, gloves should be worn and sterile swabs dampened in saline should be used. Each swab should be used only once to prevent reinfection and both eyes cleaned together if necessary. When the eye area is clean the baby's eyelids should be held open while one drop of the chloramphenicol is instilled.

Chlamydia is a sexually transmitted disease which can cause conjunctivitis and pneumonia in the baby. Conjunctivitis usually presents after the third day of birth with a purulent discharge and should be treated vigorously to prevent corneal scarring. Conjunctival swabs should be taken in a smear preparation for direct microscopy as well as routine swabs (Roberton 1993). These swabs must be directly transported to the laboratory while the organisms are still live and for this reason swabs should not be taken out of laboratory opening hours. If chloramphenicol is used, subsequent cultures for suspected chlamydia are rendered valueless.

Treatment with tetracycline eye drops must continue for one month combined with a 2-week course of systemic erythromycin. Both parents should be investigated and treated when this disease is diagnosed.

Urinary tract infection

This usually presents with poor feeding, vomiting, lethargy, unstable temperature and sometimes jaundice. Infection screening may be undertaken if it is not clearly a urinary tract infection. A sterile urine specimen, obtained from a sterile specimen bag or a suprapubic aspiration, must be sent for testing.

Urinary tract infections can develop into septicaemia if unrecognised so antibiotic treatment is necessary. Ultrasound scans of the bladder may be done to see if there is an underlying cause or defect in the urinary tract.

SYSTEMIC NEONATAL INFECTIONS

Septicaemia

This can have a dramatic onset and can develop in babies of all gestations and ages in the neonatal period. The most common bacteria are group B streptococcus. These organisms are the most frequent cause of bacterial infection in the first few days of life and up to

0.3 per 1000 births are affected in Britain (Blumberg & Feldman 1996). It has a high mortality and morbidity rate.

The group B streptococcus primarily occurs in the gastrointestinal tract of the mother but the vagina is frequently colonised leading to infection of the baby especially if there has been early rupture of membranes, chorioamnionitis or placental abruption. The infection in the baby can occur as an acute disease 2–4 hours after delivery or up to 24 hours after birth.

Clinical presentation

The baby may be in poor condition at birth, but many appear well and collapse later. The most frequent presentation is of a baby who develops respiratory distress a few hours after birth, with tachypnoea, grunting and recession. This can be mistaken for heart disease, respiratory distress or persistent pulmonary hypertension and in severe cases occurring at birth, birth asphyxia. The disease is often indistinguishable from respiratory distress syndrome and 50% of cases do show signs of this disease on X-ray. Mistaken diagnosis may lead to delay in treatment.

Infection with group B streptococcus is characterised by a history of obstetric complications and symptoms of pleural effusion and respiratory difficulties.

Management

Septicaemia is a neonatal emergency that needs urgent and effective management. The baby will be very sick and full intensive care support is needed. Antibiotic therapy will commence immediately after a full infection screen. Penicillin is the most effective drug for this disease and is used in conjunction with gentamicin. These drugs should continue for 10 days if the cultures are positive and can be prolonged for 2–3 weeks if there is meningitis. Echocardiography may be carried out to eliminate cardiac problems.

Late onset disease can occur when the baby is 7 days old or more and it presents as a neurological syndrome at up to 3 months (Blumberg & Feldman 1996). General features of poor feeding, fever, impaired consciousness and sometimes irritability are seen, with neurological signs such as seizures, bulging fontanelle, extensor rigidity. Focal signs, such as one sided paralysis, are common.

Diagnosis of late onset disease is confirmed on lumbar puncture and blood culture. Treatment and management are the same as for early onset diseases. Care should be taken to detect and treat neurological problems such as hydrocephalus, ventriculitis or brain abscess. Mortality rate is 10%, with 30% of the survivors suffering mild to moderate neurological sequelae which will be severe in 20% (Blumberg & Feldman 1996).

Prevention

Research over the last decade has addressed the need for preventing early onset group B streptococcal infection (Mohle-Boetani *et al.* 1993; Van Oppen & Feldman 1993; Blumberg & Feldman 1996). It is now known that giving prophylactic antibiotics to women during labour can significantly reduce the number of babies contracting the disease (Blumberg & Feldman 1996). Giving antibiotics to pregnant women is a controversial issue and not universally acceptable. Hospitals should have a policy aimed at preventing the infection of babies with group B streptococcus which includes:

- Antibiotics given to women with risk factors such as preterm labour or history of early ruptured membranes.
- High vaginal swabs taken for rapid screening at the start of labour in women with a considered risk factor. Antibiotics are given to those women whose swabs are positive.

Meningitis

The most common causative organism for this disease is group B streptococcus followed by *E. coli* (Synnott *et al.* 1994). Other causative organisms include *Listeria monocytogenes*, pneumococci and staphylococci (Table 11.4). Though there have been improvements in the early detection and treatment of meningitis there has been little impact on the morbidity and long term neurological outlook of the disease.

Clinical presentation

The onset is often insidious with poor feeding, vomiting and drowsiness being the only signs. Convulsions are a late sign.

Treatment

If infection is suspected a full infection screen must be done immediately and antibiotics commenced before the result is known. Antibiotics such as amoxycillin and one of the cephalosporins such as cefuroxime or ceftazidime which cross the blood-brain barrier are necessary.

Prognosis

There is a mortality rate of 25% (Kelnar *et al.* 1995) for meningitis. Complications in the survivors include, learning difficulties, hydrocephalus and deafness.

Pneumonia

This may be due to a staphylococcus or a virus, as in respiratory syncytial virus which is a nosocomial infection endemic in neonatal and paediatric units at various times of the year. This can be spread easily by staff and needs careful infection control measures.

The disease may be caused by intrapartum infection or aspiration after birth owing to poorly developed swallowing and cough reflexes. It may be a complicating factor of a serious illness resulting from hypostasis, especially in paralysed babies.

Clinical presentation

The baby will have respiratory difficulties and increasing oxygen or ventilatory needs. Chest X-ray shows patches of consolidation and infection.

Treatment

Treatment is with oxygen, antibiotics and other supportive measures as needed.

Human immunodeficiency virus (HIV).

Human immunodeficiency virus is a complicated and fatal disease that affects the immune system and which has appeared in the last quarter of this century. After infection occurs there is a period when tests are negative and there may be a 10-year gap before the full-blown disease sets in.

Many people who have the virus, although seropositive, will remain well for some time but eventually their bodies will become unable to fight off illness. At this stage they are considered to have Acquired Immune Deficiency virus (AIDS) which leads to chronic diarrhoea, malnutrition, wasting, susceptibility to opportunist infections such as candida, toxoplasmosis, pneumocystis, cancer and finally death.

Babies whose mothers have HIV but not AIDS are not normally affected by the disease in the neonatal period. Babies of infected mothers may have the virus at birth and are at risk of getting the full-blown disease, though not all will develop it (European Collaborative Study 1994).

The mother's antibodies to HIV will have been passed to the baby, so HIV testing of neonates is impossible until the baby is old enough to produce his or her own antibodies. Because HIV can be passed on in blood and urine there are significant implications for medical and nursing staff who care for these babies.

HIV testing of the mother is controversial. Public anxiety is high because there is no cure and this has led to discrimination against HIV positive people. There is also some moral righteousness as HIV is most commonly contracted through promiscuous sex, homosexual contact or from shared needles during intravenous drug abuse.

Scaremongering about epidemics and stories of persecution of people with HIV have led to protection of HIV carriers, often to the detriment of health staff. Issues of confidentiality and counselling about who has the right to know, have led to a shroud of secrecy and health care staff are often left untold and unprotected.

A national study of HIV in pregnancy in the UK found that there have been confirmed reports of 737 cases from 1989 to 1994 with 168 children being infected by 1995 (AVERT 1995). In view of the small numbers of babies infected and the difficulty in making a definitive diagnosis, owing to the time lapse from infection date to the appearance of the antibodies in the blood, it would seem unnecessary to panic. Following universal precautions as laid down by the Royal College of Nursing will protect staff from most instances of HIV infection.

Antenatal testing

Studies of HIV transmission before birth suggest that babies born to mothers who have developed AIDS will be infected before birth. There is also some evidence to suggest that women who have developed an HIV-related illness are more likely than those who are symptomless, to pass on the infection to their children before birth (Abrams *et al.* 1995).

The results of antenatal testing are not always significant as after infection HIV takes up to 3 months to appear on screening (Mercey *et al.* 1993). The tests are expensive and have not been shown to be efficacious in preventing the disease because of the uncertainty factors (Dunn *et al.* 1995). If antenatal testing were to be brought in, a counselling service for families would be essential to cope with the distress caused when positive results are obtained. At the moment the best that can be offered those women who test positive, is a termination or treatment with zidovudine a drug known to help delay the development of HIV to full-blown AIDS.

Preventing mother to baby transmission

Babies can be infected *in utero* and it has been found that a preterm baby born to a mother with the disease is more likely to have a rapidly developing AIDS disease (Abrams *et al.* 1995). This may be due to the factors that caused the preterm birth, infection, drug abuse or poor nutrition.

The most dangerous time for an uninfected baby of an HIV positive mother is during the birth. The longer the baby is protected during labour from direct contact with the mother's blood and secretions the less the risk of contracting the HIV infection. Care must be taken to keep the perineum intact if possible, and the use of fetal scalp electrodes is not advisable. Instrumental deliveries must be done carefully to prevent abrasions to the scalp and vagina and the baby should be washed as soon as possible to prevent infection of the baby and others (Verkuyl 1995).

Caesarian section has not been conclusively shown to lower the incidence of transmission (Dunn *et al.* 1994). It does increase the risk of postoperative complications to the infected mother by increasing the risk of opportunist infection and is not justified as a routine procedure (Semprini *et al.* 1995).

Breast milk is known to contain the HIV virus and infected mothers are advised not to breast feed in the Western world where suitable alternatives are available (Evans *et al.* 1995). In developing countries where a clean water supply is not available, the risk of transmission does not justify the risk of bottle feeding.

There will inevitably be pregnant women who have HIV that is not revealed, possibly because they do not know themselves or do not wish to disclose it because of the stigma. Their infants are at greater risk as no preventative measures will have been taken to help them.

Admission to neonatal unit

A baby of a woman with known HIV will not be admitted to the neonatal unit unless treatment is needed. The time of onset of signs and symptoms of AIDS in babies varies widely from within days of delivery to 18 months.

The major symptom in most infants is a recurrent bacterial sepsis.

Some babies do develop the opportunistic infections seen in adults. The most frequently noted are cytomegalovirus (CMV), *Pneumocystis carinii* pneumonia, herpes virus, candida and Epstein–Barr virus (EBV). These diseases have been known to appear as early as 12 weeks (Evans *et al.* 1995). Many babies with AIDS are preterm or small for gestational age because their mothers may be drug abusers with poor nutrition. This puts them at risk of all the complications related to these conditions (Abrams *et al.* 1995).

Babies who are HIV positive require management that involves the whole family. Apart from their mothers, there may be other members of the family who are HIV positive and multidisciplinary teamwork is needed to care for the family.

REFERENCES

Abrams EJ, Matheson PB, Thomas PA, *et al.* (1995) Neonatal predictors of infection status and early death among 332 infants at risk of HIV infection monitored prospectively from birth. *Pediatrics* **96** (3), 451–458.

AVERT (1995) National Study of HIV in Pregnancy. Royal College of Obstetricians and Gynaecologists. *Newsletter* 23. AVERT, 11 Denne Parade, Horsham, West Sussex.

Blumberg RM, Feldman RG. (1996) Neonatal group B streptococcal infection. *Current Opinion in Pediatrics*, **6**, 34–37.

Crawford D, Morris M. (1994) *Neonatal Nursing.* Chapman and Hall, London.

Drews MB, Ludwig AC, Leitis JU, Daschner FD. (1995) Low birth weight and nosocomial infection of neonates in a neonatal intensive care unit. *Journal of Hospital Infection*, **30**, 65–72.

Dunn DT, Newall ML, Mayaux MJ, *et al.* (1994) Mode of delivery and vertical transmission of HIV a review of prospective studies. *Journal of Acquired Immune Deficiency Diseases*, **7** (10), 1064–1066.

Dunn DT, Nicoll A, Holland FJ, *et al.* (1995) How much pediatric HIV infection could be prevented by antenatal HIV testing. *Journal of Medical Screening*, **2** (1), 35–40.

Eastick K, Leeming JP, Bennett D, Millar MR. (1996) Reservoirs of coagulase negative staphylococcus in preterm neonates. *Archives of Diseases in Childhood, Fetal and Neonatal Edition*, **74**, 99–104.

Eltringham I. (1996) Toxoplasmosis: why it is not a problem. *Maternal and Child Health*, **21** (6), 150–152.

European Collaborative Study. (1994) Natural History of vertically acquired human immuno deficiency virus infection. Part 1. *Pediatrics*, **94**, 815–819.

Evans JA, Marriage SC, Walters MDS, *et al.* (1995) Unsuspected HIV infection in the first year of life. *British Medical Journal*, **310** (6989), 1235–1236.

Fasano MB. (1995) Risks and benefits of intravenous immunoglobulin treatment in children. *Current Pediatrics*, **7** (6), 688–692.

Fleming PJ, Speidel BD, Marlow N, Dunn PM. (1991) *A Neonatal Vade Mecum*, 2nd edn. Edward Arnold, London.

Fowlie PW, Gould CR, Parry GJ, Phillips G, *et al.* (1996) CRIB (clinical risk index for babies) in relation to nosocomial bacteremia in very low birthweight or preterm infants. *Archives of Disease in Childhood*, **75**, 49–52.

Hristeva L, Bowler I, Booy R, *et al.* (1993) Value of cerebrospinal fluid examination in the diagnosis of meningitis in the newborn. *Archives of Disease in Childhood*, **69**, 514–517.

Jones CL. (1996) Herpes simplex virus infection in the neonate. Clinical presentation and management. *Neonatal Network*, **15** (8), 11–17.

Kelnar CJH, Harvey D, Simpson C. (1995) *The Sick Newborn Baby*, 3rd edn. Baillière Tindall, London.

Kenyon S. (1995) Oracle – an overview of the evidence. *MIDIRS Midwifery Digest*, **5** (1), 14–16.

Lamont RF. (1996) Bacterial vaginosis and adverse pregnancy sequelae. *Maternal and Child Health*, **21** (6), 150–152.

Lewis R, Mercer B. (1995) Adjunctive care of pre-term labour – the use of antibiotics. *Clinical Obstetrics and Gynaecology*, **38** (4), 755–768.

MacQueen S. (1996) Germ invasion and risk analysis. *Journal of Neonatal Nursing*, **2** (1), 20–25.

Madge P, Paton JY, McColl JH, Mackie PLK. (1992) Prospective controlled study of four infection control procedures to prevent nosocomial infection with respiratory syncytial virus. *Lancet*, **340**, 1079–1083.

Mercey D, Bewlet S, Brocklehurst P. (1993) *A Guide to HIV Infection and Childbearing*. Avert, 11 Denne Parade, Horsham, West Sussex.

Mohle-Boetani JC, Schuchat A, Plikaytis BD. (1993) Comparison of prevention strategies for neonatal group B streptococcal infections. *Journal of American Medical Association*, **270**, 1442–1448.

Roberton NRC. (1993) *A Manual of Neonatal Intensive Care*, 3rd edn., Edward Arnold, London.

Semprini AE, Costagna C, Ravizza M, *et al.* (1995) The incidence of complications after Caesarian section in HIV positive women. *AIDS* **9** (8), 913–917.

Synnott MB, Morse D, Hall SM. (1994) Neonatal meningitis in England and Wales. A review of routine national data. *Archives of Disease in Childhood, Fetal and Neonatal Edition*, **71**, 75–80.

Van Oppen C, Feldman R. (1993) Antibiotic prophylaxis of neonatal group B streptococcal infections. *British Medical Journal*, **306**, 411–412 (Editorial).

Verkuyl DAA. (1995) Practising obstetrics and gynaecology in areas with a high prevalence of HIV infection. *Lancet*, **346**, 293–296.

Wright IMR, Orr H, Porter C. (1995) Stethoscope contamination in the neonatal intensive care unit. *Journal of Hospital Infection*, **29**, 65–68.

Yoxall CW, Isherwood DM, Weindling AM. (1996) The neonatal infection screen. *Current Opinion in Pediatrics*, **6**, 16–20.

12 | Nursing Management of the Jaundiced Baby

LEARNING OUTCOMES

After reading this chapter and studying the contents the reader will be able to:

○ Identify the causes of neonatal jaundice.
○ Describe the conjugation and excretion of bilirubin.
○ Demonstrate knowledge of the treatment of neonatal jaundice.
○ Discuss the criteria for phototherapy and exchange transfusion.
○ Discuss the help families need when their baby is jaundiced.

NEONATAL JAUNDICE

As many as 50% full term babies and 80% preterm babies suffer from hyperbilirubinaemia, high levels of bilirubin in the blood, which results in jaundice (Crawford & Morris 1994). In order to perceive the effect jaundice has on the body, it is important to understand the metabolic changes that produce bilirubin and the conjugation or breakdown process needed for its use and disposal.

Bilirubin

Bilirubin is a product of haemoglobin breakdown. Haemoglobin is contained in the red blood cells and its most important function is to carry oxygen to the tissues.

As a red blood cell reaches the end of its life it is taken out of circulation by the reticuloendothelial system, which consists of the liver and spleen. The haemoglobin in the cell is then broken down, by these organs, into its two constituents of haem and globin. The globin is a protein which is conserved and re-used by the body. The haem, an iron-containing compound, which cannot be re-used, is broken down so that it can be excreted. Bilirubin is a product of this last process and accumulation in the blood causes yellow staining on the skin, jaundice.

Metabolism

Metabolism of bilirubin takes place in the reticuloendothelial system. Initially unconjugated bilirubin is formed which is fat soluble and water insoluble so it cannot be excreted in the bile or urine, which are water based. Unconjugated bilirubin has a high affinity for fatty tissue and the brain, where it causes damage. This is prevented because the unconjugated (indirect) bilirubin is bound in a plasma protein, albumin, to be carried to the liver. This binding effectively prevents bilirubin leaving the blood and entering the brain.

When bilirubin enters the liver, two carrier proteins Y and Z help convert it, by a series of enzyme reactions requiring glucuronyl transferase, to conjugated (direct) bilirubin which is water soluble and harmless to the body tissues. It is then excreted through bile into the gut and thence into faeces and urine (Table 12.1).

Table 12.1 The conjugation and excretion of bilirubin.

HAEM
↓
UNCONJUGATED BILIRUBIN (indirect)
Transported to the liver in plasma bound to albumin.
There Y, Z and glucuronyl transferase enzymes convert it to
↓
CONJUGATED BILIRUBIN (direct)
Leaves the liver in bile, enters the gut from bile duct, leaves gut by faeces and the kidneys as urine

---

Bilirubin encephalopathy (kernicterus)

If there is a failure to maintain an equilibrium between production of bilirubin and its excretion, the albumin-binding capacity of the plasma is exceeded and bilirubin will enter the bloodstream. If this is untreated the bilirubin eventually crosses the blood–brain barrier causing staining of and damage to the basal ganglia. The condition known as kernicterus or bilirubin encephalopathy may then ensue.

In the early stages of the disease the baby is lethargic and hypotonic. Later there will be hypertonia and irritability with convulsions. Untreated the condition can be fatal or result in severe brain damage to the survivors. The condition was discovered during autopsies about 40 years ago when yellow staining was found in the brains of babies who had jaundice.

The babies most likely to be affected by this disease are small sick babies. Full term healthy babies are much less liable to suffer from kernicterus, even at high bilirubin levels. This may be because in babies who suffer anoxia, hypercarbia and/or dehydration the blood–brain barrier may be affected allowing both conjugated and unconjugated bilirubin to enter the brain (Blackburn 1995).

Jaundice

Neonatal jaundice can be divided into two categories that refer to the underlying causes:

- Physiological
- Pathological

Physiological jaundice

This jaundice occurs in the first few days after birth and has cleared by 10 days. It occurs because of the physiological changes taking place during the transition from intrauterine to neonatal life.

In the fetus, the bilirubin is excreted across the placenta in the unconjugated form. At birth major changes have to take place in the baby's metabolic mechanisms to facilitate the excretion of bilirubin.

Predisposing causes of physiological jaundice

A newborn baby has a haemoglobin level of 18–19 g/dl which is necessary during fetal life to facilitate oxygen carrying capacity. As soon as the baby is born and able to breathe oxygen, the high haemoglobin level is not needed and starts to drop. The reduction in the baby's haemoglobin to about 11 g/dl will take place in the first week of life and this breakdown of fetal red blood cells by the reticuloendothelial system may cause unconjugated bilirubin to exceed the plasma carrying capacity of the blood.

The liver of the neonate may be immature and deficient in the enzymes Y, Z and glucuronyl transferase which are responsible for conjugating the bilirubin into an excretable product.

A preterm baby's red blood cells have a life span of about 40 days and a term baby's about 70 days, compared with the 120 days of an adult's blood cells. This means that as well as reducing the haemoglobin the reticuloendothelial system has to deal with more used up red blood cells.

Late clamping of the umbilical cord allows more blood into the fetus which then has to be reduced. There may be bruising and/or cephalhaematoma at delivery releasing more blood into the tissues that has to be dealt with by the reticuloendothelial system.

Delay in establishing breast feeding causes

a form of dehydration which alters bilirubin metabolism (Blackburn 1995).

Pathological jaundice

This refers to jaundice that arises from factors that alter the usual process involved in bilirubin metabolism in the liver. This includes blood group incompatibility, hypoglycaemia, hypoxaemia, sepsis, endocrine or metabolic disorders and bile duct obstruction (Blackburn 1995).

Pathological jaundice may be significant in the first 24 hours of life in rhesus incompatibility. It may persist for more than 2 weeks in some conditions when the baby will be jaundiced all over and may appear a muddy yellow colour.

MANAGEMENT OF JAUNDICE

The aim of management is to prevent bilirubin encephalopathy (kernicterus) developing as a result of high levels of serum bilirubin.

Investigations

Investigations should begin when:

- The jaundice is significant in the first 24 hours.
- If jaundice persists after 10 days of age.
- If there is a serum bilirubin level above 250 µmol/l or less in a preterm baby.
- If jaundice is present in a baby who is already ill.

Bilirubin estimation

Serum bilirubin level must be estimated in any baby with a significant jaundice. This is usually done by capillary blood sampling. The use of icterometers which measure skin colour will give a reasonable guide to the levels without resorting to invasive techniques. However, blood must be sent for serum bilirubin assessment, if the levels are rising and the baby is obviously yellow.

Unconjugated bilirubin levels
Unconjugated bilirubin has not been processed by the liver. The levels measured in the blood are those that have exceeded the plasma carrying capacity of the blood and have the potential to cause kernicterus when high levels are reached.

Conjugated bilirubin levels
Conjugated bilirubin is the 'harmless' bilirubin that has been processed by the reticuloendothelial system ready for excretion. If this is higher than 30 μmols/l further investigations should be made. High levels mean that the bile is not being excreted efficiently, which may be the result of rhesus incompatibility, bile duct obstruction, or an inborn error of metabolism.

Mother's blood group

This needs to be known to ascertain compatibility and rhesus antibody status. The antenatal history of antibody levels can be checked if not known.

Baby's blood group

This should be checked for rhesus status, the Coombs' antibody test result should be obtained from the mother's notes or assessed from a blood specimen.

Baby's haemoglobin

This must be checked at the same time as the bilirubin as it will be low if the jaundice is caused by haemolysis that is causing anaemia.

Infection screening

Blood cultures, cerebrospinal fluid and sterile urine samples should be sent for laboratory testing if infection is suspected. A chest X-ray should also be taken and any abrasions or wounds swabbed for culture.

Further tests

These may be undertaken if the cause of the jaundice is not clear and may include:

- Liver function tests
- Thyroid function tests
- Liver ultrasound scan
- Liver biopsy

Treatment

Once the cause of the jaundice has been established, treatment can begin. There may be an underlying cause such as infection or inborn error to be treated but specific therapy to reduce the level of unconjugated bilirubin in the blood should be started immediately if the level of serum bilirubin is high.

Levels of bilirubin

There is a great deal of controversy as to the serum bilirubin level likely to cause damage. Newman & Klebanoff (1993) in an American trial found that neonatal bilirubin levels seem to have little effect on intelligence or neurological abnormalities and that higher bilirubin levels are associated with only minor motor abnormalities. Ahlfors in 1994 agreed that there is no correlation between neurological sequelae and the level of serum bilirubin concentration. It is also known that physiological jaundice with higher serum bilirubin levels is normal in healthy breast fed babies and appears to do no harm. This is thought to be because of the delayed clearance of meconium and the enhanced fat absorption (Hey 1995a).

In practice, however, when the level of bilirubin in the blood reaches 230 µmol/l in a term baby, lower in a preterm baby, treatment is often instigated. Treatment at this level is based on reports from the late 1950s which showed a strong correlation between serum bilirubin concentrations and clinical kernicterus in babies with severe haemolytic disease. It was found that exchange transfusion produced dramatic reduction in serum bilirubin and abolished kernicterus as long as the serum bilirubin was kept below 340 µmol/l. This is now contested by some who use a much lower level for treatment for sick and preterm babies and a higher level for healthy newborn infants. There have been no documented cases of kernicterus developing in an otherwise healthy term baby, in the absence of haemolysis, until the serum bilirubin exceeds 500 µmol/l (Maisels & Newman 1994).

Roberton (1993) suggested the approximate starting point for treatment should be a serum bilirubin level of 90 µmol/l for a 24 week baby with an exchange transfusion carried out at a level of 150–190 µmol/l. This figure increases to about 150 µmol/l for a 32 week baby with exchange transfusion at 160–280 µmol/l.

Dodd (1993) carried out a survey of paediatricians in the UK and found that generally serum bilirubin levels used as criteria for treatment never exceeded 250 µmol/l for phototherapy and 400 µmol/l for exchange transfusion in preterm babies and 350–500 µmol/l for term babies without haemolytic disease of the newborn.

Reducing the levels of bilirubin

Neonatologists will have their own protocols for treatment to reduce bilirubin levels. All babies with significant jaundice should have at least daily assessment of serum bilirubin and this should be done more often if the level is high or has risen rapidly over a short time.

There are currently three methods of treatment for reducing the levels of unconjugated bilirubin in the blood of a newborn baby: drug therapy; phototherapy and exchange transfusion.

Drug therapy

Phenobarbitone in low doses has been shown to stimulate glucuronyl transferase activity in the liver and has been tried with varying success rates. Prenatal use in mothers with known rhesus incompatibility has been successfully used to stimulate enzyme activity in the baby (Blackburn 1995). It can be given from the 32nd week of pregnancy and needs to be given for 3–10 days and results in babies who are less jaundiced (Kelnar *et al.* 1995). If used postnatally the drug takes 48 hours to work and makes the baby sleepy and feed poorly so is not commonly used.

Intravenous albumin acts by increasing the bilirubin binding capacity of the blood and can be given as an emergency measure if there is a delay in obtaining blood for exchange transfusion. The albumin does not reduce the serum bilirubin levels but reduces its toxicity.

It has been noted that preterm infants often have a lower serum bilirubin level once they have had their bowels open, though this does not justify the use of laxatives in these cases (Roberton 1993).

Phototherapy

In the 1950s natural sunlight was found to reduce jaundice, so a device was patented that used electric fluorescent strip lights to imitate natural sunlight. Phototherapy does not treat the cause of the jaundice but reduces the amount of unconjugated (indirect) bilirubin in the plasma photochemically in three ways:

- Lumirubin
- Photoisomerisation
- Photo-oxidation

Lumirubin

This is formed when phototherapy changes the structure of unconjugated bilirubin into lumirubin, which can then be excreted through bile and urine without the need for conjugation.

Photoisomerisation

Photoisomerisation occurs where the light energy converts the unconjugated bilirubin into a soluble isomer which can be safely carried by the albumin into the liver to be slowly excreted in the bile.

Photo-oxidation

This occurs where the bilirubin molecules absorb light energy which is transferred to oxygen, forming a reactive oxygen molecule. The bilirubin is then oxidised, producing water-soluble products that can be excreted in urine (Blackburn 1995).

Phototherapy should not be given to babies with high levels of conjugated bilirubin as it has no effect on this type of bilirubin. If phototherapy is given the babies are likely to turn a deep brown colour and the urine will be very dark. This change is harmless and will resolve in a couple of months but is very disconcerting to parents.

Methods of use

Phototherapy is used for babies whose bilirubin levels are rising to possibly toxic levels. These include:

- Babies with haemolytic diseases, incompatibilities, or red blood cell abnormalities.
- Small sick babies including those with sepsis whose bilirubin levels are high.
- Full term healthy babies with levels of over 340 μmol/l.

The traditional way of giving phototherapy is by overhead striplights using 20–40 watt bulbs. Usually white fluorescent tubes provide the nearest spectrum to sunlight and make it easier to judge the colour of the baby accurately. Narrow-spectrum blue lights are effective but are disturbing for the staff and make it impossible to check for cyanosis.

Lamps become less effective over time so there should be a timer on the equipment that records and displays the number of hours use. The tubes are usually replaced after about 200 hours use to ensure maximum efficiency.

Administering phototherapy

When using phototherapy treatment, distance from the light, temperature control, dehydration, eye care, skin care and parental reactions need to be taken into consideration.

Distance from the light

There is a direct relationship between the amount of light given and the speed at which the bilirubin level falls. The amount of light is influenced by the number and wattage of bulbs used and by their distance from the baby. Halving the distance doubles the amount of light received by the baby (Hey 1995b). If the baby has a high level of bilirubin that must be reduced quickly, two lamps can be used both overhead, or one tilted sideways and the other overhead.

Temperature control

As much skin as possible must be exposed to the light so the baby has to be unclothed and turned regularly to ensure maximum exposure. This may cause problems with temperature control as if the baby is in an incubator, the lamps may warm the incubator top and increase environmental temperature causing overheating. The baby may get cold, especially if in a cot. In these cases a waterproof thermal blanket can be used underneath the baby. If a cot is used, a Perspex top can be fitted over the top to control temperature.

Eye care

It is standard practice to protect babies' eyes from the intensity of the light and the possibility of retinal damage, by the use of eye pads. These pads can be bought commercially or made on the unit with gauze padding over a foil strip. They are secured round the eyes by strapping on to a knitted bonnet or tubegauze hat. There is a slight danger of the mask slipping and obstructing the nose and there may be corneal abrasion and increased intercranial pressure if fitted too tightly. The pad should be removed for inspection at each nappy change to allow the baby to look around and to check for eye infections.

Dehydration

Phototherapy increases insensible water losses from the skin and stools, especially in preterm babies because of the increased metabolism needed for the breakdown of bilirubin. Loose stools are probably the result of stimulation of the intestinal secretions by the bile salts and bilirubin excreted into the gut.

Though there is no documented evidence that this fluid loss needs replacing there is a need for additional energy requirements to achieve and maintain enzyme activity for the degeneration of the bilirubin. Many units increase fluid intake to counter these problems. Fleming *et al.* (1991) advocate 1 ml per kilogram per hour increase in fluid, other authors advise an increase of 25–30% of daily fluids (Blackburn 1995; Edwards 1995).

Skin care

There may be skin rashes and irritation owing to the action of the light. No cream or oil should be used on the skin or lips while the baby is having phototherapy as blisters or burns could result.

Babies will naturally pass urine and faeces while under the light. Urine will burn the skin so needs to be thoroughly washed off and dried each time. Faeces will dry out and become difficult to remove if not cleaned frequently.

There have been reports of genetic damage from phototherapy treatment (Edwards 1995) and it has been advocated that the gonads should be covered in very small babies. This presents a problem as maximum skin exposure is necessary. A possible solution may be to use a small piece of gauze or a theatre mask to cover the area.

Parents reactions to phototherapy

When their baby appears jaundiced the parents are naturally anxious as to the outcome. They often feel very isolated from their baby if, during treatment with phototherapy, they are not be allowed to feed or cuddle the baby.

There is no evidence that taking the baby out for feeds interferes with the process of bilirubin breakdown.

There is a case for using intermittent phototherapy, which can be given one hour out of every four (Dodd 1993). This would allow the parents more access to their baby and help with the parent–infant interaction. Many parents are distressed at the sight of their baby blindfolded and the pads should always be removed for feeding and handling.

No studies have yet been done on the possible adverse psychological effect on the baby of continuous visual occlusion for days. The baby may be miserable missing the security of wrappings and the constant disturbance for hygiene purposes. This fretting upsets the parents and makes them anxious. It is difficult to rationalise to the parents that their baby must stay under the light and not be cuddled, so nurses should advocate for intermittent phototherapy as it has now been shown that this is effective (Edwards 1995; Hey 1995b).

Results of phototherapy

Phototherapy causes reactions in the bilirubin molecules immediately, starting the breakdown that leads to safe excretion. After about 12 hours of treatment 20% of the bilirubin is in a non-toxic form from the photochemical action of the light (Roberton 1993).

Bilirubin levels should be assessed 6–12 hourly with blood tests taken when the lamp is switched off. If it is left on, the light will act on the blood sample and a falsely low level may result. Phototherapy is most effective in the first 48 hours but should be continued until the bilirubin level shows a continuous fall and has reached a safe level. There may be a rise in the bilirubin levels when it is stopped.

The icterometer, which gauges the colour of the skin to assess jaundice level, should not be used on babies who are having phototherapy as the skin will be pale due to the action of the light and not reflect the correct bilirubin level.

Newer types of phototherapy treatment

Fibreoptic phototherapy blankets

These are a recent introduction and consist of bundles of fibreoptic fibres woven into a pad. The baby lies on the pad and can be dressed as long as the pad is inside the clothes. There is no need to protect the eyes. Another advantage is that if the bilirubin level is high and needs to be reduced quickly these blankets can be used in conjunction with striplight lamps.

Halogen spot lights

These too are a recent innovation and produce an intense beam. They have a narrow beam range which is impossible to focus on the whole baby, so that if the baby wriggles away they are rendered ineffective. The lights also generate heat and, as yet, there is no evidence that they are any more effective than the traditional strip lights (Hey 1995b).

Exchange transfusion

The use of phototherapy has drastically reduced the frequency of exchange transfusion but if the bilirubin level is not controlled by phototherapy, exchange transfusion will be necessary. Treatment consists of giving aliquots of donor blood and removing the same amount of the baby's blood. This not only washes out bilirubin but also removes haemolytic antibodies and corrects anaemia. It is the treatment of choice in severe haemolytic anaemia and is the only technique that can be used when the bilirubin level of the blood has to be reduced urgently.

Exchange transfusion can be used for treating other conditions such as sepsis, non-haemolytic anaemias, the removal of toxic drugs and factors causing coagulation disturbances and to help babies with inherited metabolic disease.

Kelnar *et al.* (1995) suggest that the level of bilirubin at which exchange transfusion takes place is 380 µmols for a full term baby dropping to 340 µmols for a 30 week baby. For small sick babies the exchange criteria level is lower as there is slower maturation of the glucuronide transferase enzyme and a faster haemolysis of red blood cells (Ergaz & Arad 1994). This gives the baby a high bilirubin level with a slow clearance from the blood.

Parental consent

The treatment will be discussed with the parents and a consent form is signed when they understand the procedure and its reasons. If there are religious objections to their baby's treatment these will need to be discussed. Doctors may seek legal help under the auspices of the Children's Act 1989 if the treatment is necessary to save the baby from serious handicap or death (Department of Health 1991). Before legal assistance is sought parents should be given as much notice as possible to enable the court to hear both sides. Non-blood medical management can be suggested and all the factors heard before a decision is reached. This is a difficult situation creating hostility and mistrust between parents and staff. There is often the risk of the child being rejected by the family if treatment goes ahead so clear and honest communication is necessary on both sides to ensure that the best treatment is given.

Nursing care of a baby undergoing exchange transfusion

Exchange transfusion involves removing the baby's blood in aliquots of 10–20 ml and replacing it with an equal amount of matched donor blood. The usual amount exchanged is twice the baby's volume of blood, approximately 160 ml per kilogram of body weight (Fleming *et al.* 1991).

Pre-exchange care

Blood for the procedure is obtained by sending a sample of the baby's blood to the blood bank for cross matching. Enough blood must be ordered to prime the blood warmer and giving set. Whole blood should be used that is not more than 2 days old. Blood that has been stored in citrate phosphate dextrose (CPD) for longer than this degrades having a low pH and a high PCO_2 which could cause metabolic stress. Rhesus negative blood that is negative to CMV, HIV, hepatitis B and C must be used.

Equipment and sterile packs for the procedure are set up in readiness.

Equipment needed for exchange transfusion

- Blood and blood giving set
- Blood warmer and warming coil
- Volumetric pump if used
- Umbilical catheters or intravenous cannulas
- Cut down set
- Scalpel
- Aqueous chlorhexidine
- Ampules of saline
- Ampules of calcium gluconate
- Blood specimen bottles
- 20 ml, 5 ml and two 1 ml syringes

- Three-way taps
- Sterile gloves

The exchange

If the baby is ventilated the airway is suctioned. The baby's stomach is aspirated to prevent vomiting and inhalation. Temperature control is essential throughout the procedure so an overhead warmer on servo-control mode or an incubator with the temperature module on servo-control can be used.

Cardiopulmonary monitoring must be carried out during the whole procedure as there is risk of arrhythmias and possible cardiac arrest. Blood pressure and oxygen saturation monitoring should also be used. The limbs should be gently restrained to prevent the baby knocking out cannulas and haemorrhaging.

Pain relief should be given before cannulating the baby. If the baby is ventilated an opiate drug may be already in use and this can be increased slightly. If not a paracetamol suppository can be given and possibly a dose of chloral hydrate sedative. It should be borne in mind that exchange transfusion will wash out these drugs once the cannulas are in place,

but the actual removal and infusion of blood is painless.

Cannulation

The umbilical vein is often used, if the cord is not too shrivelled, as blood can be removed and infused through this vessel (Fig. 12.1). Some units also cannulate the umbilical artery so that blood can be removed from this line and then given through the umbilical vein. The procedure is always done using aseptic techniques to minimise the risk of sepsis. If the umbilical cord cannot be used, a peripheral blood vessel will be cannulated.

The equipment should be set up and, once cannulation has taken place, the system primed with blood which is prewarmed as it goes through the warmer. There are two common ways to give an exchange transfusion, both using prewarmed blood:

- The withdrawal and injection of aliquots of 10–20 ml of blood through a central vein, usually the umbilical (Fig. 12.3).
- The continuous removal of blood from the umbilical or a peripheral artery, balanced by continuous infusion into the umbilical or a peripheral vein (Fig. 12.2).

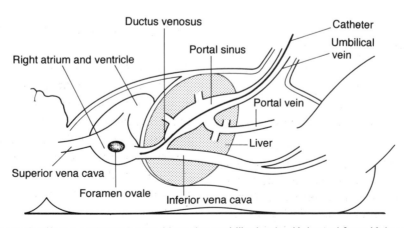

Fig. 12.1 Diagram showing a catheter passed into the umbilical vein. (Adapted from Kelnar *et al.* (1995).)

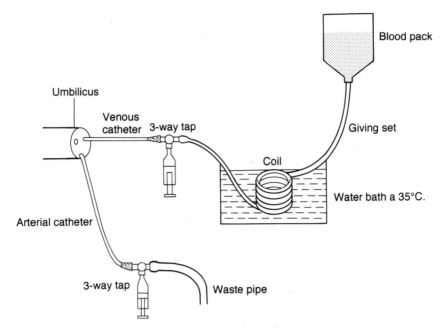

Fig. 12.2 Circuit for isovolumetric exchange transfusion. (Adapted from Halliday *et al.* (1989).)

The second method is safer, less invasive and less likely to cause necrotising enterocolitis (Todd 1995). There is also less risk of changes in blood pressure because of the evenness of the transfusion. Fluctuations in the blood flow in the brain that might predispose to intravenous haemorrhage are less of a problem. This method cuts down the risk of air embolism in the tubing and takes less time so mitigating the risk of cold and systemic stress.

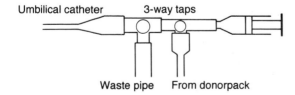

Fig. 12.3 Single vessel venous exchange transfusion. Blood is drawn into the syringe from the umbilical vein and discarded into the waste bag. Blood is then drawn from the reservoir of fresh blood, through the warmer and injected into the baby. (Adapted from Halliday et al. (1989).)

Once the cannulas are in place a specimen of blood should be taken from the baby to ascertain:

- Serum calcium
- Serum electrolytes
- Blood gases
- Serum bilirubin, conjugated and unconjugated
- Full blood count, platelets and haemoglobin

Caring for the baby during the exchange

The baby should be comfortable, settled and warm after cannulation. Blood should be removed from the baby first to risk overloading the circulation. If the exchange is manual the actions of withdrawing and replacing should be done slowly to prevent fluctuations in blood pressure and vital signs. Roberton (1993) recommends 4–5 minutes for each action. Thus, using this method could take 2–2½ hours depending on the size of the baby. The continuous method where there is less likelihood of reactions, takes about an hour (Todd 1995). A record must be kept of all infusions and removals and drugs as they are given.

If the exchange is continuous the volumetric pump is set to give the amount needed through the venous line and the doctor or nurse practitioner removes blood from the arterial line at the same rate. Blood is not given into the artery as it may cause spasm, blocking the catheter and endangering blood supply to the limb. It is important that blood is evenly given and removed to prevent fluctuations in blood pressure. The baby's vital signs are recorded every 10 minutes or as blood is given and extracted.

Complications during exchange

The catheter

Disconnection or displacement of the catheter could result in significant haemorrhage. There is also the risk of clotting in the catheter or air embolism.

Haemodynamic complications

Care must be taken not to remove or give too much blood to overload or deplete the system. Too rapid an exchange may lead to cardiorespiratory deterioration from shock or acidaemia as citrated blood has a pH of 7.1. Gases should be monitored and metabolic acidaemia corrected during the exchange before major problems present. This is especially important if the baby is small or sick.

Electrolyte disturbance

Hypocalcaemia
The cardiac trace must be continuously monitored for arrhythmias associated with

hypocalcaemia. This can be corrected with intravenous calcium gluconate given slowly.

Hyperkalaemia
The potassium in donor blood increases the longer it is stored and may cause sudden severe cardiac disturbance and death. Hyperkalaemia is treated by calcium gluconate infusion and with sodium bicarbonate if the first is not successful.

Stopping the exchange

In view of the seriousness and rapidity of onset of problems there should be no hesitation in stopping the exchange if there is persistent tachycardia, bradycardia, cyanosis or arrhythmias. Nursing observations are vital throughout the exchange as complications can occur at any stage of the transfusion.

At the conclusion

If there are no problems, the calculated amount of blood will be exchanged. A sample from the last blood removed is sent for assessment of bilirubin levels, with the pretest sample. Catheters or peripheral cannulas are then removed, secured against bleeding and an antibiotic spray used on the umbilicus. If another transfusion is likely, the cannulae may be left in place.

After-care

The baby should be made comfortable and left to rest. Temperature should be monitored and rewarming measures taken if necessary. Cardiorespiratory monitoring should continue for a few hours to check for cardiac arrhythmias. Blood sugar is monitored hourly for 4–6 hours afterwards to prevent rebound hypoglycaemia. Citrated blood has a high glucose level which may raise the glucose level to above 10 mmol/l during the exchange, provoking insulin release with a following rebound hypoglycaemia.

Phototherapy will be continued and the serum bilirubin level will be estimated 2–4 hours after the exchange. A severely affected baby may need more than one exchange.

Parents, if they have not been present during the exchange, will want to see their baby and speak to the staff about the result of the procedure.

Risks associated with exchange transfusion

Mortality rate from this treatment is 2–3 per 1000 exchanges (Maisels 1994). It used to be a common procedure in neonatal units but has declined since the success of phototherapy. This decline in use has also meant a decline in the clinical skills of the staff and it is thought that the morbidity and mortality rate may increase in the future as the need for exchange falls even more (Maisels 1994).

CONDITIONS CAUSING JAUNDICE IN THE NEWBORN

As jaundice in the neonatal unit is so common it is necessary to look into the conditions that predispose to it (Table 12.2).

Physiological jaundice

The most common jaundice in the neonatal unit is physiological jaundice which affects more than 60% of babies. It usually appears during the second day of life and reaches its peak at 3–7 days. The baby is not ill and will not normally refuse feeds though some

Table 12.2 Common conditions that cause jaundice in the new-born.

Physiological jaundice
Haemolytic disorders
Infections
Polycythaemia
Breast milk jaundice
Inborn errors of metabolism
Hepatitis
Extrahepatic obstructions
High intestinal obstructions

preterm babies may be slightly lethargic. For jaundice to appear on the skin of a baby the bilirubin levels must exceed 80 μmol/l (Kelnar *et al.* 1995).

Jaundice appears on the face before reaching the trunk and is seldom seen over the lower legs and tibiae until the bilirubin level reaches 250 μmol/l. By now stage serum bilirubin assessment should have begun (Hey 1995a).

If the bilirubin levels reach the unit's protocol for treatment, phototherapy will be started. In these days of early discharge, a well, term baby may have been discharged before the jaundice appears. If the baby needs treatment, the use of fibreoptic pads in the community prevents re-admission while breast feeding is being established.

Preterm sick babies will have a high level of jaundice earlier than full term and will usually need treatment. Physiological jaundice rarely needs exchange transfusion but may need phototherapy and fades without adverse effects over the first 7–10 days of life.

Prevention

Physiological jaundice can be lessened by a number of measures in a healthy term baby. Care should be taken at delivery to clamp the cord early. If the baby is to be breast fed, early and unrestricted feeding must be allowed. If energy intake is inadequate babies meet their energy needs by increased fat metabolism which interferes with hepatic function and slows bilirubin metabolism (Blackburn 1995).

Breast feeding does not cause jaundice and should not be stopped during this time as this will only add to the anxiety of the mother. Giving extra water does not improve matters and could prevent breast milk intake. There is no clinical evidence that healthy term babies will become dehydrated if not fluid supplemented during the first few days of life (Hey 1995b).

Haemolytic disorders

These include rhesus incompatibility, ABO incompatibility, spherocytosis and glucose-6-phosphate dehydrogenase deficiency (G-6-PD).

Haemolytic disease may result from incompatibility between the baby's blood and the mother's. The commonest of these is rhesus incompatibility.

Rhesus incompatibility

This disease occurs when the mother and baby have different rhesus status in their blood. Untreated babies have a high mortality rate with death occurring before birth in some cases. Severely affected babies are born with ascites, pleural effusions, severe anaemia, heart failure and the prognosis is poor.

The rhesus antigen

Red blood cells carry three sets of antigens which are labelled by the letters Cc, Dd and Ee and denote dominant (large letters) and recessive (small letters) genes. When the blood cells contain only antigens denoted by small letters c, d and e the blood is rhesus negative. When the cells contain antigens denoted by the large letters C, D and E or any combination of them with the small letters, the blood is rhesus positive.

The majority of people carry the rhesus antigens in their blood that classify it as rhesus positive. Those with rhesus negative blood have no problems until a blood transfusion needs to be given and during pregnancy.

If rhesus positive blood is given to a rhesus negative person, the positive blood produces rhesus antibodies in the negative blood. This causes haemolysis of the red blood cells in which haemoglobin is released from the blood cells and is broken down by the reticuloendothelial system. In some cases severe anaemia and jaundice is caused which may require urgent treatment with an exchange transfusion of rhesus negative blood.

Rhesus isoimmunisation during pregnancy

If a woman with rhesus negative blood has a partner who is rhesus positive, their baby may be rhesus positive. If there is then a spontaneous miscarriage, termination of pregnancy or small antepartum haemorrhages during pregnancy, small amounts of blood from the fetal circulation leak into the mother's blood. The mother then develops a mild antibody response, the specific antibody that causes the problem is the large D of the rhesus positive group.

When the baby is born there is often another leak of fetal blood into the mother's circulation provoking further antibody response in the mother. As blood from the mother mixes with the baby's, haemolysis of fetal red cells is caused. The disease will become more severe with each pregnancy and in the past many babies died from this disease either *in utero* or after birth. Preventative measures now begin antenatally for all rhesus negative women.

Prevention of rhesus haemolytic disease

Since 1969 the incidence of rhesus haemolytic disease has fallen dramatically as a result of preventative measures taken to ensure that the rhesus negative mother does not get sensitised and produce antibodies that harm the baby.

This is achieved by giving the non-sensitised mother hyperimmune gammaglobulin within 60 hours of any procedure which may cause sensitisation. This includes amniocentesis, giving birth to a rhesus positive infant, miscarriage or a termination of pregnancy. The gammaglobulin binds to the fetal cells in her blood enabling their safe removal and excretion. This must be repeated each time a sensitising procedure occurs in every pregnancy.

Antenatal care

When a woman books into antenatal clinic one of the first checks will be on her blood group and rhesus status. It is helpful to know her partner's rhesus status too. If his blood is also rhesus negative there should be no problems with antibodies though staff should not be too complacent about this, as paternity is sometimes falsely assigned for the mother's own reasons.

There should be no complications with a first pregnancy but maternal antibody status will be assessed throughout. The antibody level will be plotted and if showing a rising titre, an amniocentesis or fetal blood sampling will be carried out to assess the disease in the fetus. The earlier haemolysis starts in the baby, the more severe the results. The baby may incur hydrops fetalis which is gross anaemia, enlarged spleen, liver damage, pleural effusions, cardiac failure and generalised oedema with ascites. Women who are likely to be severely affected are usually referred to a regional centre for treatment and delivery.

An at-risk pregnancy is followed from 20 weeks with 2-weekly sampling of the mother's blood. The aim is to keep the fetus healthy, by intrauterine infusions of fresh blood, until it is at least 28 weeks. Intrauterine transfusions will continue until the baby is born. The baby will have a series of ultrasound scans to look for ascites, pleural effusion or hydropic features.

Intrauterine transfusion

This is done under ultrasound screening with a cannula aimed through the fetal abdominal wall. Rhesus negative blood compatible with that of the mother is then injected into the fetal peritoneal cavity where it is rapidly absorbed (Kelnar *et al.* 1995). This temporarily corrects fetal anaemia by providing red blood cells which are not haemolysed and may have to be repeated several times during the pregnancy. The procedure can result in fetal bleeding causing intrauterine death. Results are good with survivors having fewer complications and a good prognosis.

At birth

Severely affected infants will be very pale at birth from the anaemia. This means that there will be no cyanosis making any degree of hypoxia difficult to judge. An umbilical arterial catheter can be passed in the labour ward for urgent blood gas sampling in case respiratory support is necessary.

When the baby is born the cord must be

clamped immediately and cut to a short stump of about 5 cm to ensure that the baby has as little of the mother's blood as possible. Cord blood should be subjected to the direct Coombs' test for antibodies and checked for blood group, bilirubin level, haemoglobin and packed cell volume. This will give an indication of the severity of the disease and confirm the diagnosis.

If the baby has received intrauterine infusions then the cord blood tests may not be accurate. There may be a lower level of bilirubin and higher haemoglobin from the transfused blood. A capillary sample from the baby should be tested in these cases.

Treatment

Phototherapy should be started as soon as possible after birth in all babies with rhesus incompatibility. If the haemoglobin is less than 10 g/dl this is an indication for immediate exchange transfusion (Fleming *et al.* 1991).

Serum bilirubin levels should be estimated every 6 hours and plotted on a graph. If the bilirubin is rising at the rate of 1 µmol/l per hour then an exchange will almost certainly be needed (Roberton 1993). If the baby is sick or small a lower rate of increase must be accepted for exchange level.

If the disease is severe, the baby will be very sick with ascites and pleural effusions which have to be drained. There may be cardiomegaly with some degree of heart failure. There may be platelet problems and DIC may ensue (Chapter 8).

Prognosis

Following severe haemolytic disease, an obstructive jaundice might develop which usually clears by 3–4 weeks of age. Babies may also become anaemic at a few weeks of age,

before their bone marrow starts producing red blood cells, and they may need top-up transfusions.

Babies who have had a milder disease with a positive Coombs' test at birth may develop anaemia later at a few weeks of age from slow haemolysis. These babies may need top-up transfusions and possibly iron supplements.

Parents

The parents of a baby with rhesus antibodies will have had a worrying time throughout the pregnancy. If intrauterine transfusions have taken place frequently they are likely to have spent much time travelling back and forth to the regional centre. There was also the added anxiety that they might lose the baby at every transfusion. The birth is a relief especially when they see the baby looking well.

They may have been to the neonatal unit and met some of the staff there before the birth. The treatment their baby needs may have been explained by the obstetricians and they will anxiously await the results of bilirubin assessments to see whether an exchange transfusion is needed.

If bilirubin levels are satisfactory the baby will be allowed home after the first week as long as feeding is adequate and the weight is at least 2 kilograms (4 lb 6 oz). The general practitioner (GP) will then follow up the family.

ABO incompatibility

This is a common disease caused by a mother with blood group O, who is carrying a baby of group A or B, passing an antibody across the placenta that causes haemolysis in the baby's blood. This passage of antibodies affects each pregnancy equally and will occur regardless of rhesus status of mother or baby.

The antibodies are gammaglobulin G which

destroy group A and B blood cells causing haemolysis in the baby. The disease is usually mild, jaundice appearing within 24 hours of birth. Occasionally the serum bilirubin levels will rise high enough to require exchange transfusion.

Glucose-6-phosphate dehydrogenase deficiency (G-6-PD)

This is an inherited condition common among people from Africa, the West Indies, the Mediterranean countries, East Asia and African Americans. It is a sex-linked, genetic disease with males affected and females being the carriers, though occasionally female infants are affected.

There is an enzyme deficiency in red blood cells, leucocytes and other blood cells which causes red blood cells to haemolyse in certain situations. Drugs such as sulphonamides, aspirin, quinine, vitamin K (aqueous) are known causative agents. In some cases food such as broad beans triggers the same reaction – a condition known as favism. Episodes of infection can also trigger the disease in susceptible individuals. There is often haemolysis enough to warrant exchange transfusion.

Care must be taken when giving drugs to mothers who are carriers if they are breast feeding, as the drugs will be excreted through her milk into the baby causing the haemolytic reaction. When discharging these patients, a list of drugs liable to affect the baby should be given to the mother and her GP.

Congenital spherocytocis

This is an hereditary disease in which the red cells are small and spherical. It usually presents later in life but may sometimes appear in the new-born period. The symptoms are usually mild but occasionally exchange transfusion is required.

Infection

Bacterial infection causes red cell destruction which leads to jaundice. This should always be suspected when the baby does not have haemolytic disease and/or the jaundice occurs more that 7 days after birth. Blood cultures are taken and antibiotics given. Phototherapy and exchange transfusion are used when necessary.

Polycythaemia

In polycythaemia there are extra red cells to be dealt with by the reticuloendothelial system resulting in a slower clearing of the bilirubin. Polycythaemia occurs when there is delayed clamping of the cord giving extra blood to the baby, in cold stress or hypoxia at delivery, in infants of diabetic mothers, and during twin to twin transfusion when one twin has an accidental infusion of blood from the other *in utero*.

Breast milk jaundice

Breast milk jaundice is due to the beta-glucuronidase in the milk which causes already-conjugated bilirubin to become unconjugated and remain in the blood. It is of no significance to the baby and the mother should be reassured that breast feeding can continue.

Prolonged jaundice

Jaundice that persists beyond the seventh day is considered prolonged. It may result from unconjugated or conjugated hyperbilirubinaemia.

Unconjugated hyperbilirubinaemia may be the result of delayed feeding in the preterm infant leading to decreased bile flow so that unconjugated bilirubin is reabsorbed instead of excreted.

Conjugated hyperbilirubinaemia may be caused by damage from severe haemolytic disease, metabolic disease or bile flow obstruction. These problems prevent the secretion of conjugated bile which then builds up in the blood. It can also occur because of intestinal stasis in babies who have had a prolonged period of parenteral feeding, in this case the baby makes a full recovery. Babies with conjugated hyperbilirubinaemia, whatever the cause, should never be given photo-therapy as it turns the skin to an alarming grey-brown colour which may take many weeks to clear.

Investigations

Once the common causes of prolonged jaundice are excluded there remain possibilities which include hepatitis and biliary obstruction.

Hepatitis

This may be caused by one of several organisms which include hepatitis A and B, cyto-megalovirus, rubella, toxoplasma and herpes simplex. The infection is usually acquired *in utero* and the jaundice may be a part of a syndrome, but often the cause cannot be found. The diagnosis of hepatitis is made when jaundice is marked and prolonged with an enlarged liver and markedly abnormal liver function tests.

Many babies recover spontaneously although they may be left with a malabsorption of vitamins A, D and K (Fleming *et al.* 1991). A few will go on to develop cirrhosis

and hepatic failure, or cancer of the liver and some will retain chronic carrier status.

Babies with hepatitis will often be miserable and fretful and may have rashes in response to irritation of the skin from the prolonged raised bilirubin in the blood. Management will consist of keeping the baby comfortable by ensuring the skin is clean and dry. Gentle washing with warm water is soothing and cool cotton clothing should be used to dress the baby. If the hepatitis is caused by infection, gloves must be used for handling to minimise the risk of contaminating other babies and staff. Laboratory specimens should be clearly marked to protect pathology staff.

Breast feeding is not contraindicated. Active and passive immunity with HBV vaccine is given, at birth, to babies of HBV positive mothers.

Biliary atresia

This type of jaundice is difficult to distinguish from hepatitis. The baby will have increasing jaundice and a large firm liver. It is important to diagnose this condition as soon as possible, as even though the prognosis is poor, early surgery during the first 2 months of life may be successful in some cases. After this time irreversible liver damage will have occurred. Nursing management will be similar to that of the baby with hepatitis.

REFERENCES

Ahlfors CE. (1994) Criteria for exchange transfu-sion. *Pediatrics*, **93** (3), 488–492.

Blackburn S. (1995) Hyperbilirubinemia and neo-natal jaundice. *Neonatal Network*, **14** (7), 15–25.

Crawford D, Morris M. (1994) *Neonatal Nursing*. Chapman and Hall, London.

Department of Health. (1991) *The Children's Act*

1989: An Introductory Guide for the NHS. Department of Health, London.

Dodd KL. (1993) Neonatal jaundice, a lighter touch. *Archives of Disease in Childhood, Fetal and Neonatal Edition*, **68**, 529–533.

Edwards S. (1995) Phototherapy and the neonate. *Journal of Neonatal Nursing*, **1** (5), 9–12.

Ergaz Z, Arad I. (1994) Hyperbilirubinaemia in premature infants; relevance to blood transfusion. *Biology of the Neonate*, **66**, 71–75.

Fleming PJ, Speidel BD, Marlow N, Dunn PM. (1991) *A Neonatal Vade Mecum*, 2nd edn. Edward Arnold, London.

Halliday HL, McClure G, Reid M. (1989) *Handbook of Neonatal Care* 3rd edn. Baillière Tindall, Philadelphia.

Hey EN. (1995a) Neonatal jaundice – how much do we really know? *MIDIRS Midwifery Digest*, **5** (1), 4–8.

Hey EN. (1995b) Phototherapy; a fresh light on a murky subject. *MIDIRS Midwifery Digest*, **5** (3), 256–260.

Kelnar CJH, Harvey D, Simpson C. (1995) *The Sick Newborn Baby*, 3rd edn. Baillière Tindall, London.

Maisels MJ. (1994) Jaundice. In: *Neonatology*, (eds G. Avery, MA Fletcher & MG McDonald), 4th edn. pp. 687–696. JB Lippincott, Philadelphia.

Maisels MJ, Newman TB. (1994) Kernicterus occurs in full term healthy newborns without apparent haemolysis. (Abstract No. 1419) *Pediatric Research*, **35** (4), 239A.

Newman TB, Klebanoff MA. (1993) Neonatal hyperbilirubinaemia and long term outcome. *Pediatrics*, **92** (5), 651–656.

Roberton NCR. (1993) *A Manual of Neonatal Intensive Care*, 3rd edn. Edward Arnold, London.

Todd NA. (1995) Isovolaemic exchange transfusion of the neonate. *Neonatal Network*, **14** (6), 75–77.

13

Discharge Planning and the Community Outreach Service

LEARNING OUTCOMES

After reading this chapter and studying the contents the reader will be able to:

○ Identify when to begin discharge planning.
○ Demonstrate a knowledge of discharge planning tools.
○ Identify the importance of the neonatal outreach service.
○ Discuss the discharge learning needs of parents.
○ List the babies likely to need nursing support at home.
○ Describe the teaching needs of parents with a baby on home oxygen.

PREPARATION FOR DISCHARGE

The discharge home of a previously sick neonate is an anxiety-provoking event for parents because of the physical and emotional trauma they have been through with the baby. According to Merenstein & Gardner (1993) the parents of a sick preterm baby have five psychological tasks to work through before they are ready to take their baby home. These are:

• Working through traumatic events concerned with labour and delivery.
• Grieving for and withdrawal from the baby they had dreamed of during pregnancy.
• Acknowledging feelings of guilt and failure.
• Adaptation to the intensive care environment.
• Making a relationship with the new baby.

Failure to complete these tasks can contribute to poor parenting and a poor outcome for the baby, which could include failure to thrive, emotional deprivation and possible physical abuse (Merenstein & Gardner 1993).

Most parents work through the first three tasks with the help of family members and supportive staff. In some cases support may be needed in the form of counselling and parents can, if they wish, be referred to the family support sister if there is one, or other counsellor for help.

Initially the nurse focuses on helping parents to feel comfortable in the unit by a welcoming informative attitude. Unit routines that affect parents are explained and available written material about the unit given to reinforce this. Parents can be encouraged from the admission of their baby to help with the physical care. Some may feel unable to care for their baby emotionally or physically due to their lack of knowledge about hospital policy and the needs of a sick baby. If parents are reluctant to give care to their baby this fear needs to be recognised so that the nurse can work towards overcoming it.

Regular communications of medical findings and treatment options are given to the family. Their questions and concerns are discussed openly and when decisions are made by the medical staff, the nurse helps parents to understand the options and reasons for the choice of treatment (Laurie 1995).

To emphasise their role as primary carers, parents are encouraged to perform basic physical care such as nappy changing and mouth care. As they become more familiar with the baby's needs they are encouraged to rely less on staff supervision. Developmental care can be enhanced by bringing in toys that stimulate vision and hearing, such as bright soft toys, musical toys and tapes of family members' voices. Parents need to be consulted when planning the baby's routine to allow them maximum participation, for example feed and bath time schedules.

Ideally if the above factors are implemented, the progression to total parental care after discharge will be easier for them.

DISCHARGE PLANNING TOOLS

The increasing complexity of treatment and the shortened lengths of stay in today's units require efficient and effective methods of discharge planning and teaching (Drake 1995). Parental anxiety often centres around not remembering all that is learnt, and making a mistake in the treatment. Worry about coping in a crisis if their child becomes ill is often paramount, so knowing who will be available for support is essential.

The search for a discharge planning tool to help parents and alleviate such worries has led to research into ways of improving teaching and communication (Robinson 1994; Drake 1995; Vecchi *et al.* 1996). Most units now employ a system of helping parents learn to care for their baby in the hospital and at home. This system will involve parents, siblings and other family members and work towards the discharge home of the baby (Table 13.1).

Table 13.1 Components of a good learning plan for parents.

Teaching, demonstration and supervision of standard tasks
Time allowance for repeat teaching and communication
Discussion with parents about what they wish to learn
Family support structures taken into account
Working with a time plan of expected discharge

A system such as this gives the parents confidence in their skills and enables them to deal safely with the baby at home. It is an advantage if there is written material to reinforce the information and for future reference.

People learn in different ways and some will have few difficulties with the physical care of their baby while others do not gain confidence until they have performed a task many times under supervision. Learning pace must be taken into account if it is to be successful (Robinson 1991).

Many units have psychosocial meetings to discuss the dynamics of individual family functioning and the likely effect of a sick baby on the family. These meetings are usually attended by social workers and unit staff. There are opportunities for both sides to discuss and understand the feelings and reactions of the families involved. The purpose is to evaluate and assess families, to provide support and counselling services and to co-ordinate discharge planning and follow-up care for the baby.

Predictive planning

It is generally agreed that parents need advance notice of the discharge date so that they can prepare physically and mentally for the event (Vecchi *et al.* 1996). It is not always possible to predict this with accuracy as pre-term babies often acquire infections and set backs that throw plans into confusion.

Development of critical or clinical pathways reflects attempts to control costs and estimate discharge dates by predicting the length of hospital stay. The predictive planning method works by calculating the shortest time and the longest time each stage of treatment takes. This is worked out on the statistics or averages of previous babies.

A plan such as this can be worked out for all aspects of the baby's treatment, for oxygen therapy, phototherapy, intravenous fluids, oral feeds, weight gain and expected discharge (Vecchi *et al.* 1996). This method

appears time consuming but such plans can be generated on computer. It is not in common use at the time of writing but may have its place in the future.

Checklist planning

Many units use this method to ensure that parents have a basic knowledge of their baby's needs. It consists of a checklist of standard tasks for nurses to help parents work though. If the baby has special requirements such as home oxygen administration then an additional teaching and support programme is needed.

The previous experience of the parent must be taken into account. It is unnecessary to give a demonstration bath to an experienced mother or to show her how to make up feeds. Though even experienced parents may need to go through these procedures to gain confidence caring for their previously sick baby (McKim 1993). If the mother is physically disabled she may need special equipment or help from occupational therapists to learn the best way of handling the baby. If the mother has learning difficulties that mean she needs extra support, a family worker may be assigned to help if there is no other able person in the household.

The checklist

Different units will have different priorities but all help new parents learn about nappy hygiene, bathing, making up feeds and administering medicines. Each task will be demonstrated, discussed and reinforced by rationale. Health and safety advice about home environment and equipment is usually given (Table 13.2) (Figs 13.1 and 13.2).

Table 13.2 A standard learning plan for parents.

Skill	Demonstration	Practice
NAPPY HYGIENE Nappy, cotton wool, water, cream Cleaning of area Hygienic disposal of nappy		
BATH Room temperature Water temperature Towels, cotton wool, soap Skin care Safe handling of baby		
BREAST FEEDS Positioning of baby Nipple care Expressing and storing milk		
ARTIFICIAL FEEDS Making up powdered feeds Checking temperature of feed Position of baby Winding Times of feeds		
MEDICINES Method of administration Purpose of giving Side-effects Timing of doses Missed doses or vomiting Safe storage		
PREVENTION OF COT DEATH Positioning Prevention of smoking near baby Room temperature Bedding and appropriate clothing		
HEALTH Immunisations date due Date of Guthrie test Eye or hearing test, if necessary Outpatient follow-up		
ENVIRONMENT Toy safety Plastic bags Smoking People with colds Warmth When to go out		
EQUIPMENT Advice on cots Avoid pillows Leaflets on car seats		

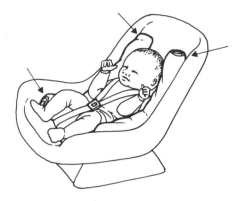

Fig. 13.1 Preterm infant properly positioned in car seat. Rolls at the side and under legs improve head and body support.

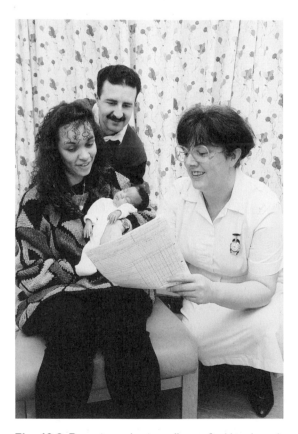

Fig. 13.2 Parents and nurse discussing treatment. (Printed with kind permission of Mr and Mrs Grey.)

DISCHARGE PLANNING AND THE OUTREACH SERVICE

The advances in medical technology and nursing practice have meant an increase in the number of babies needing extended periods of hospitalisation. These babies also have a high morbidity and mortality rate in the first year leading to frequent readmissions (Kurdahi Zahr & Montijo 1993).

Increasingly babies are being discharged home while still needing medical treatment. This is as a result of various studies, which have shown that the benefits of early discharge with home support are advantageous to baby and family in terms of physical and psychological development (Wakefield & Ford 1994; Foden 1996). Studies have also shown that supervised community care of these babies can reduce the frequency of readmission and the utilisation of hospital facilities, so making early discharge a cost-effective, beneficial exercise.

The outreach service

Many neonatal units have now implemented specialised outreach services, consisting of experienced neonatal nurses who plan the discharge and mobilise support for the family in the community. This ensures that parents are supported at home and enables discharge weeks or months earlier than would otherwise have been possible.

The philosophy of the neonatal outreach service is to ease the transition from hospital to home of babies who have a health-care need, so promoting family-centred care as well as acting as a resource for general practitioners (GPs), health visitors and community nurses. The neonatal outreach service provides a link between hospital and community services. Education and support of parents, follow-up of babies and specific nursing care are provided where needed.

Discharge planning

The discharge of a baby who needs medical and nursing care, can only come about if parents are provided with relevant skills, knowledge and community support to care for the baby safely. It is an enormous commitment for parents and the outreach service must safeguard their well-being to ensure the baby is not discharged before parents feel able to cope.

Ideally discharge planning will begin when the baby is recovering from the critical phase and is making satisfactory progress. Many outreach services are ward based enabling the first meeting between parents and outreach staff to be on an informal basis. Follow-up meetings before discharge may take place on a weekly or monthly basis depending on unit policy. As a discharge date becomes feasible the outreach sister may visit the parents at home to discuss discharge arrangements and assess conditions there, such as adequate heating and facilities that may need modification. This visit is also to ensure teaching programmes are being implemented and to gain parents' confidence in the service that will be provided.

The baby's discharge requires careful planning, organisation and attention to individual family needs. It is important to remember that not all families want or need such support and that a barrage of health care workers descending on a family can cause confusion and be looked upon as an unwelcome invasion of privacy.

Care must be taken to select the babies who require home visits so as not to overload the outreach service with babies that could be cared for by the health visitor (see Table 13.3). Criteria for individual hospitals are independently set but many have similar categories of care.

Table 13.3 Criteria for neonatal outreach visiting.

Babies on tube feeds
Poor feeders
Those needing apnoea monitoring
Babies under 2 kg at discharge
Oxygen dependent babies
Babies who need withdrawal treatment from
    maternal drug abuse
Babies who require terminal care
Poor parenting ability
Babies on home total parenteral nutrition
Babies needing ostomy care

DISCHARGE OF BABIES WITH SPECIAL NEEDS

A routine learning programme that covers basic hygiene, health and safety needs should be worked through with every parent and if the baby has special needs other topics need to be covered. Special teaching will be needed if the baby is going home with:

- Home oxygen administration
- Apnoea monitoring
- Nasogastric tube feeding
- Gastrostomy feeding
- Intravenous feeding
- Colostomy/ileostomy care
- Tracheostomy care

Discharge of a baby needing oxygen administration

Some of the most challenging babies to be cared for in the community are those with chronic lung disease requiring home oxygen therapy. The numbers of these babies are increasing with the survival of early gestational age and very low birth weight babies. Such babies may already have spent weeks in hospital undergoing treatment and the need for oxygen may continue for many more months. In order to maximise and normalise their development, early discharge has been initiated where there are services to teach and support parents and oversee treatment (Foden 1996).

Babies who go home on oxygen have lung disease which will put them at risk of chest infections and failure to thrive. Looking after such a baby can be a frightening experience for parents and their commitment and understanding of the need for oxygen treatment is vital.

Timing of discharge

Discharge planning will begin when the baby is well, gaining weight, sucking feeds are becoming established and oxygen requirements are stabilising. This may be 3–4 weeks before discharge. Parental ability and willingness to take the baby home on oxygen will be ascertained. A planning meeting is held during this time, attended by the general practitioner, health visitor and district nurses to ensure that the discharge is formalised effectively and that all medical and nursing supplies are ordered and delivered to the baby's home.

Learning needs encompass, recognising when the baby is hypoxic, the use of home oxygen equipment such as nasal cannulas, flow meters, oxygen concentrator or cylinders and safe use of oxygen. Some units teach parents cardiopulmonary resuscitation (CPR) skills especially if the baby is prone to apnoeic attacks.

Recognising hypoxia

If the baby is allowed to remain hypoxic, lung damage may be caused, which could result in increased oxygen requirements and a longer time spent in oxygen. Lack of sufficient oxygen can cause pulmonary hypertension and heart failure leading to a fatal condition called cor pulmonale. Weight gain and growth will also be affected as the baby will be using energy in the struggle to breathe. Oxygen should not be decreased or stopped without assessment from the community nurses.

A hypoxic baby may be pale or slightly cyanosed, lethargic, breathless and not be able to finish feeds, and oxygen must be increased until there is an improvement. If oxygen needs stay high the baby may have a chest infection needing antibiotics, the outreach nurses must be informed.

Use of equipment

Topics covered by the outreach service include familiarisation with equipment to be used, nasal cannula, low flow meter, oxygen tubing, tape used to secure cannulae and the correct positioning of a nasal cannula.

Methods of providing home oxygenation

There are two methods of providing oxygen at home; the concentrator machine or cylinders.

The concentrator
This is used if the baby is likely to need long term oxygen. It is an electrically operated machine the size of a small fridge which separates a high proportion of nitrogen and other components out of the atmosphere. It then pipes oxygen rich gas to two points, in the house, where a flow meter and oxygen tubing can be attached. This method costs

approximately £500 (1996 prices) to install and the oxygen company pay for the electricity used. It requires very little weekly maintenance, just a simple filter change once a week but it can be noisy and does require the extra room. The family health service administration (FHSA) meet the costs of this method.

Cylinders

Oxygen cylinders can be delivered on a regular basis and this costs approximately £165 a month (1996 prices) regardless of how much oxygen is used. The cost of this method is met by the GP or the hospital.

For use outside the home portable oxygen cylinders are available with both these methods. Cylinders should be stored in an outhouse or garage.

Advice on safety and care of equipment

As oxygen increases the risk of fire, it may be necessary to have central heating installed by Social Services instead of open coal, electric or gas fires. Smoking should be banned in the house while the oxygen is turned on and fire insurance policies reviewed and the company informed of the extra risk in case of accidents (Bernbaum & Hoffman-Williamson 1991). A telephone is essential to summon help and this will either be installed or checked to ensure it is in working order.

Resuscitation skills

These skills (see below) will be taught at the discretion of the neonatologist.

Discharge of a baby needing apnoea monitoring

Babies who are at risk of apnoeic attacks are often those who have chronic lung disease,

had extremely low birth weight or have a sibling that succumbed to sudden infant death syndrome (SIDS). There is a risk that repeated episodes of apnoea may lead to hypoxic brain injury (Spinner *et al.* 1995) so if the baby is considered at risk, apnoea monitoring is continued after discharge.

Timing of discharge

The baby will be discharged when feeding 3–4 hourly and gaining weight. Parents may have requested a monitor for home use if the baby has been prone to apnoeic attacks but more often home monitoring is carried out at the discretion of the neonatologist.

Learning needs will encompass use of the monitor and cardiopulmonary skills (CPR).

Learning to use the monitor

Monitoring is carried out using a machine and sensor which will detect apnoea within the first few seconds and give parents the opportunity to resuscitate the baby. There are sophisticated electronic devices on the market but these give rise to safety concerns such as power cuts, sibling curiosity or electrical faults (Spinner *et al.* 1995). The easiest monitors to manage at home are the small battery types with a lead and sensor which can be placed in the cot or pram. The sensor is attached to the baby's lower abdomen under clothing in a position that picks up all respirations and set to ring 20 seconds after the last breath. The monitor itself should not be covered with clothes as this will mute the alarm. Battery checks must be made daily and every alarm call attended even when the baby is obviously breathing as the monitor may have become detached or the battery may be low.

During the first few weeks at home the alarm may ring a few times during the night.

This may be because the baby sleeps more heavily due to the lack of noise and takes shallow breaths which do not register. The sensor can be moved until a place on the abdomen is found that picks up shallow breathing.

When the baby first goes home the monitor must be used at all times. As the baby grows and sleep time diminishes this can be adjusted to when the baby is asleep or unattended. At home, life may be totally disrupted as there is always the fear that the alarm will not be heard. This makes normal activities for the parents such as showering or cooking a meal, a problem. Commercial baby alarms could be set up in bathroom or kitchen if this helps.

CPR skills

Parents are taught cardiopulmonary resuscitation (CPR) skills (Bruce 1995) in case the baby is found apnoeic.

First the mouth must be cleared of vomit or mucus and this itself may cause the baby to restart breathing, if not a few sharp pats can be given on the back being careful not to shake or injure. If this does not restart breathing the emergency services should be contacted and resuscitation begun while awaiting their arrival. Ideally two people should carry this out.

The baby is placed supine, on a firm surface, with the chin supported and neck extended, one person will inhale, cover the baby's nose and mouth with their mouth and blow gently while watching to see if the chest inflates. Ten breaths can be given with 2 to 3 seconds between each, removing the mouth with each breath. If respirations have still not recommenced, the pulse in the groin or neck should be checked. If this beats in the region of 60 a minute, heart massage will not be necessary. But if it is very slow or absent then chest compressions should begin (Chapter 8).

After every 30 seconds during resuscitation, the pulse should be checked. Resuscitation is continued until the ambulance crew arrive. If recovery occurs before then, the baby is wrapped warmly, nursed in the side position. He/she should not be left unattended and needs to go to the hospital for a check up.

Discharge of a baby needing nasogastric feeding

Babies who are slow to feed or unable to take sufficient nutrition by sucking can be discharged weeks earlier if parents are taught how to give nasogastric feeds. These babies include very preterm babies, those with cerebral impairment or congenital abnormalities.

Timing of discharge

Discharge planning begins when the baby is feeding 3-hourly and may be able to take a proportion of feed by bottle or breast. The baby's condition will be stable with a steady weight gain. Parents will understand the need for nasogastric feeding and see the necessity for continuing.

Learning needs encompass measuring and passing tubes and giving the feed.

Passing the nasogastric tube

The baby is measured from the tip of the sternum to the bridge of the nose and across to the top of the ear. When the tube is passed through the nose to this length it will be in the stomach. Ideally the tube should be replaced in the same nostril, as the trauma and rubbing of the tube can erode the nares causing narrowing and blocking (Kelnar *et al.* 1995).

The tube is passed up into the nostril then downwards into the stomach gently but quickly. It is impossible to pass the tube when the baby is screaming so wait until the baby is calm. To check that it is in the stomach, a small amount of fluid is withdrawn by syringe and tested for an acid reaction with blue litmus paper. Some babies on long term tube feeding get sore cheeks so for skin protection a plastic dressing such as Comfeel can be used under the tube before securing it.

Administering the feed

Equipment used for tube feeding must be sterile as for bottle feeding. The tube is checked with litmus paper, to ensure it is in the stomach, before each feed. Before starting the feed the tube must be well secured and the baby comfortable and calm, or being cuddled.

The feed is poured into a 50 ml syringe or other type of funnel for the purpose, which may be held or balanced on a holder. The feed may need a slight push with the syringe barrel to start but should never be syringed in quickly as this may cause vomiting or reflux. The baby must not be left unattended during a tube feed as milk inhalation or asphyxia could occur if the tube becomes displaced. If there is vomiting during the feed, it should be stopped and the baby given a short rest before continuing.

When to give breast/bottle feeds

Weaning the baby to all breast or bottle feeds can be frustrating and time consuming. When bottle or breast feeds are being given as part of the regime, any feed left in the bottle at the end must be given through the tube so that the baby will gain weight. This is important as exhausting the baby by insisting on too long at the breast or bottle may result in a poor weight gain and failure to thrive.

Discharge of a baby on gastrostomy feeding

If a baby has a condition affecting the upper intestinal tract that precludes normal oral feeding, a gastrostomy, an opening into the stomach, may be performed. There may be an oesophageal defect, vomiting and reflux problems, an inability to suck or swallow due to neurological or congenital problems or intestinal malabsorption causing nutritional problems.

Timing of discharge

The baby will be discharged when temperature and vital signs are stable, 3-hourly feeds are tolerated with a steady weight gain, and parents feel confident and safe giving the gastrostomy feeds.

Learning needs will encompass care of the gastrostomy site, skin care, displacement of tube, method of giving the feed and general handling.

Care of the stoma

The stoma is different from a colostomy/ileostomy in that it does not protrude. It is an opening in the abdominal wall to the stomach into which a catheter is placed and used for feeding purposes. The area must be kept clean and dry to prevent infection, washing with mild soap and water and gentle drying is sufficient. If the skin becomes sore, this may be due to stomach acids, which excoriate the skin, and cleaning needs to be carried out more frequently. Barrier cream or plastic dressing can be used as a protection.

If there is a discharge around the gastrostomy tube medical advice should be sought as there may be an infection requiring antibiotics. Bleeding may occur around the stoma which can be treated by direct pressure but if bleeding persists it may be due to hypertrophic granulation tissue around the edges of the stoma that needs to be cauterised (Bernbaum & Hoffman-Williamson 1991).

Leakage of stomach contents can be a problem caused by a gradual enlargement of the stoma from the action of the gastrostomy tube. Taping the tube at a 90° angle from the skin so that there is no gap around the stoma, may help prevent this happening. If leaking persists, the baby may have to be readmitted and the tube removed for a few hours to allow healing and contraction of the edges before repassing the same size tube.

Displacement of tube

There are different types of gastrostomy tube depending on the internal apparatus to prevent the tube falling out; some have a mushroom shape others a balloon. Later on these may be replaced with a button catheter that has an antireflux valve to prevent leakage.

The length of external tubing should be measured daily as if the length has decreased the tube may have migrated to the small bowel which could lead to diarrhoea or vomiting. The tube can be pulled gently back to its original length. If this cannot be done with gentle pressure medical help should be sought.

Babies often inadvertently pull at the tube and remove it. A balloon type gastrostomy tube can easily be put back at home, but other types must be replaced by a surgeon. All types should be renewed within 24 hours of removal to prevent the stoma closing.

Method of giving feed

Feeds are made up in the usual way and all equipment must be kept sterile. The baby should be comfortable, calm and preferably lying down to facilitate the passage of the feed without leakage. The feed is usually given through a syringe or funnel which is attached to the tube. Milk is poured into the syringe or funnel and left to run into the baby's stomach. If the baby struggles or cries, the feed will not go down and may bubble over the top. Nonnutritive sucking in the form of a dummy may help by letting the baby associate sucking with a feeling of fullness, a dummy also helps to keep the mouth clean and assist buccal muscle development. After the feed it is important to put the spigot firmly back on the end of the gastrostomy tube to prevent spillage.

General handling

The baby can be bathed normally, there is no fear of soapy water getting into the stomach. Dressing the baby in a one piece outfit prevents pulling on the tube. The baby can be taken out and handled normally.

Discharge of a baby on intravenous nutrition

Babies are discharged on total parenteral nutrition (TPN) if they have a gastrointestinal problem that causes serious malabsorption. This may have resulted from surgery for necrotising enterocolitis leaving a short intestine, congenital obstructions, intestinal anomalies or congenital gut stasis (Wise 1992). Intravenous nutrition is given through a central venous line cannulated by a catheter such as a Hickman or Broviac which has been inserted under general anaesthetic.

Timing of discharge

Discharge will take place when the baby's condition is stable with a satisfactory weight gain on the feeding regime. Discharge planning will begin several weeks before the event to allow parents to become experienced with the complex skill of managing a central line.

Learning needs will encompass safety and hygiene when dealing with fluid bags and line connections, clean storage of fluids, management of the pumps to give the fluid, recognising problems with the line and surrounding skin and general handling.

Changing the bags

The fluid bags will be provided by the hospital and delivered approximately once a week. They are stored in a refrigerator in a drawer or shelf designed for the purpose.

The bag of fluid is changed daily. When there is a filter in the line the giving set may need changing only every 3–4 days. Everything that comes into contact with the equipment and bags must be clean.

Two people are needed to carry out the change with one being 'clean' and the other helping. Both wash and dry hands thoroughly. Sterile gloves may be worn by the clean person, though this depends on the hospital policy.

For a bag change, the helper clips off the giving set and detaches the bag. The clean person then attaches the new bag. When changing the whole set this must be primed with fluid from the new bag, with great care taken to eradicate air bubbles. It is vital that the line close to the baby is clipped off to prevent air being sucked into the vein when changing the set.

The bags must be covered with their dispensing dark bags at all times, whether in use or not, to prevent changes in the constituents of the fluid caused by light.

Priming the line

The baby may be allowed some hours of the day free of infusions for outings. The line is flushed with saline after stopping the infusion to clear it of fats and TPN contents, and when the solution is restarted, it is again flushed with about 2 ml of saline to check its patency. These procedures must be done in a clean or sterile manner.

Managing the machinery

An hourly volume is set on the pump and pressure readings checked frequently while the baby is having fluid. If the pressure alters substantially it could mean the line is blocking or displaced and the community team should be phoned for advice. The pumps run on battery in case mains power fails.

Redressing the site

Transparent plastic dressings are usually used and are only changed when soiled or peeling off to reduce the risk of accidental dislodgement of the line (Trotter 1996). Dressing changes are a sterile procedure and can be done after bag or set changes. Great care must be taken to prevent dislodgement of the line during dressing changes.

These lines are precious and the number of successful sites limited. Loss of the line means an admission to hospital for reinsertion under general anaesthetic. When changing the dressing the area round the catheter site is inspected for leakage, swelling, reddening or discharge and the GP or outreach team informed if this is found.

General handling

Maintaining the line is of prime concern as it is

the baby's lifeline. When bathing, the site must be kept dry to prevent infection. If the site becomes moist from any source, the dressing must be changed. Dressing the baby in a one piece suit may solve the problem of accidental removal by the baby pulling on the line.

Discharge of a baby with a colostomy or ileostomy

Babies born with a congenital abnormality such as imperforate anus, gastroschisis, exomphalos or obstruction such as Hirschsprung's disease may often be discharged with a stoma. If there has been a neonatal disease such as necrotising enterocolitis or meconium ileus, surgery may have been necessary to remove the affected area and a stoma formed to rest the intestine.

Appliances are usually fitted in the first 24 hours after surgery when the intestine starts to produce faeces. Parents are involved, as soon as possible in the care of the stoma to accustom them to meeting their baby's needs and reinforce their role as primary carers.

Timing of discharge

Discharge will be considered when the baby is feeding well, gaining weight and the parents are competent at dealing with the stoma.

Learning needs will encompass fitting the appliance, skin care, hygienic disposal of faeces and bags, observance of stoma condition and colour and monitoring stoma output.

Fitting the appliance

Plenty of time is needed for this even when well practised to make sure the appliance is comfortable and leakproof. To ensure a good fit, a template is made of the size and shape of the stoma and the appliance cut using this as a guide. The new appliance should be ready before the old one is taken off to avoid too much messy leakage from the stoma. The skin is carefully washed and dried and the stoma inspected for changes in size, colour or shape that may need medical or nursing attention.

Skin problems may occur from contact with the effluent from the bag. Skin needs to be cleaned with soap and water and barrier creams such as Coloplast cream used sparingly so as not to affect the adhesive properties of the appliance. Skin problems may also occur from the appliance itself and it may be necessary to try a different one (Black 1994).

When fitting the bag the fingers can be run around the edge of the cut hole to stretch it slightly so that the edges will shrink back when in position ensuring a snug fit around the stoma. The appliance is changed when it leaks, otherwise changes may be dependent on the amount and type of effluent. Usually 2 to 4 days can go by without changing if there is a good seal and no other problems.

Emptying the bag

Drainable bags are emptied by removing the clip, milking the contents into the nappy and then securing afterwards. Drainage is briefly examined for change in consistency or the presence of blood. For ease of handling and disposal, the bag can be emptied into the used nappy before being removed. The nappy is then wrapped in newspaper and put in a plastic bag before disposal in a dustbin. Some local authorities operate a collection service for dressings and appliances and the appliance company may provide disposal bags (Parry 1998).

Condition of stoma

The stoma normally looks pink and healthy, any change in size or colour should be reported to the stoma nurse, community nurse or doctor as soon as possible.

The stoma does not have sensory nerve endings and is therefore painless even when knocked. Problems such as bleeding following washing or a knock may often occur and quickly stop. Bleeding from inside the stoma should immediately be reported to the doctor.

If the stoma protrudes more during coughing or crying and does not return to its normal position it may have prolapsed and need surgical revision. A different size stoma bag may be needed when this happens until the problem is dealt with. The stoma may retract as the baby grows making the bag difficult to apply, surgical revision may be the only solution.

Problems

Diarrhoea

Babies with diarrhoea, especially those with ileostomies, quickly become dehydrated and need to be investigated by their local hospital. Sodium levels should be monitored and sodium replacements may be needed (Johnson 1992).

Some babies get diarrhoea from sugar intolerance and if this occurs may need a change of milk to one that contains pre-digested sugar, such as Pregestimil. This problem usually resolves after the stoma is resected.

Constipation

If there has been no drainage into the bag for 12–16 hours medical help should be sought as there may be an obstruction.

Obtaining supplies

Although the hospital will see that there are enough supplies for the first few days at home, an order should be given to the local pharmacy a week before discharge in case there is any delay in getting the appliances. In some cases it is possible to order directly from the suppliers.

Community support

Community support of a baby with a stoma is often given by a specialist stoma nurse who will be introduced to the parents during the baby's stay on the neonatal unit. There are organisations for parents with children with a stoma who have helpful leaflets, friendly advice and contacts for the family if needed. Families can be given these addresses for contact when they feel ready (Appendix 1).

Discharge of a baby with a tracheostomy

A tracheostomy is performed in babies to manage the upper airway in those who have needed prolonged ventilation for chronic lung disease, which has left them with malacia (softening) of trachea, larynx or bronchus. It may also be done for congenital obstruction of the upper airway which occurs in Pierre Robin syndrome and other malformations. Generally the baby will have the tracheostomy until the airway has grown sufficiently to allow adequate ventilation or a surgical correction has been made and nasal respiration is possible.

Preterm babies with a tracheostomy have a high mortality and morbidity rate owing directly to problems relating to the tracheostomy and to the underlying disease that necessitated its formation (Schlessel *et al.* 1993). It is thus important not to pressure parents towards early discharge as management of the tracheostomy is complicated and often critical (Mok & Whincup 1994). Complete commitment on the parents' part and good community support is essential to promote the survival of the baby.

Timing of discharge

The baby will usually stay in hospital for at least 10 days after the tracheostomy is performed for the stoma to mature. This ensures that there is a well established tract for easy recannulation if the tube is dislodged (Duncan *et al.* 1992). Most babies will stay in hospital for much longer while they are being stabilised for home. During this time parents will be familiarised with all aspects of care. Discharge home will be planned when the baby is gaining weight on 3 hourly feeds and the chest condition is stable. The actual discharge will take place when the parents are confident and willing to look after their baby at home, and equipment and community support are ready.

Learning needs will encompass tracheal suction, changing tubes, neck tape changes, skin care, dealing with tube obstructions and general handling advice.

Suctioning

The frequency of suction will depend on the chest secretions. As a rough guide, when the secretions sound 'rattly' or if the baby is distressed, suction is needed. The procedure must always be performed in a sterile manner to prevent chest infections. Hand washing and the use of gloves are essential and the catheter should only touch the inside of the tube.

The size of suction catheter depends on the size of tracheostomy tube. Usually a 6 Fr catheter is used for small babies and 8 Fr for large. The depth of suction will depend on the length of tube; if the catheter meets any obstruction it should be withdrawn 0.5 cm before suction is applied to prevent mucosal damage. Recommended vacuum pressure is no more than 50–100 mmHg (Young 1995) to prevent mucosal damage. Raising the pressure does not increase the volume of the secretions removed.

The whole procedure must be done quickly as it occludes the airway, causing hypoxia. Vacuum pressure must not be applied to the catheter until being removed. Secretions are inspected for any change of amount or colour that may be a sign of infection. Blood in the secretions may be due to harsh suctioning, but if it continues medical help needs to be sought to rule out granuloma, which is a growth in the trachea from tubal irritation.

A clean catheter must be connected to suction equipment at all times in case of emergency and suction equipment should be checked daily.

A humidifying filter, which fits into the tube, collects the baby's expired moisture using it to humidify inspired air and prevent secretions getting thick and sticky. Filters need to be changed 24–48 hourly, according to the manufacturer's instructions. Nebulisers are often used to keep secretions moist and free flowing.

Changing tubes

This is a traumatic procedure to learn and needs two people to do it until well practised. The tracheostomy tube is removed from the baby each day for cleaning or renewal to prevent build-up of secretions. The old tube is removed and the new one quickly inserted to prevent hypoxia as the tracheostomy channel collapses without the support of the tube. This is a sterile procedure that needs hand washing and gloves. Many tubes are disposable and just need replacing. Non-disposable tubes are soaked in sodium bicarbonate solution to loosen clinging mucus, then scrubbed and rinsed before being put to sterilise in sodium hypochlorite. The tube is then rinsed with sterile water before use. There should be at least two spare tubes ready in case of accidental dislodgement.

Changing neck tapes

Cotton tapes hold the tracheostomy tube in place and are usually threaded through the holder each side of the tube. Tapes must be kept dry to prevent chafing of the neck and need to be changed, when damp with perspiration, vomit or saliva, a few times a day. Ideally the change is done with another person helping as the baby usually wriggles and squirms and the tube could become dislodged. The tapes should not be tied too tightly as this can contribute to erosion or cellulitis of the stoma (Schessel *et al.* 1993). While the tapes are being changed, skin care of the neck and stoma can be carried out.

Skin care around stoma and neck

The skin of the neck and around the stoma is washed with warm water and mild soap and carefully dried. No powder is used because of the risk of inhalation. Protective nappy creams can be used on the neck, taking care not to get them in the stoma. A foam collar to hold the tapes can prevent chafing. There may be excoriation round the stoma from drooling, perspiration or tracheal secretions. The best prevention is to keep the area cool and dry with soft gauze pads under the flanges of the tube, which can be changed when dampened. If excoriation does occur, routine cleaning of the area can be increased and the baby positioned with the neck slightly extended when sleeping so that air will dry secretions. A topical antibiotic can be tried or the area can be covered by a plastic dressing, e.g. Comfeel, taking care not to occlude any part of the stoma.

Aspiration and obstruction

Obstruction of the tube results in cyanosis and apnoea and if it is unrelieved the baby may die. Obstructions may occur from inhaling vomit, thick or copious secretions or parts of clothing or other objects in the tube. If the baby shows signs of distress such as coughing, spluttering, changing colour or sudden floppiness quick action is needed to find and remove the cause.

Resuscitation skills

An apnoea alarm is issued on discharge and basic cardiopulmonary skills (CPR) taught (see above). The difference when doing CPR on a baby with a tracheostomy is that air has to be breathed into the tube not the nose and mouth. The baby should always be checked over in hospital after stopping breathing at home.

General handling

No fluffy garments or toys that could shed fibres into the tube must be used. High necked or close fitting clothes round the neck can obstruct the stoma. The humidifying appliance should be worn at all times to prevent thickening of the mucus. When taking the baby out, a portable suction unit with a supply of catheters is needed. The baby must never be left alone without the apnoea monitor attached and working, and someone close enough to take action if the alarm activates.

When bathing, care will be taken to prevent

water entering the tube. If there is a humidifying unit on the tube this will prevent accidental splashes. Talcum powder is never used as there is the risk of inhalation.

The baby may need to sleep in a chair or with head extended if there is vomiting, excoriation of the neck or stoma skin. People with colds are kept away and smoky atmospheres avoided to prevent irritation of the mucosa causing greater mucus production.

If the baby is prone to vomiting this can be relieved by allowing rests between suctioning and feeding, frequent winding, elevating the head of the cot, sitting in a baby chair and minimal handling after feeds. If these measures do not work and there is failure to thrive it may be necessary to refer the baby to the hospital for further assessment.

Using equipment

Portable and mains home suction machines will be provided and training given in their use and maintenance. Supplies for the tracheostomy can be obtained from pharmacists but may need to be ordered well in advance of need.

Conclusion

When any baby is discharged from the neonatal unit, the parents must be confident in the care of their baby and have access to support services such as general practitioner, health visitors, neonatal outreach nurses or a specialist team treating their baby. Support in the community will be available for families as long as the baby has a health need. Where the need is long term, the family is referred to specialist centres where their children's development will be monitored. The outreach service is an important step forward in the care, support and education of neonatal graduates and their families. Though not every neonatal unit has such a service it is to be hoped that in future this challenging and expanding role will become more widespread.

REFERENCES

Bernbaum JC, Hoffman-Williamson M. (1991) *Primary Care of the Preterm Infant*. Mosby Year Book, St Louis.

Black PK. (1994) Common problems following stoma surgery. *British Journal of Nursing*, **3** (8), 413–417.

Bruce M. (1995) Teaching parents CPR skills. *Journal of Neonatal Nursing*, **1** (3), 27–30.

Drake E. (1995) Discharge teaching needs of parents in the NICU. *Neonatal Network*, **14** (1), 49–53.

Duncan BW, Howell LJ, de Lorimer AA, Adzick AS, Harrison MR. (1992) Tracheostomy in children with emphasis on home care. *Journal of Pediatric Surgery*, **27** (4), 432–435.

Foden P. (1996) Preterm care in the community. *Neonatal Nurses Year Book*. CMA Medical Data, Cambridge.

Johnson H. (1992) Stoma care for infants, children and young people. *Paediatric Nursing*, **4**, 8–11.

Kelnar CJH, Harvey D, Simpson C. (1995) *The Sick Newborn Baby*, 3rd edn. Baillière Tindall, London.

Kurdahi Zahr L, Montijo J. (1993) The benefits of home care for sick premature infants. *Neonatal Network*, **12** (1), 33–37.

Laurie J. (1995) Family centred care. *Journal of Neonatal Nursing*, **1** (2), 11–14.

McKim E. (1993) The difficult first week at home with a premature infant. *Neonatal Network*, **12** (4), 72.

Merenstein GB, Gardner SL. (1993) *Handbook of Neonatal Care*, 3rd edn. Mosby Year Book, St Louis.

Mok Q, Whincup J. (1994) Tracheostomy in children – indications and management. *Pediatric Respiratory Medicine*, **2** (3), 15–20.

Parry A. (1998) Stoma care in neonates. *Journal of Neonatal Nursing*, **4** (1), 8–11.

Robinson TMS. (1991) Teaching parents in the NICU. *Neonatal Network*, **10** (2), 73–74.

Robinson TMS. (1994) Discharge teaching: sending babies home safely. *Neonatal Network*, **13** (5), 77–78.

Schlessel JS, Harper RG, Rappa H, Kenigsberg K, Khanna S. (1993) Tracheostomy: acute and long-term mortality and morbidity in very low birth weight premature infants. *Journal of Pediatric Surgery*, **28** (7), 873–876.

Spinner S, Gibson E, Wrobel H, Spitzer AR. (1995) Recent advances in home monitoring. *Neonatal Network*, **14** (8), 39–45.

Trotter CW. (1996) Percutaneous central venous catheter related sepsis in the neonate. *Neonatal Network*, **15** (3), 15–27.

Vecchi CJ, Vasquez L, Radin T, Johnson P. (1996) Neonatal individualised predictive pathway (NIPP). A discharge planning tool for parents. *Neonatal Network*, **15** (4), 7–13.

Wakefield J, Ford L. (1994) Nasogastric tube feeding and early discharge. *Paediatric Nursing*, **6** (9), 18–19.

Wise BV. (1992) Neonatal short bowel syndrome. *Neonatal Network*, **11** (7), 9–15.

Young J. (1995) Endotracheal suction and the intubated neonate. *Journal of Neonatal Nursing*, **1** (4), 23–28.

14

Stress in the Neonatal Unit

LEARNING OUTCOMES

After reading this chapter and studying the contents the reader will be able to:

○ Describe the way the neonatal environment stresses babies.
○ List the possible causes of stress to parents.
○ Demonstrate a knowledge of alleviating problems for parents.
○ Identify the issues causing staff stress.
○ Discuss ways in which stress to babies, parents and staff can be alleviated.

STRESS INTERACTIONS

The birth of a small sick baby affects all who are involved: the nurses who strive to ensure the survival; the parents and family trying to cope with events; and the baby – vulnerable, defenceless and often very sick.

The stress that these three groups encounter is interactive and reactive, affecting daily relationships and possibly enduring psychologically for a long time (Redshaw & Harris 1995; Orford 1996). This chapter will look at what causes such stress and how it can be mitigated.

THE STRESS OF THE BABY

Various studies (Sparshott 1991; Becker *et al.* 1993; Als *et al.* 1994) have shown that the way babies are treated in the neonatal unit directly affects their responses to their environment. By paying more attention to alleviating stress their potential development is enhanced and family relationships are improved (Becker *et al.* 1993; Als *et al.* 1994; Mouridian & Als 1994). Studies to examine the relationship between care-giving and the growth and development of sick neonates have shown that the neonatal environment is overstimulating, unpredictable and too complex for the new born baby to cope with (D'Appolito 1991; Peters 1996).

Causes of stress

The babies in the neonatal unit are often very ill from birth. They need ventilatory support, possibly surgery, many different drugs, arterial, intravenous and central venous lines inserted, chest drains positioned, lumbar punctures performed and sometimes peritoneal dialysis. They are subjected to frequent suctioning, probe removals for re-calibration, heel pricks and tube changes. Intravenous infusions are resited, often daily, stabbing and needling already bruised limbs. Babies are turned, prodded and disturbed almost every minute of the day when they are at their most vulnerable.

The baby cannot differentiate between good and bad stimuli so reacts physiologically to all stimuli in a variety of ways that can be personally damaging. Heart rate drops or speeds up, there may be apnoea and/or skin colour changes. Blood pressure rises and there are increased bowel actions. Vomiting, gagging or yawning are common signs of stress and there may be hiccoughs or sneezing (Sparshott 1991). These are all variations of the 'fight or flight' syndrome that affects humans in stressful situations. The sick baby's situation is so stressful that this uncontrolled panic state may be experienced many times a day (Sparshott 1989; Peters 1996).

The environment and incubator are unsettlingly noisy, alarms go off and loud staff voices interrupt sleep; radios play, bin lids crash down and lights are constantly bright (Fig. 14.1). The world up to now has been unpredictable and mostly unpleasant.

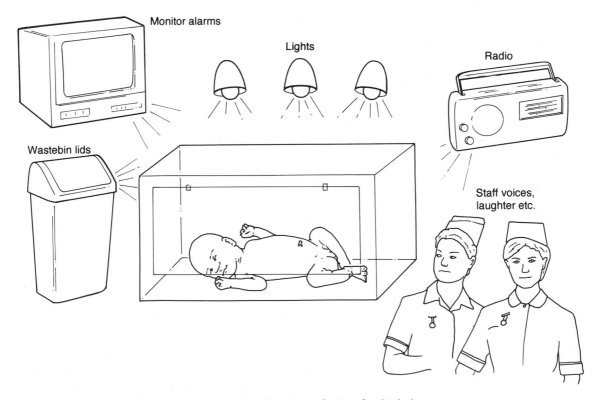

Fig. 14.1 The neonatal unit environment showing stress factors for the baby.

Coping strategies

In an attempt to self-regulate these responses the baby either becomes active, fussy and irritable or opts out by becoming limp and sleepy. These behavioural changes are made in an endeavour to shut out disrupting stimuli, changes that may cause long term harm. The baby may be awake and distressed for long periods after being disturbed, or very quiet. Babies who get distressed can be difficult to comfort and may need sedation to settle (Sparshott 1989; Peters 1996).

Results of stress

As a result of these conditions the baby's physiological and behavioural systems are not integrated. They are unable to interact with parents or provide clear clues to indicate needs – both facets of establishing a strong family relationship. If this relationship is not properly established developmental outcomes may be poor as parents are unable to understand when the baby needs comfort, food, play, cuddles or stimulation. This negative feedback tends to minimise parental interactions (Olson & Baltman 1993).

Interventions to prevent stress

The baby

Adjustments in the environment and handling often help to alleviate stress and improve behavioural reactions. Wake–sleep patterns can be observed and interventions carried out when the baby is awake. A policy of minimal handling for all but emergency procedures can be used.

Non-urgent procedures performed by doctors, X-ray technicians and physiotherapists should be carried out when the baby is awake

though this can be difficult to achieve, especially where other departments and specialities are involved and their time is limited.

If the baby has to be woken for essential non-emergency procedures, it can be done gently allowing time to come to the alert state. Pouncing on a sleeping baby with some uncomfortable activity will disrupt an already compromised sleep pattern (Slota 1988). Comfort should be offered after each painful stimulus, talking softly, patting the back or smoothing the brow. Adequate pain relief should be given if appropriate. Moving the baby's hands towards the mouth or letting the feet brace against something firm helps to comfort and establish boundaries (Sparshott 1991).

Attention paid to positioning, with a nest of sheets tucked firmly around, makes the baby feel secure. The aim should be to get the baby smoothly back to sleep without major changes in vital signs.

Environment

Noises from radios, loud voices or tapping on the incubator should be reduced. A study in a neonatal unit showed that babies startled and cried when linen bin lids slammed shut (Cote *et al.* 1991), padding of lids could solve this problem (Table 14.1).

Table 14.1 Ways of easing babies' stress.

Reduce noxious environmental effects
Ensure comfort
Good positioning and 'nesting'
Pain relief
Periods of undisrupted sleep
Non-nutritive sucking

A study done into the use of earmuffs for preterm babies showed that those who wore them had improved behavioural and physiological responses with higher oxygen saturation levels, fewer fluctuations in these and a longer time spent asleep or quiet (Zahr & de Traversay 1995).

A period when lights are dimmed helps establish sleep patterns (Weibley 1989). If this is impossible in the intensive nursery, a folded sheet or blanket could be put over the top of the incubator to shield the light (Mouridian & Als 1994).

Systems of care

In America a system of individualised developmental care for low birth weight babies has been shown to be successful in reducing adverse medical and neurodevelopmental sequelae (Als *et al.* 1994).

The programme involves observations by nurses of baseline recordings during and following care-giving. These recordings are used to gauge each baby's response to stress and to create a care plan to address needs (Tribboti & Stein 1992). It is a complex, time-consuming programme requiring extensive staff training and can be aimed at as the ideal.

Studies on preterm babies have shown that those subjected to individualised care programmes had improved neurobehavioural and motor skills compared with those who had not (Mouridian & Als 1994; Buehler *et al.* 1995).

A study in America (Tribboti & Stein 1992) showed that infants who had received a specifically designed system of care had fewer crises in the course of treatment and as a result they:

- Spent fewer days on the ventilator.
- Needed oxygen for fewer days.
- Had reduced incidence of pneumothorax.
- Had reduced incidence and severity of intraventricular haemorrhage.
- Had reduced severity of bronchopulmonary dysplasia.
- Were wholly breast fed earlier.

THE STRESS OF THE BABY'S PARENTS

The birth of any baby is a transitional stage in the parents' lives. It turns people into parents, maybe for the first time, and is a stressful event (Orford 1996).

The birth of a preterm or sick baby may precipitate a crisis as joyous hopes and plans are plunged into confusion. Many parents find their small baby and the loss of their hopes for a cuddly full term baby overwhelming. Grief reactions such as denial, anger, bargaining, depression, acceptance may occur as parents try to come to terms with their experience (Orford 1996).

Not all parents will have the same reactions but all will have had a serious psychological setback. Stress alone does not provoke a crisis situation but a prolonged level of anxiety about the baby coupled with the shock and feeling of loss can often overwhelm parents to the extent of their not being able to cope with normal life (Orford 1996).

Causes of stress

The admission of a sick baby into the neonatal unit causes emotional stress to the parents, apart from the other problems with family relationships, finance and housing that may beset them during the time their baby is in the unit. There are a number of stress factors that affect all parents (Table 14.2).

Table 14.2 Factors which cause parents' stress.

Maternal illness or diagnosed fetal abnormality
Feelings of helplessness
Fear of the baby
Fear of the unit
Being transferred to a regional unit
Problems with visiting

Maternal illness or diagnosed fetal abnormality

There may have been problems during pregnancy such as high blood pressure, diabetes, rhesus incompatibility or the diagnosis of an abnormality which caused anxiety about the health of mother and baby and outcome of delivery.

Feelings of helplessness

The helpless inevitability of birth that accompanies preterm labour may be compounded with guilt at not being able to help the baby. After the birth, parents may glimpse the baby briefly before admission to the neonatal unit and they do not know what will happen there.

Parents may feel that a chain of events has been set in motion that has taken the baby out of their control, forcing them to relinquish their role as primary care givers to medical and nursing team, leaving them powerless and frightened.

Fear of and for the baby

Parents may find difficulties in accepting their sick preterm baby. The chubby rounded baby they dreamed of is a thin, tiny scrap who cries like a kitten, making formation of a relationship difficult. The incubator is a barrier and often the baby is surrounded by equipment and covered in tubes and wires. Alarms ring, monitor readings are incomprehensible and parents may be terrified to touch the baby for fear of disturbing equipment and causing harm. Often they are frightened to come to the unit for fear of bad news. For many parents the dread of disability or death of the baby is foremost in their minds at all times (Graham 1995).

Fear of the unit

The unit itself is full of high-tech equipment and busy efficient staff, making parents feel inadequate and in the way. Doctors flood them with information, using words they do not understand, when they are shocked and frightened. These factors contribute to feelings of low esteem and lack of control of the situation (Farrell & Frost 1992).

Being transferred to a regional unit

Research has shown that a baby born very prematurely, with low birth weight or with a life-threatening disease has a greater chance of survival if delivered in a hospital with a specialist unit (Roper *et al.* 1988). But though the baby benefits from being in such a unit, the parents often feel very vulnerable as they may be far from home without the normal support network of family and friends to help them.

If the baby has to be transferred to a regional unit, it is sometimes impossible for the mother to go so soon after delivery. The father then has to visit the mother in one hospital and the baby in another. Emotional and physical stress occurs as the father commutes between the two hospitals with the possible addition of financial problems from travelling expenses and child care problems if there are other children in the family.

Problems with visiting

Many parents find the burden of visiting emotionally, financially and physically difficult. Some parents want to stay on the unit as much as possible providing the care they can. Others may be reluctant to establish a relationship with their baby in case the baby should die. A lack of confidence in providing care for their baby makes some parents reluctant visitors (Graham 1995).

It is well known that many families with sick or preterm babies often come from social classes 4 and 5 (Kogan 1995, Wilcox *et al.* 1995) Visiting, for them, will be a financial burden as, if they have no transport of their own, they have to rely on friends, family, neighbours or expensive public transport.

However open the visiting is, it is not always possible for parents to stay with their baby as much as they wish. In most neonatal units parents are asked to leave when doctors' rounds or staff handovers are taking place, or for privacy for another baby and family. This may cause distress to parents who wish to stay or those whose visiting time is limited by other family commitments.

Coping strategies of the parents

Although not all parents are stressed to the same degree, many do have reactions that are not their normal way of expressing themselves. As parents are not known to the staff of the unit, it may be difficult to distinguish which is normal behaviour and which reactions are caused by the stress of the situation. It is helpful to know that certain types of reaction can be attributed to stress and then measures can be taken to alleviate the problem (Orford 1996). Stress reactions can cause physical or psychological symptoms as parents attempt to cope with their situation (Table 14.3).

Sometimes parents react with aggression and rudeness to cover up their helplessness and to seem in control. Others may be extremely quiet appearing uncaring or unaware of how sick the baby is in an attempt to protect themselves emotionally. Some may attempt to suspend their feelings in case the baby dies (Orford 1996). Some react by talking incessantly and being hyperactive. They may rush around redecorating the house, busying themselves with life outside the unit, anything

Table 14.3 Common anxiety reactions of stressed parents.

Reaction	Manifestation
Unusual behaviour	Aggression, rudeness
Quiet and withdrawn	Appear uncaring
Talking incessantly	Hyperactive, shutting out the situation
Frightened	Anxious, tearful, nervous
Physical symptoms	Feeling cold Indigestion Irregular breathing

to avoid dwelling on the baby. Some parents will not leave their baby in case anything happens This may lead to other family members being neglected.

There may be problems between the parents. Perhaps they are not able to talk about their emotions, possibly to protect the other. This may lead to estrangement as each thinks the other uncaring.

Some parents are very tearful and sad the whole time their baby is in the unit and have difficulty seeing any hope. Others will have vague symptoms of illness such as headaches, shivering, indigestion, breathlessness and poor sleep.

Fathers' problems

Fathers often have to break the news to the rest of the family that the baby is ill. They will be worried about their partner, the baby and problems at home. Those in employment may have to arrange leave for themselves or risk losing a precious job. There may be arrangements to be made for other children to be looked after. Problems within the extended family may arise if the couple are unmarried or if either side does not approve of the relationship.

Fathers usually are the main support for the family and have to ignore their own needs to grieve. In the mostly female environment in which his partner and the baby are nursed the father may find increasing difficulty in expressing feelings and may appear aggressive and rude as a result.

Results of parental stress

If parental stress is not alleviated it may reach crisis point. At this stage parents often act out of character as they struggle with the different emotions produced by their situation.

Emotional or financial problems that are already within the family often seem to surface at this time (Orford 1996). Parents can make life difficult and miserable for themselves and the staff on the unit by becoming hostile and unco-operative with each other and not coping with their own needs or those of the baby.

Interventions to relieve the stress of parents

The delivery of a small baby is a significant and often traumatic event in family life. A visit from a member of the neonatal team when the mother is in the labour ward helps foster a positive attitude towards the outcome of labour and the understanding attitude of the staff. Parents will realise that their baby is expected to live, will be cared for and that they are important as parents. If there is to be a planned delivery a visit can be arranged to see the unit and meet staff beforehand.

After the birth, a warm welcome on the first visit will help put them at ease. A friendly attitude with information carefully given and questions answered openly allows opportunities for parents to express themselves. An early interview with the doctor who is treating the baby is essential. Parents often remember this first talk with the medical staff for a long time, and some phrases will be engraved on their minds forever (Jupp 1992).

Nursing support for parents is essential during the early days when everything is a blur of shock, bewilderment and fear. Parents feel vulnerable and rely on the confident authority of the medical staff for reassurance (Farrell & Frost 1992). Good communication with parents is essential to promote their confidence as parents. The aim should be to empower them as much as possible. From the start they should be involved in the care of their baby and in any decisions made about treatment. Mothers will be encouraged to express their milk for the baby, even if they are not going to breast feed in the long term. A photograph of the baby for the mother is essential (Graham 1995). The aim is to increase parents' morale and enable them to feel accepted and empowered. An informative and friendly attitude on the part of the staff enables the parents to start working through their stress and grief (Farrell & Frost 1992).

Family-centred care is vital as the baby will eventually take a place in the extended family. Grandparents are often main supporters and are grateful to be involved. The mother may be a single parent and her parents are the main financial and emotional supporters. Siblings are made welcome in the unit and encouraged to enjoy the baby. Brothers, sisters and relatives of the parents as well as friends, are welcomed.

Visiting should always be open for parents and their families but there are times when they may be asked to leave the unit. Asking visitors to leave during doctors' rounds and nursing handovers is a contentious issue and sometimes lead to the suspicion that the parents are not being given all the information on their baby's condition (LaMontagne & Pawlak 1990). Confidentiality of the other babies has to be preserved and in open intensive care units there is no way of preventing parents overhearing details of other cases.

For those parents who need it, accommodation should be available. Parents with financial difficulties may be eligible for help from social workers. Social workers can often help with other problems such as poor or non-existent housing or with difficult family relationships.

Support groups and counsellors

Nurses and medical staff have always been traditional supporters. They are still seen as the most important source of information and reassurance (Affonso *et al.* 1992). Support by other parents also has its place and often occurs informally among parents with babies on the unit.

There may be a support group on the unit set up by another parent or the nursing staff. These groups often have the advantage of having fathers among their members. Neonatal units and maternity wards are female dominated and fathers may be glad to talk to a man who has had a similar experience. Not all parents feel the need for or welcome this kind of support and some may resent it, feeling they can cope alone (Yeo 1994). Often the unit will have addresses of parents or groups dealing with special conditions. These can be given, to be contacted later, to those who are not yet ready for this kind of help. Choosing the right time to introduce the parents to support groups is important as different families will have different needs. The nurse looking after the baby can usually judge if the parents have such a need.

Stress changes people and parents of sick babies are not the same as they were before the delivery and admission of their baby (Orford 1996). Their life plans have gone astray at a very vulnerable time. Often they hide psychological problems from the staff and think that they will not be able to help. Some units have a counsellor trained in parent support who can encourage the parents to look at their experiences and come to terms with them. Where no counsellor is available on the unit a referral to a counselling service can be offered if it appears to be needed.

Effects of the stressed baby on stressed parents

Even when parents get used to having their baby in the neonatal unit, they will still be anxious. Many of these babies do not have a smooth course through the unit and often, just when they seem to be making good progress, they have an infection that causes a set-back. The parents thus feel they can never completely relax. The nurse has to maintain open communication at all times and work with the parents towards their baby's discharge.

Babies who have been in neonatal units have been shown to have a high risk of behavioural problems in childhood (Olson & Baltman 1993). This is thought to be partly due to the tension that parents feel with the baby, which creates a barrier between them that is never wholly overcome. Also parents may try to compensate by becoming over anxious or having unrealistic ideas about the baby's progress.

From the time of admission parents should be encouraged to begin looking after their baby. Small tasks such as changing the nappy and mouth care are introduced gradually to suit the parents' abilities.

Sometimes because of the responses of the baby, such as bradycardia or cyanosis which causes monitors to alarm, parents get disheartened. They become afraid of causing this disturbance and distance themselves physically and emotionally. Some parents overhandle their baby in a determined effort to overcome this problem. Both reactions cause anxiety and tenseness in the relationship (Graham 1995).

It is difficult for parents to know how to treat their baby, they cannot interact or stimulate their baby if there is no recognisable response. Parents have been shown to interact much more with babies who are active and responsive (Olson & Baltman 1993) than with their quiet or irritable, still or fussy, sick neonates. This leads to a vicious circle for the relationship. The baby does not evoke the usual responses, so the parents tend not to interact with the baby and if responses do not improve a difficult relationship ensues. Difficulties in behaviour, irritability and feeding problems are then more common. There is then a greater likelihood of readmission with feeding problems or failure to thrive.

How parents can interact with their stressed baby

They can be helped to observe signs that mean their baby is ready to interact with them. This is when the baby is relaxed and comfortable, eyes open, intent and alert, head and eyes turning to sounds and movements smooth and calm. There might be attempts to get a thumb or hand in the mouth and colour will be even with calm breathing (Sparshott 1991).

Parents can be encouraged to talk or sing with their face about 25 cm (10 inches) away. This is the ideal field of vision for new-born babies and the distance at which they are held for breast feeding. The baby should be held firmly, but not tightly, and not moved suddenly. Soft toys that can be grasped, bright designs for the cot or musical lullaby toys are all enjoyed by parents and babies.

When the baby starts crying or is not responding, gentle talking in a soft voice can help or holding the baby's hands together or giving a finger to grasp. If these actions fail the baby should be returned to cot or incubator. Most babies have a preferred position, most like being tucked into a blanket. If parents wish they can keep a record of their baby's behaviour so that they get to know reactions and preferences.

There may not appear to be a great deal of

success at first but preterm neonates improve as their nervous systems mature (Weibley 1989) and with patience their responses will be strong enough to evoke a good parental relationship.

Kangaroo care has been shown to be comforting to mothers and beneficial to their babies. It involves placing the nappy-clad baby upright between the mother's breasts for skin-to-skin contact (Luddington-Hoe *et al.* 1994). Results show that apnoea and periodic breathing stop for the duration of this care. Babies nursed this way should be relatively well, stable and should have had breathing tubes removed at least 24 hours previously.

Nurses' role in relieving stress between parents and baby

The neonatal nurse takes a major role in promoting good family relationships from admission to discharge by giving parents confidence to acknowledge their anxiety and negotiating ways they can learn to take care of their baby. The nurse will teach the skills needed if the baby has special needs and show the parents how to recognise stress signs in their baby and themselves.

The mother makes an important emotional and physical commitment when she agrees to express breast milk, and later breast feeding, which gives a proactive outlook for her. The pleasure and excitement parents have over every new development, such as transfer out of the intensive care room, or transfer from cot to incubator, will be shared by staff.

First bath and bottle feeds should be given by parents or at least watched by them. A plan can be made of the baby's daily needs and parents are encouraged to write the times they will visit and carry them out. Some parents of long-stay babies can be encouraged to write a diary of their baby's stay. If they live some distance from the hospital and cannot visit every day, the staff can write in the diary for them.

A friendly and welcoming attitude is essential for good communications to take place. Parents should feel as soon as possible that they have control over their baby and that staff will always listen to problems and help work through them (Callery & Smith 1991).

THE STRESS OF NEONATAL STAFF

Stress is a common feature of many job situations but those working in hospital environments seem more vulnerable due to the nature of work undertaken. Over the last decade neonatal nurses have needed an ever increasing technical knowledge and clinical expertise to keep pace with research developments in the neonatal field. They have also had to develop skills to address the psychosocial needs of families and the ability to cope with the ethical issues inherent in saving babies at the edge of viability. Staff on neonatal intensive care units work in complex settings where there is a constant threat of crisis.

Causes of staff stress

There are a number of factors that cause stress to the staff of the neonatal unit (Table 14.4).

Shortage of staff and poor skill mix

A major stress factor for neonatal nurses is the ever increasing workload of very sick babies requiring more complicated technical care. This often has to be done with limited staff, resources and equipment. A 4-year study carried out by the Department of Health into

---

Table 14.4 Causes of staff stress.

Shortage of staff and poor skill mix
Taking on other roles, counsellor, technician
Ethics of treating sick babies
High death rate of babies
Accepting more babies than unit capacity
Dealing with relatives

---

nurse stress and staffing in 56 neonatal units in England found that stress levels were often directly related to staff shortages and that most units did not have the staffing levels recommended in various reports from the Department of Health issued between 1971 and 1992 (Redshaw *et al.* 1996). This report found that the staffing skill mix was often unsatisfactory and many units were taking more intensive care patients than their funds allowed (Redshaw *et al.* 1996).

Skill mix refers to the experience and skill of staff within different grades. It is an important factor in the neonatal unit where there are many learners and grades of staff, from nursery nurses to the clinical nurse specialist (Dunbar 1995). Nurses rely greatly on support from each other and if there are too many inexperienced staff working particular shifts, the stress level rises as there is no one to turn to for help with difficult decisions.

Taking on other roles

Nurses are often expected to take on time-consuming roles for which they may not have received training, for example taking bloods, dealing with computers, budgeting, ordering, auditing, counselling. The reduction in junior doctors' hours and the altered functioning of technical departments mean that nurses' roles are changing in the clinical area and there is pressure to take on tasks that used to be the province of other specialities. There is not always adequate training given for these extra tasks or recognition of the time and effort needed. If something goes wrong blame may be too easily apportioned to the nurse (Redshaw & Harris 1995).

Some trusts run courses to educate nurses for the role of advanced neonatal nurse practitioner (ANNP). On these courses experienced neonatal nurses are taught to perform tasks that are normally done by a junior doctor. However the UKCC code of conduct for nurses is much less forgiving than those rules for practice imposed on doctors, so that those taking on these extended roles need to be aware of their accountability as nurses. It can also be said that this extended role takes nurses out of 'nursing' as the advanced practitioner's role is to provide immediate and direct care and, once the baby is stabilised, to hand over care to an 'ordinary' nurse (Doherty 1996). The major advantage of the ANNP is that, whereas junior doctors normally rotate on a 6-monthly basis, the ANNP stays so that the level of skilled care is maintained. This makes the role of the ANNP valuable and essential, and one that will surely become more common in neonatal units.

Ethics of saving small and malformed babies

Today's technology permits the saving of very small and early gestation babies. These babies often have residual serious handicaps which cast doubts on the technology involved in their survival and raise questions as to the morality of such treatment (Chapter 16). The mortality rate is high among these babies and the cost in terms of finance, staff and family emotional trauma is high.

Regional units have seriously ill and malformed babies referred from other hospitals and have to make decisions about their treatment. The cost of treating these babies is very high and requires a multidisciplinary approach, skilled doctors, specialised equipment and experienced, qualified nursing staff capable of providing the complicated care. Often these babies die, or if they live their quality of life may be poor, raising ethical questions about treatment. Morale may be low if nurses are not involved in team decisions and feel strongly about certain ethical aspects.

High death rate of babies

There is always a high death rate on neonatal intensive care units owing to congenital birth defects, complicated deliveries and very low birth weight babies. The emotional toll on nurses is great as they support families through the grief process many times a year.

Taking on more babies than funds allow

Excessive workload and understaffing are potential stress factors. For individual nurses these are a prime concern and a central issue in their working lives (Redshaw *et al.* 1996). Taking on more intensive babies than the unit is funded for often means that nurses feel they cannot give the best care possible.

Job satisfaction is low and there is the constant worry that in the rush mistakes will be made or something important overlooked. Sometimes a busy or stressful shift is relived over and over in a futile attempt to find possible errors.

A survey into the neonatal unit as a working environment in England discovered that more than half of the nurses employed had worked extra shifts to provide staff cover for the unit. Nursing shortages were typically responded to in this short term fashion causing the existing staff more stress-related problems (Redshaw *et al.* 1996).

Dealing with relatives

Parents and their relatives are under stress and may see nurses as not doing enough for the baby. Conflicts can arise over, for example visiting – if parents wish to be with the baby constantly and unit policy requires them to leave during doctors' rounds and nursing handovers. If relatives are rude or insulting nurses have to remain calm and politely professional whereas they may feel like reacting differently (Farrington 1997). If there is a personality clash with a family, especially if the baby is likely to be a long term patient, staff will get stressed dealing with the family over the length of the baby's stay.

Poor coping strategies

The traditional way nurses have always dealt with stress is to turn to each other. Bottled up emotions are often defused by exploding to friends and talking over problems. In these days of shortened breaks and heavy work load there is often no time for this. When staff have no means of release they tend to become tense and have an adverse coping reaction that could affect all aspects of their lives. This is sometimes referred to as 'burn-out'.

The burn-out victim is exhausted on all levels – physical, emotional and attitudinal. Some nurses turn to habits injurious to their long term health such as excessive coffee drinking, smoking or alcohol. These may have short term benefits in that they promote relaxation at first but continued use leads to more extravagant consumption and health problems.

Some stressed nurses find even a mild illness in themselves too difficult to overcome adding to higher sickness rates on the neonatal unit.

Results of stress

The physiological link between stress and illness is in the activation of the adrenal glands by the pituitary and hypothalamus. This is clearly indicated by the flight or fight reaction to emergencies. Rises in adrenaline level result in obvious symptoms – raised heart rate and blood pressure, rapid breathing, fluttering in the stomach – a natural response to help the person cope in emergencies. However, repeated rises in the adrenaline level put enormous strain on the cardiovascular system and immune function. The responses can be sustained long after the trauma by the person continuing to dwell on the event (Roger & Nash 1995b). By reliving events, these feelings are reproduced time and time again evoking the stress response each time.

Stress is a threat to mental and physical health. The sickness rates increase and there is unnecessary staff wastage. There may be 'burn-out' where the staff become apathetic, lose confidence in themselves and cannot give of their best (Astbury & Yu 1982). Some have sleep problems leading to permanent fatigue and some staff are constantly angry, irritable and difficult to work with or apathetic and unmotivated. In extreme cases stress can lead to suicide (Roger & Nash 1995b).

Personality and stress

Stress is determined by the way an event elicits a response and can be the result of preoccupation with emotional upset. Events are not in themselves stressful but act as a focus about which to feel anxious. It is the way of thinking about the event and the process in the mind that causes the stress. The personality often affects the manner in which this is handled (Roger & Nash 1995b).

Some nurses are highly motivated to achieve but have a low self-esteem and cope badly with stress as they dwell on their own failures. Nurses with higher self-esteem will take the situation in their stride and ascribe it to an 'off day' or an extrinsic factor such as staffing levels, not to a total failure of their capabilities. These are the people that cope best with stress as they can rationalise it.

It has been found that the way some nurses deal with the situations that arise can actually cause more anxiety (Roger & Nash 1995b). The personality and self-esteem of the person can influence the emotional mechanism that leads to stress.

Interventions to help deal with staff stress

Many units acknowledge that stress affects their staff and organise staff support meetings where everyone can air their views. There may be a member of staff trained to support parents and staff on the unit or a counselling service that offers help. Some units have a strong social life with outings and breaks together to foster a supportive and protective attitude that helps staff feel able to relax. This helps staff to 'off-load' stress to each other in a friendly supportive atmosphere (Farrington 1997).

Attention by ward managers to ensure a good skill mix is of considerable practical use. In-service training of inexperienced staff builds their confidence to deal with stressful situations. Monitoring the workload of neonatal staff is needed (Dunbar 1995) to ensure the unit and its resources are not dangerously overloaded. Staff undertaking new roles should get adequate training (Table 14.5).

New staff need to be initiated carefully into the work of the unit to cut down on losses due

Table 14.5 Measures to counteract staff stress.

Good skill mix
Monitoring workload
In-service training of new staff
Support for those undertaking new roles
Clinical supervision
Networking with other colleagues
Classroom teaching about stress
Reflective practice
Supportive unit atmosphere
Staff counsellor
Social life

to inability to cope. Many nurses coming into the neonatal unit will never have seen small babies or the technology needed. A mentor from among the experienced staff can help them over those first exacting months. Ongoing clinical supervision of all grades of nurses allows discussion and development of roles and exploration of the boundaries of their practice and involvement in decision making (Derbyshire 1997).

Classroom and ward teaching can help nurses recognise the effects of stress and networking with other colleagues outside the unit in organisations such as the Neonatal Nurses Association allows exchange of ideas and views as well as professional updating. Reflective practice is a good way of looking at a situation in a more positive way. Valuable lessons can be learnt for handling the next occasion without dwelling on the adverse emotional effects.

It is often difficult for staff to acknowledge their own stress or even recognise it. If they are seen to be unable to cope with the work, they may incur career damage, and so they struggle on. Recognising stress in oneself and in others can be the greatest help in combating it. The neonatal unit is a stressful place to work for many reasons and nothing will change that. The effects can only be mitigated by careful attention to the known stress factors by nurses and their managers (Dunbar 1995).

REFERENCES

Affonso DD, Mayberry LJ, Hurst I, Haller L, Lynch ME, Yost K. (1992) Stressors reported by mothers of hospitalised premature infants. *Neonatal Network*, **11** (6), 63–70.

Als H, Lawhon G, Duffy FH. (1994) Individualised developmental care for the very low birthweight preterm infant. *JAMA*, **272** (11), 853–858.

Astbury J, Yu VYH. (1982) Determinants for stress for staff in a neonatal intensive care unit. *Archives of Disease in Childhood*, **5** (7), 108–111.

Becker PT, Grunwald PC, Moorman J. (1993) Effects of developmental care on behavioral organization in very low birth weight infants. *Nursing Research*, **42** (4), 214–220.

Buehler DM, Als H, Duffy FH *et al.* (1995) Effectiveness of individualised developmental care for low risk pre-term infants. *Pediatrics*, **96** (5, 1), 923–932.

Callery P, Smith L. (1991) A study of role negotiation between nurses and the parents of hospitalised children. *Journal of Advanced Nursing*, **16**, 772–781.

Cote JJ, Morse JM, James SG. (1991) The pain response of the post operative newborn. *Journal of Advanced Nursing*, **16**, 378–387.

D'Appolito K. (1991) What is an organised infant. *Neonatal Network*, **10** (1), 23–29.

Derbyshire F. (1997) Implementing clinical supervision in a neonatal unit. *Journal of Neonatal Nursing*, **3** (1), 8–9.

Doherty L. (1996) The advanced neonatal nurse practitioner. *Journal of Neonatal Nursing*, **2** (4), 23–28.

Dunbar CP. (1995) Quality within neonatal nursing; getting the skill mix right. *Journal of Neonatal Nursing*, **1** (5), 19–22.

Farrell MF, Frost C. (1992) The most important

needs of parents of critically ill children. *Intensive and Critical Care Nursing*, **8**, 130–139.

Farrington A. (1997) Strategies for reducing stress and burnout in nursing. *British Journal of Nursing*, **6** (1), 44–50.

Graham S. (1995) Psychological needs of families with babies in the neonatal unit. *Journal of Neonatal Nursing*, **1** (5), 15–18.

Jupp S. (1992) *Making the Right Start.* pp. 9–12. An Opened Eye Publication, Cheshire.

Kogan MD. (1995) Social causes of low birth weight. *Journal of the Royal Society of Medicine*, **88** (11), 611–615.

LaMontagne LL, Pawlak R. (1990) Stress and coping of parents of children in paediatric intensive care. *Heart and Lung*, **19** (4), 416–421.

Luddington-Hoe SM, Thompson C, Swinth J, Hadeed AJ, Anderson GC. (1994) Kangaroo care. Research results and practice implications and guidelines. *Neonatal Network*, **13** (1), 19–27.

Mouradian LE, Als H. (1994) The influence of NICU caregiving practices on motor functioning of preterm infants. *American Journal of Occupational Therapy*, **48** (6), 527–533.

Olson JA, Baltman K. (1993) Infant mental health in occupational therapy practice in the neonatal intensive care unit. *American Journal of Occupational Therapy*, **48** (6), 499–504.

Orford T. (1996) Psychological support for parents whose children require neonatal intensive care. *Journal of Neonatal Nursing*, **2** (1), 11–13.

Peters KL. (1996) Selected physiologic and behavioral responses of the critically ill premature neonate to a routine nursing intervention. *Neonatal Network*, **15** (1), 74.

Redshaw M, Harris A. (1995) Quality and quantity: staffing and skill mix in neonatal care. *Nursing Times*, **91** (27), 29–31.

Redshaw M, Harris A, Ingram JC. (1996) *Delivering Neonatal Care*. pp. 196–200. HMSO, London.

Roger D, Nash P. (1995a) A threat to health. *Nursing Times*, **91** (22), 27–29.

Roger D, Nash P. (1995b) Cracking points. *Nursing Times*, **91** (25), 44–45.

Roper LP, Chiswick MI, Sims DG. (1988) Referrals to a regional neonatal unit. *Archives of Disease in Childhood*, **63**, 403–407.

Slota M. (1988) Implications of sleep deprivation in the pediatric intensive care unit. *Focus on Critical Care*, **15** (3), 35–44.

Sparshott M. (1989) Minimising the discomfort of newborns. *Nursing Times*, **85** (42), 39–42.

Sparshott M. (1991) *This is Your Baby*. South Western Regional Health Authority Printing Department, Plymouth.

Tribotti S, Stein M. (1992) Implementing the NIDCAP. *Neonatal Network*, **11** (2), 35–40.

Weibley T. (1989) Inside the incubator. *American Journal of Maternal Child Nursing*, **14** (2), 96–100.

Wilcox MA, Smith SJ, Johnson IR, *et al.* (1995) The effect of social deprivation on birthweight excluding physiological and pathological effects. *British Journal of Obstetrics and Gynaecology*, **102** (11), 918–924.

Yeo H. (1994) Support from people who know. *Child Health*, **2** (1), 32–35.

Zahr LK, de Traversay J. (1995) Premature infant responses to noise reduction by earmuffs: effects of behavioral and physiologic measures. *Journal of Perinatology*, **15** (6), 448–455.

15 | Transcultural Nursing in the Neonatal Unit

LEARNING OUTCOMES

When this chapter has been read and the contents studied the reader should be able to:

○ Compare the problems faced by racial minority families with those of other families in the neonatal unit.
○ Identify the particular needs of such families.
○ Describe the way direct and indirect racial discrimination can work.
○ List the ways in which nurses can improve the service given.

THE BABY FROM A RACIAL MINORITY FAMILY

The birth of a sick baby causes a major psychological upheaval for parents. They have to come to terms with the loss of their dreams and expectations for the baby and face the reality of the neonatal intensive care unit (NICU). They go through a variety of emotions akin to grieving as they come to terms with their small, fragile baby. Neonatal nurses use many resources to help and support parents at this time.

When the parents come from a different racial background from the prevailing one, there can be perceived or actual difficulties that lead nursing staff to believe that these parents do not need, deserve or want the usual help. These difficulties encompass racial discrimination, cultural differences, language problems and racial stereotyping. Research has proved that when help and support is offered by nurses it is welcomed and improves the outcome for parents and baby (Sen 1996).

This chapter will attempt to examine the difficulties multiracial families and nurses face when interacting in the neonatal unit.

Current health care policy

The National Health Service was set up to provide a comprehensive range of health services for everyone on the basis of individual need. It is not discriminatory to recognise that a family from an ethnic minority might have different needs and face different problems from those of the ethnic majority. The recognition that there are significant differences in racial and ethnic groups is important in the delivery of health care.

Different groups are subject to different illnesses, for example thalassaemia in Mediterranean and Asian families; and glucose-6-phosphate dehydrogenase (G-6-PD) deficiency is an inherited condition common among people from Africa, West Indies, Mediterranean and among African Americans.

Health needs of a multiracial society

Research has shown that families from ethnic minority groups experience difficulties gaining access to appropriate and adequate health care (Richardson *et al.* 1994; Hempel 1995; Roberts *et al.* 1995). The reasons for this could be that:

- Many people have migrated to this country and find themselves financially impoverished with poor housing, unemployment, ill health and educational disadvantages. It is well known that these factors cause health problems, particularly in pregnancy (Wilcox 1995; NCH Action For Children 1995).
- Some families do not understand how to obtain good health care or may have problems finding out what is available. It is well established that poor families of whatever racial origin have difficulty

accessing appropriate health care (Mares *et al.* 1985; NCH Action For Children 1995).

These factors can be further compounded by racial prejudice and harassment (Mares *et al.* 1985).

Aspects of existing care may be culturally specific. For example hospital diets, washing and bathing facilities and chaplaincy services are geared to the needs of the indigenous Christian population. This may present problems to others whose values and normal practices are different. For example some cultures regard sitting in a bath as 'dirty' and would prefer to shower. Dietary advice given during pregnancy may not be culturally appropriate and therefore useless. Some women cannot allow examination by a male doctor for religious and cultural reasons.

Racial recognition

Ethnic origin

This is a term used to identify people who have certain cultural characteristics in common. This may be language, religion or race, which provides the group with a distinct identity. The term 'ethnic' is often used to describe black or minority racial groups even though white people also belong to an ethnic group (Mares *et al.* 1985).

Discrimination

Direct discrimination occurs when a person is given less favourable treatment on racial grounds. Racial grounds are those of colour, race, nationality, citizenship, ethnic or national origin.

Indirect discrimination happens when policies and practices unintentionally or unconsciously disadvantage a particular group of people. This is the most difficult type to perceive and prevent, as it is built into the system and accepted as unchangeable.

The Patient's Charter states that the patient has the right to be given detailed information on health services and to have access to a health service that has respect for privacy, dignity and religious and cultural beliefs (Department of Health 1995).

Cultural differences

Culture refers to the life-style of a group of people and includes the values and beliefs carried on from one generation to another. Everyone belongs to some sort of culture which includes family, religion and life-style.

Theoretically most people use three health care systems (Wenger 1993):

- The professional service provided by doctors and nurses.
- The lay system of treatments commonly shared among the public.
- Traditional care within a specific culture.

When neonatal nurses meet the families of their patients they interact and respond partly through shared values about these three systems of health and care. When background is not shared this interaction seems fraught with pitfalls for both sides. If there are added complications with language differences, the difficulties seem almost overwhelming. Often problems are explained away as cultural problems that cannot be solved. This is a culture-blind approach resulting in less effective care that is negligent to needs.

Stereotyping

Customs and religious beliefs are sometimes portrayed in the literature in a way that makes people from different cultural backgrounds seem backward or bizarre. Background information on, for example, Muslim families or Chinese culture is too generalised to be of any real help. Does 'British culture' mean Scottish, Irish, Welsh, working class, upper class? The variations between social groups within one culture are enormous and generalisations may cause stereotyping.

Everyone is judged consciously or unconsciously on the image they present and decisions are made, possibly subconsciously, on how much help will be offered to the individual concerned. This is a human trait that often leads to stereotyping of people. Stereotyping is typical and damaging, leading to false expectations and immediate barriers. An example of stereotyping was seen in a study into the delivery of maternity care to women of South Asian descent (Bowler 1993). The women were perceived to be lacking in maternal instincts because of the preference some had for male children and their reluctance to hold or feed their baby immediately after birth. Communication difficulties were regarded as the patient's fault.

Another stereotyping factor may be the expectation of language difficulties where none exist. It may be thought that information will not be understood, so it is not given.

Language difficulties

Communicating health information may be difficult if there are language difficulties. There may be stress on the part of the patient or nurse over past misunderstandings, so that even if there is no language problem, information on what is available may not be asked for or given. Most people, even from the prevailing culture, often have to be assertive and articulate before obtaining the care and information they want (Chesterton 1994).

A study published by the Royal College of

Nursing called 'The Unpopular Patient' looked at factors that might influence a nurse's care of a particular patient (Stockwell 1972) or her baby. It was seen that popular patients:

● Communicated readily.
● Knew the nurses' names.
● Laughed and joked with nurses.

Patients who were not English-speaking thus lacked the characteristics of the popular patient. This study suggests that nurses can wrongly interpret behaviour and attitude as awkward when in fact it may be due to language barriers and lack of confidence.

PROMOTING TRANSCULTURAL CARE IN THE NEONATAL UNIT

After looking at the reasons why some families have difficulties in accessing and benefitting fully from health services it is interesting to look at the neonatal unit to see how the problems affect parents and nurses there and how they can best be managed.

Studies have shown a direct link with the social status of the mother and the health of the baby (Kogan 1995; Lumme *et al.* 1995; Wilcox *et al.* 1995). As long ago as 1980 the Short Report identified perinatal and neonatal mortality among ethnic minorities as a major problem (House of Commons Social Services Committee 1979–1980). The adverse socio-economic factors that prevail for many of these families put them in a high risk group for problem births. The OPCS survey in 1995 found that the perinatal and neonatal mortality rate for babies of immigrant mothers was generally higher than those of women born in the UK. This suggests that the babies of these mothers are likely to be admitted to the neonatal unit.

For an immigrant mother, having a baby may be the first contact with the health service and she may feel very frightened, bewildered and isolated by the experience. If she has recently come from a small village in her home country, she may be homesick and be suffering from culture shock at being in a different country. Such emotional and sensory overload may cause her to appear unresponsive and uninterested.

Problems encountered

If the mother speaks little English her problems in the neonatal unit are likely to be magnified. Measures that have been developed to support parents and their baby appear useless and nurses feel they cannot give of their best. This atmosphere can lead to parents feeling ill informed, lacking in confidence and unable to take an active part in caring for their baby (Miller 1994). Teaching parents to care for their baby and giving health and safety advice as to future welfare will be difficult.

If the baby has special needs some cultures may find this more difficult to accept than others. It can reflect on their prestige in the community, the mother may be blamed or there may be guilt if the parents are first cousins. Some parents may feel they are being punished for some misdeed in a past life (Miller 1994). These facts may lead parents to refuse treatment that causes pain to the baby or will prolong the baby's life.

Communicating the baby's needs and follow-up care is difficult when the parents speak little English and many of these families may not get the support they need in the community as a result (Miller 1994).

The main aspects of transcultural care in the neonatal unit are:

- Possible difficulties with communications and language.
- The need to give culturally and religiously acceptable care.
- Helping parents come to terms with their baby's illness.
- Ensuring that all families are adequately followed up and supported in the community.
- Nurse education on how to help parents from racial minorities.

Communication and language

Parents often have a grief reaction after the baby is born especially if the baby is very small or sick. They have emotional and psychological difficulties coming to terms with their baby's illness which will not be helped by the technical aspect of the neonatal unit surroundings. Added to this, they feel their role as primary carers has been taken over by the staff of the unit. These feelings are usually talked through and information and advice given. When there are language problems the distress and difficulties of the parents are compounded.

Good communication with parents is essential to promote their confidence and to reassure them. The aim should be to empower them as much as possible and involve them in the care of the baby and discussions about treatment. Medical staff must make sure that agreement for treatment and procedures is informed consent.

Language difficulties may make parents who speak little English feel overwhelmed by helplessness and depression. They cannot express themselves to the staff and may find it difficult to judge what is best for their baby.

Interpreters

Many inner city areas use the services of link workers for pregnant women and their families who do not speak English. These workers can interpret and help families obtain the care they need. They may be available if the mother has a baby in the neonatal unit and agree to translate for the family. Finding interpreters may be difficult as there are many different languages spoken even by people of the same race. On the Indian subcontinent there are about 20 major languages with many more dialects.

In some cases the family may refuse the offer of an interpreter as this is seen as an invasion of privacy. The interpreter's role should be sensitively explained to them but if this help is refused this must be respected.

Siblings as interpreters

If the children go to school in Britain they will speak English and may act as interpreters for the family. This state of affairs is not satisfactory as the interpreter may only give information that is judged to be necessary, or the information may be very difficult to explain to a young child. Interpreting can be potentially harmful for these children, by making them assume adult reponsibility at too young an age.

Working without an interpreter

If there is no interpreter, for whatever reason, the nurse caring for the baby must take this into account and plan how to proceed when there is only a limited common language (Table 15.1).

Communication problems can be a combination of lack of confidence or fear of disapproval on both sides. The nurse caring

Table 15.1 Communicating with a limited common language.

Allow plenty of time
Encourage relaxed interaction
Give non-verbal signals, smiling, pointing
Use simple phrases repeated in the same words
Check comprehension
Give any literature available in the language

for the baby should plan what is to be taught to the mother and allow plenty of time for any interaction. A relaxed friendly atmosphere should prevail, frequent smiles help relieve the tension for everyone.

Simple words and phrases must be used, spoken slowly and clearly but not louder. Words that the family are likely to know should be used and phrases repeated using the same words. Simple unambiguous gestures can be used to help. To check if the communication has been understood, the mother can be asked to give a demonstration, where appropriate. Understanding should be checked at each step and no embarrassment shown if either side misunderstands.

Parents should not be interrupted when they speak and the nurse should carefully observe their reactions to the communication. If the parents become rude or aggressive, they may have misunderstood or taken offence. It may help to go over what has been said to find the cause of the problem.

If the parents or staff feel that there is a difficulty with the care of the baby it may be essential to obtain the services of an official interpreter.

Working with interpreters

Interpreters are needed wherever there is a limited understanding of English by the family of a baby in the neonatal unit. Even if the day-to-day care of the baby and family can be competently exercised using the above measures, it may be necessary to use an interpreter if sensitive information or informed consent to an operation or procedure is needed.

It is not easy conducting vital verbal transactions through a third party and when using an interpreter, whether an official one or a member of the family, there are pitfalls for the unwary. To help counteract these:

- It should be checked that the interpreter and the parents speak the same language or dialect. Asian people, for example, speak a variety of languages and dialects. Introduce both parties and give them time to talk together before starting.
- The interpreter should be briefed about the content of the interview/discussion and told to interrupt if necessary to clarify points.
- The staff should use straightforward, jargon free language and allow plenty of time for the interaction. Then they must listen to the interpreter and the family carefully.
- The interpreter should be asked at the end to check whether the family wish to know more.
- After the discussion the interpreter should be asked if all is well.

If the discussion is not going favourably, it may be that the interpreter is not acceptable to the family in respect of age, sex or class. There may be too much responsibility on the interpreter if he/she does not seem to be getting the intended message across. It could be that the English used is too difficult or that the family do not understand the interpreter's role.

Pictures, demonstration packs and videos in the family's language may help but these are not readily available. This is usually because of the cost of producing such material and the fact that it has to be funded by district health authorities struggling with stringent budgets (Hayes 1995).

Giving culturally and religiously acceptable care

Nurses should bear in mind that the delivery of a small baby is a very traumatic event in family life. The stress of the situation often affects the behaviour of parents causing them to be, for example, aggressive, hostile, withdrawn or talkative (Orford 1996). When the parents have a different culture and religion from the prevailing majority it is difficult for nurses to discover whether the reactions of the parents are due to psychological and emotional problems or cultural and religious ones and so the nurses are not sure how to react (Murphy & McLeod-Clark 1993).

Care plans

The nursing process encourages nursing staff to treat all patients as individuals and care plans are made to suit the individual's needs. When making a care plan for a baby with parents from an unfamiliar background discussion with the parents is even more essential. They should be consulted as to their wishes for breast feeding, visiting, family access, when they will name their baby or if they want a naming or religious ceremony.

They may want the baby to have or wear a religious symbol, for example some Muslim families like their baby to wear a specially prepared and blessed black ribbon called a *tah-weez*, just as some Catholic families like their baby to have a rosary in the incubator or cot.

If the family fasts on special days they may

not want to visit until the evening. This could cause problems with ward regulations or the establishment of breast feeding and should be discussed in a relaxed and non-judgemental way, when making care plans.

Visiting may be a problem with some families if they believe that the baby's mother should stay indoors for a few weeks after the baby is born. Other mothers may have transport only in the late evening when the father has finished work and this should be considered to prevent any problems.

To teach the parents to care for their baby effectively, neonatal nurses need to understand the role of the parents and extended family members. In some cultures the opinion of the paternal grandmother is very important in feeding practices and health care decisions so she should be involved in the teaching sessions if they are to be productive. It is important that every family receives individual help and support geared to their own needs and wishes, be they cultural, religious or customary.

Referral to Social Services

Parents in the neonatal unit often suffer from financial constraints. These may be due to housing problems, unemployment, difficulty getting benefits or educational difficulties. Many parents from the multiracial community are often not referred to the Social Services because they do not ask for referral, or do not know their rights, or because staff believe that the extended family will provide for them. This can be an erroneous assumption as often there may be no extended family if the parents have recently settled in Britain. The mother may in fact be isolated and lonely (Gatrad 1994).

The extended family may also be in financial need as many black and Asian families are known to be poor and to work in low paid jobs. Any family whose baby stays in the unit for more than a few days will probably need help with, at least, visiting. A referral to the social worker for an informal chat will help discover their needs.

Referral to other services

There is a higher incidence of handicap and learning difficulties among Asian children. This is thought to be due to the higher incidence of congenital rubella and the high rate of consanguineous marriages (Miller 1994). These are first cousin, or other near relative, marriages arranged to ensure wealth is kept within the family. It is estimated that 75% of marriages in the British Pakistani population are consanguineous. A study in 1993 showed that the offspring of consanguineous parents had a threefold increase in postnatal death and serious genetic and chronic diseases compared with all Europeans (Bundey & Alan 1993).

Support groups can be helpful to some parents and the unit should have addresses of groups dealing with special conditions. Choosing the right time to introduce the parents to such a group is important as different families will have different needs. Parents from ethnic minorities may not use such groups fearing they will not be accepted and may prefer to contact a family of the same racial and cultural background as themselves.

Nurse training in transcultural management

Racial, cultural and religious matters can arouse strong personal feelings which may have a psychological or physical bias and the hospital community is not immune to them. Doctors and nurses can exhibit negative attitudes towards ethnic minority patients which lead to suspicion and unease on both sides and an unsatisfactory provider–user relationship.

In 1990 a policy for equal opportunities and anti-racism was included in the guidelines for courses run by the English Nursing Board. The need to adopt a practice that reflected a multiracial society was emphasised. Although some institutions have made efforts to implement this policy, in general there has been little impact on professional practice (Neile 1997).

Inadequate training is given to students about understanding cultural diversities and providing effective and safe care to these groups (Papadopoulos & Alleyne 1995). Nurse education should aim to develop a set of principles that equip the nurse to care for people not just of one culture but of many different ones. It should also provide an environment in which discrimination at all levels can be challenged.

At a practical level

During training, nurses should be given an awareness and understanding of the multicultural and multiracial nature of today's society. Practical information on various cultures will assist the understanding of other cultures but should not be used to stereotype people. This information could include:

- The dietary patterns of cultures and how they affect health.
- Religious beliefs and practices and their implication for health care.
- Recognition of physical symptoms such as jaundice in dark skinned babies.
- The naming systems of different cultures so that records can be kept efficiently and people can be addressed correctly.

- Family values, concepts of responsibilities, male and female roles, expectations of children, old people and sick ones.

Opportunities to discuss, examine and understand their own expectations, assumptions and attitudes about multiracial groups can be made. There should be an awareness of how direct and indirect racial discrimination works and an ability to identify and counteract racial stereotypes, racist myths and propaganda.

The role of ethnic minority staff

Often staff in inner city hospitals will be of the same race as their patients. These nurses may be in the lower grades and can often be regarded by colleagues as less competent and less qualified (Mares *et al.* 1985) because of racial differences. They may be frequently called upon to interpret for those who do not speak English and may be under pressure from the local community to advocate for patients.

These nurses have their own problems with racial prejudice, lack of understanding, and respect, which can occur even from their own culture if the work is regarded as demeaning. They may not want to be continually identified with patients from the same ethnic groups, especially if they come from a different social or educational background.

Improving the care given in a multiracial society

Factors that have been identified in this chapter that need thought, education and application are those of:

- Family–nurse relationships in a transcultural setting where cultural or racial background causes negative feelings.

- Communication and overcoming language barriers.
- Nurses' feelings of frustration, stress and helplessness due to lack of knowledge.

These are also the needs identified by Neile (1997) in a research report enquiring into the content and quality of multicultural education in the midwifery curriculum. This recommended that education for nurses should urgently address the issues of race and culture to give the knowledge base needed for care of culturally diverse families (Neile 1997).

Rule 7 of the Code of Professional Conduct of the UKCC states that a nurse in the exercise of professional accountability must 'recognise and respect the uniqueness and dignity of each patient and client, and respond to their need for care, irrespective of their ethnic origin, religious beliefs, personal attributes, the nature of their health problems or any other factor'.

Implementing the care

Caring for the baby is not just a matter of learning particular religious observances or cultural habits. The most important factor is the individuality of needs, anxieties, problems and wishes.

When making care plans for the baby, parents' wishes should be ascertained and documented. These should be gathered by friendly relaxed questioning and careful listening. If there is no common language, the use of interpreters is sometimes essential but often body language, gestures and sensitive observation can be used. A sympathetic, friendly presence is recognised and welcomed. Individualised and appropriate care will go a long way to smoothing the difficulties on both sides.

Professional nurse education should play

an important part in the dissemination of culturally sensitive nursing care. Teaching and learning about differing cultures is not easy due to lack of research into the provision of a culturally sensitive service that addresses the users' and the providers' perspective.

Many nurses in the Health Service share the ethnic and cultural background of their patients. These nurses should be empowered to make a positive contribution not only towards the care of their patients but also in the education of their peers (Papadopoulos & Alleyne 1995).

REFERENCES

Bowler I. (1993) They're not the same as us; midwives' stereotypes of South Asian descent maternity patients. *Sociology of Health and Illness*, **15** (2), 157–177.

Bundey S, Alan H. (1993) A five year prospective study of children in different ethnic groups with particular reference to the effect of inbreeding. *European Journal of Human Genetics*, **1**, 206–219.

Chesterton A. (1994) Antenatal education – catering for all women? *Maternity Action*, **65**, (July–August), 8.

Department of Health. (1995) *The Patient's Charter*. HMSO, London.

Gatrad AR. (1994) Attitudes and beliefs of Muslim mothers towards pregnancy and infancy. *Archives of Disease in Childhood*, **71**, 170–174.

Hayes L. (1995) Unequal access to midwifery care: a continuing problem? *Journal of Advanced Nursing*, **21**, 702–707.

Hempel S. (1995) Race relations. *Nursing Times*, **91** (41), 62–64.

House of Commons Social Services Committee. (1979–1980) *Second Report; Perinatal and Neonatal Mortality*. (The Short Report) HMSO, London.

Kogan MD. (1995) Social causes of low birth weight. *Journal of the Royal Society of Medicine*, **88** (11), 611–615.

Lumme R, Rantakallio P, Hartikainen AL *et al*. (1995) Pregnancy weight in relation to pregnancy outcome. *Journal of Obstetrics and Gynaecology*, **15** (2), 65–75.

Mares P, Henley A, Baxter C. (1985) *Health Care in Multiracial Britain*. Health Education Council/National Extension College, Cambridge.

Miller S. (1994) Disability in Asian communities. *Paediatric Nursing*, **6** (1), 16–18.

Murphy K, McLeod-Clark J. (1993) Nurses' experience of caring for ethnic minority clients. *Journal of Advanced Nursing*, **18**, 442–450.

NCH Action For Children. (1995) *Poor Expectations: Poverty and undernourishment in Pregnancy*. NCH Action For Children, 85 Highbury Park, London, N5 1UD.

Neile EE. (1997) Multicultural education in midwifery. *Midwifery Matters*, **71** (winter), 14–16.

OPCS. (1995) *Mortality Statistics; Perinatal and Infant (Social and Biological Factors)*. OPCS, Series DH3. HMSO, London.

Orford T. (1996) Crisis and crisis intervention. Psychological support for parents whose children require neonatal intensive care. *Journal of Neonatal Nursing*, **2** (1), 11–15.

Papadopoulos I, Alleyne J. (1995) The need for nursing and midwifery programmes of education to address the health care needs of minority ethnic groups. *Nurse Education Today*, **15**, 140–144.

Richardson J, Leisten R, Calviou A. (1994) Lost for words. *Nursing Times*, **90** (13), 31–33.

Roberts A, Cullen R, Bundey S. (1995) The representation of ethnic minorities at genetic clinics in Birmingham. *Journal of Medical Genetics*, **33**, 56–58.

Sen D. (1996) Newcastle Bangladeshi Midwifery Project. *MIDIRS Midwifery Digest*, **6** (2), 225–229.

Stockwell F. (1972) *The Unpopular Patient*. Royal College of Nursing, London.

Wenger AFZ. (1993) Teaching families from diverse cultural backgrounds. *Neonatal Network*, **12** (1), 69–70.

Wilcox MA, Smith SJ, Johnson IR, *et al*. (1995) The effect of social deprivation on birthweight excluding physiological and pathological effects.

British Journal of Obstetrics and Gynaecology, **102** (11), 918–924.

SUGGESTED READING

Small M. (1995) Perinatal and neonatal mortality in ethnic minorities. *Professional Midwife,* **4** (5), 29–31.

Schott J, Henley A. (1996) *Culture, Religion and Childbearing in a Mutliracial Society: a Handbook for Health Professionals.* Butterworth-Heineman, Oxford.

16 | Ethical Issues in the Neonatal Unit

LEARNING OUTCOMES

When the this chapter has been read and studied the reader will be able to:

○ List the attributes used to describe personhood.
○ Discuss the argument for and against nurse advocacy.
○ Identify the decision makers and their roles.
○ Describe the steps needed to obtain informed consent from parents.
○ Describe the qualities needed to help empower parents.

ETHICAL ISSUES

In analysing the ethical issues inherent in the nature of neonatology, it is imperative to remember that at the centre of the argument is a tiny human life (Brykczynska 1994).

Extremely preterm babies and their parents are offered hope in the form of modern technological equipment and the latest medications. However, 'while new technology can sustain life, it does not always restore health' (Harrison 1986). Medical ethics must be repeatedly revised to stay aligned with technological advancement and its implications.

While each baby is unique, the ethical issues raised during the care fall into general categories. One moral issue stemming from the baby's premature status concerns personhood.

PERSONHOOD

Engelhardt (1977) emphasised the importance of persons and personhood in defining the moral community. Deciding the meaning of personhood is morally significant as it determines what duties and obligations are owed. But, at what stage of life does personhood begin? Is a newborn baby a person? (Merenstein & Gardner 1993).

No other nursing discipline has the question of personhood thrust upon it so blatantly from the outset. To some nurses personhood is synonymous with human life, while to others it is the ability to survive. What constitutes personhood is a matter of moral decision. One conservative view, taken by the Catholic Church, holds that personhood begins at conception (Mason & McCall Smith 1991). However, according to Jewish Rabbinical law, the fetus is morally entitled to protection, as soon as the pregnancy is visible (Mason & McCall Smith 1990).

Ultimately, it is society's burden to uphold the meaning of personhood. Nurses caring for infants on the edge of viability find themselves questioning arbitrary definitions of personhood. While all babies are entitled to protection from suffering, they do not all command the right to life (Wells 1989). Ultimately, it appears that the legal status of personhood is not defined.

Defining personhood

Consider the proposal that all humans are of equal value. What criteria then can be used to distinguish between those babies who deserve protection (care) and nurturing and those who do not? To distinguish between humans and persons, certain criteria can be used. All babies have 'human' characteristics but they lack certain attributes of intelligence. This does not mean they should be treated differently but may mean that different moral obligations are owed to them. Every human life has the potential to become a person. The fetus may not be a person but has the potential and capacity to become one and therefore has rights (Watt 1996).

This concept is contentious, suggesting that the fetus is not of value, only what it will eventually become (Watt 1996). This potential should not be dismissed completely, as it can provide a reason for regarding the killing of a fetus or a new-born baby as different from killing a fully fledged person (Wells 1989). It can also act as a constraint on the circumstances in which that killing is appropriate. In other words, potentiality is the leveller.

According to Grobstein (1981), personhood is reached at 12 weeks gestation when the fetus is recognisable as alive by others. In contrast, Tooley (1983), adopts the physiological approach and views the concept of a person in terms of rationality and self-awareness.

Being human does not confer an intrinsic value to the individual. Humans have human characteristics such as the ability to communicate, to reason and to be self-conscious. These qualities are diminished in neonates, so does this mean that they are not persons? It could be argued that the personhood of babies is held in trust by their parents who must decide their moral stance when decisions are to be made for their baby.

Contentious issues

Assigning characteristics to humans and making these characteristics qualifications for personhood is a dangerous practice (Whyte 1989). For as we become judge and jury, individuals are stripped of all rights. For nurses to separate characteristics or categorise individuals is the antithesis of humanistic approach to care (Derbyshire 1989). Nurses must therefore have a clear idea how they perceive the patient. Also by conferring characteristics of personhood we immediately create two societies – one of persons and one of non-persons. We then have reason to deny weaker, defenceless persons the right to protection and life, raising echoes of the holocaust in Nazi Germany.

In essence, to support the theory that personhood is synonymous with certain characteristics is to support the diminution of human rights and degradation of human life. Nurses working with preterm and sick babies identify and experience the development of their individual personalities. 'Pigeon-holing' babies confers a sliding scale of respect for those of lesser ability. Vulnerable individuals are excluded from the 'personhood club'.

However, should not the fact that individuals are vulnerable imply that they should be protected and nurtured to enhance their personhood status? What of anencephalic babies and those who die soon after birth; are they to be denied care on the grounds of non-personhood? It may be argued that these babies do not have the potential for personhood because of their short life expectancy. These babies must, however, be accorded full rights of care offered to a dying baby.

Personhood and the law

Legally, the boundaries of personhood in terms of rights to protection are widening. For according to Taylor (1995), the Court of Appeal ruled that murder or manslaughter can be committed where unlawful injury is deliberately inflicted on a child *in utero* and causes death.

In considering personhood the most important facts are not that the status of personhood and consensus of definition is reached but that the meaning of personhood is continually evaluated.

ADVOCACY

In establishing babies as persons, nurses seek to protect them by acting as advocates on their behalf. Advocacy for babies obviously presents nurses with many problems, notably the fact that they will never know if they are right. They can only exercise professional and clinical judgement combined with knowledge.

Respect for patient autonomy stems from respect for their decision-making ability. Autonomous individuals define their own boundaries for what is good and what is harmful. The baby, however, is a non-autonomous being, unable to assert rights of freedom and relying on others to access and meet needs.

Nurses as advocates

There is a debate as to whether a nurse can ever truly represent the patient's views and interests, especially when dealing with neonates and sick babies.

The proposition that nurses are, or should be, patient advocates now seems to be part of the nursing role (Allmark & Klarzynski 1992). Although not specifically mentioned in the Code for Professional Conduct (UKCC 1992), the principles of beneficence (the moral duty to do good) and non-maleficence (the moral duty to avoid harm) are well outlined. The code is firmly rooted in the philosophy of deontology (the science of duty) which urges the individual to respect another's needs and desires and to view each as an individual. Tschudin (1992) views advocacy as fundamental to an ethic of caring.

Developing advocacy

Development of a nurse–patient relationship is essential to the expression of patient needs. Thus whether it is evolutionary or revolutionary in nature, patient advocacy should become the cornerstone of ethical guidelines for practice. As patient advocates, nurses seek to protect the patient and to nurture self-determination in the form of empowerment. Thus patients are encouraged and assisted to voice their concerns and wishes.

Assessing the silent cues of the new-born may be difficult. The advocacy role is not easily carried out in the neonatal unit. The difficulty is obvious, dealing with babies unable to choose for themselves is the norm. How then are nurses to advocate on an infant's behalf? Can the parents be the advocates or do they too need an advocate?

Jennings (1988) observed that the language of rights is inadequate as a basis for advocacy for infants. Penticuff (1989) echoes this and states that the language of rights is not germane to the reality of the new-born. Traditionally the self-determining adult is protected by the language of rights. For the non-autonomous infant however, Penticuff (1989) suggests that nursing advocacy arises not from ethical theories of rights but ethical theories of good. Ethics of good to the neonatal nurse means alleviation of pain in the neonate and examination of whether prolongation of treatment results in unnecessary suffering for a baby who will soon die.

Advocacy in conflict

Nursing advocacy for babies could be questioned. If advocacy for infants is based on what nurses see, hear or feel, what about those infants who are too weak to object, thus not displaying any signs of distress? Experienced neonatal nurses observe infants closely for subtle cues. If the nurse is inexperienced in assessing infants' hidden pain reaction, then the advocacy role is inadequate.

Advocacy is seen to be in conflict with nurses' other roles of health promotion (Allmark & Klarzynski 1992). Nurses can only plead what is in the patient's best interest and not the patient's cause and sometimes these are in direct conflict – the small baby may not want an intravenous drip resited or the pre-operative fasting baby may want a feed. This issue is seen to limit nurse advocacy.

The role of the nurse advocate

Part of the role of nurse advocate is the ability to communicate effectively. Thus, dealing with problems thoughtfully will alleviate patient anxiety. For the neonate needing to have blood samples taken, the nurse can gently stroke the affected limb, while offering gentle sympathy by holding the vulnerable baby. Parents as surrogates are offered reassurance.

The progression from a subservient role to a doctor's representative is not the essence of advocacy; nor is the adoption of a lawyer-theologian-psychologist-family counsellor and dragon-slayer role.

Formal education enhances the level of ethical thinking and moral judgements giving the nurse the ability to communicate knowledgeably and intelligently when advocating for new-born babies. This leads to greater influence among peers and medical staff.

The more influential the nurses, the more likely they are to request regular analgesia, periods of rest and minimal handling with grouping of procedures. Credibility and expertise enhance professional relationships and promote a co-operative working environment. According to Penticuff (1989) the attention given to care plans, alleviation of an infant's discomfort and involvement of parents in the planning of the infant's care are indicators of nurse advocacy on the neonatal unit.

DECISION MAKING

In the neonatal unit, from birth onwards, the central issue is determining the appropriate treatment and in some cases non-treatment. The role of determining appropriate treatment usually falls to the neonatologist dealing with the baby. As the law currently stands doctors legally determine what is in the baby's best interest even if this disregards parents' wishes. It is legally permissible to obtain a protection order giving doctors these rights if necessary.

In practice, decisions regarding the baby are made in conjunction with parents. If parents are to be treated as autonomous individuals, health care professionals must provide them with appropriate information and obtain informed consent where required. Recognition of trust and respect will build the bridges of communication.

Treatment without consent

According to Harrison (1986) professionals discuss issues of treatment among themselves and the parents' right to information is not always recognised. Parents are therefore hostage to circumstance and the concept of choice becomes a misnomer. Some health care professionals adopt a paternalistic approach and decide to withhold information to avoid upsetting parents. This non-disclosure supports the fact that parents are not seen as partners in the decision-making process. Nurses become accessories to the conspiracy when information about treatment is withheld.

Neonates frequently undergo invasive and non-invasive treatments without parental consent. Treatment or procedures initiated are deemed necessary to improve the infant's health outcome and are beneficial in the long run. Treatments can, however, have harmful side-effects thus limiting the beneficence. Parents should be informed, therefore, of treatment effects and involved in the decision-making process to decide if treatment is appropriate.

Recently blood transfusions have been perceived by the media as potential disease carriers. Justifiably so as in isolated cases, patients who received blood transfusions in the early to mid eighties became infected with the human immunodeficiency virus (HIV). Blood transfusions can be greeted with negative response by some parents and there may be a cultural or religious taboo in some communities.

Occasionally, ill infants are transfused as a life-saving measure. Usually, routine type transfusions are administered to increase the oxygen carrying capacity of the baby's blood, thus minimising the need for oxygen therapy or, if the infant has become infected, a dramatic decrease in red cells may indicate a transfusion. Thus, the prevalence of treatment with blood transfusions has led to an almost cavalier approach to administration of blood and parents are not always informed nor consent sought.

Obtaining consent

The UKCC (1992) states that if it is accepted that clients have a right to information about their condition then it must be accepted that health care professionals involved in giving the care have a duty to provide the correct information. It further suggests that truth is a crucial factor in the public's trust and confidence in health care professionals.

The Council suggests that when dispensing medication the administering practitioner can reasonably expect that the prescription has been written with the patient's understanding and consent (UKCC 1992). Since the parents act on behalf of the infant this must imply that parental understanding and consent should be sought. Furthermore, the nurse must always act in a manner to promote the interests of the patient. The nurse has a duty to ensure that parents understand the implications of treatment and consent should be sought at all times.

To obtain informed consent:

- All relevant information for a decision should be given.
- Risks and side-effects explained fully.
- The parents should be given the help that any 'reasonable person' could expect.

The 'reasonable person' reflects an ideal composite of what a reasonable person is in society.

Consent can be given verbally or in writing. Written consent is required when the investigation or treatment involves a degree of risk; for example, blood transfusions carry risks of infection, cardiac failure and volume overload (Merenstein & Gardner 1993).

According to the Children's Act (HMSO 1989), parents may do what is reasonable to safeguard and promote their child's welfare. If, however, the treatment is deemed urgent and necessary and the parents refuse treatment, a doctor may obtain a protection order to act in the best interest of the baby. This means that babies can in some cases be treated without informed consent supporting a paternalistic approach to health care and eroding parental autonomy (Forshaw 1995).

EMPOWERING PARENTS AS DECISION MAKERS

Parental responsibility should be initiated from the admission of the baby and parents empowered to see clearly their role in the baby's care. Initially a visit to the unit before delivery, if elective, helps alleviate anxiety. Parents are introduced to staff, and are shown around the unit and parental role is loosely established. One goal of nurses is the initiating of responsible parenting in the neonatal unit (Pinch & Spielman 1990).

On admission parents are orientated to the unit and necessary explanations offered from health care staff. Nurses attend discussions or meetings with doctors and parents so that they can discuss the conversations later with parents. Parents often do not remember what has been said and may need to be reminded. The nurse offers explanations to enhance parents' understanding and often arranges for another meeting with doctors at the parents' request.

There are many ways to help parents understand treatments in the neonatal unit. Discussion of their baby's particular problem with the help of pictures of past infants' progression through the unit helps parents understand the condition and offers them hope. Handout leaflets reiterate what parents have been told. Information provided should be delivered in an easily understood, compassionate manner. This lays the groundwork for open communication and good relationships, promoting understanding of the goals that are being set for their baby.

Parents are advised of the support services available to them – the parent support sister, social worker and clergy to name but a few. Parents are encouraged to question treatment and are frequently asked 'do you have any questions?' Every effort should be made to inform parents of procedures and adequate explanation offered.

In the neonatal unit a high level of respect is maintained between staff and parents. Confidentiality is a priority and often discussed with parents. Truth telling similarly is given high priority borne out of respect for parents from admission. Recognising that the family will be affected by the outcome, parental involvement is sought with shared decision making.

Confidentiality

Confidentiality should prevail in the health care professional to patient/parent relationship. Information gained by both parties is confidential. There may be cases in which confidentiality is justifiably breached, i.e. to preserve or protect a patient's life. The value of human life outweighs the duty of confidentiality even though it violates a person's privacy and autonomy. Instances of breach of confidentiality may include child abuse, neglect and certain communicable diseases.

The integrity of health care professionals' relationships relies on respect for patient and parent autonomy. This relationship is enhanced by truth telling, confidentiality and fidelity and forms a basis for the decision-making process.

Fidelity

The moral rule of fidelity may be derived from the principle of autonomy (Beauchamp & Childress 1989). Whether implicitly or explicitly, professionals promise to seek their patients welfare (Merenstein & Gardner 1993). Health professionals act primarily in the patient's best interest, not necessarily the family's.

In no other health care area are conflicts of fidelity more morally troubling. Revision of nursing codes reflects changes in the profession, but their implications are not fully clarified. Consequently, nurses may have to choose between their obligations to doctors and institutions or their obligations to patients (Beauchamp & Childress 1989).

Veracity

Veracity is derived from several principles – autonomy, beneficence, maleficence and justice. It is commonly agreed that people have an obligation to tell the truth. The obligation of veracity is the respect owed to others. Based on the principle of autonomy, veracity depends on truthful information. This has implications for consent to treatment since the act of consent cannot be autonomous unless the patient or parent is informed.

Relationships developed between health care professionals and parents rely on trust. Non-disclosure is a failure to acknowledge respect for families and threatens the bond of trust. In some cases non-disclosure and lying can be justified where deception has been shown to be justifiable if it is of benefit to the patient, or in this case parent (Beauchamp & Childress 1989). In contrast, Merenstein & Gardner (1993) propose that respect for persons acknowledges patient autonomy to know the truth of a particular situation.

Although parents should be provided with adequate information, this is not always the case. Discussion of the infant's prognosis is often couched in euphemisms – 'developmental delay' instead of the more easily understood 'retardation'. Since it is difficult to predict outcomes, evasive comments are passed, e.g. 'you can never tell with babies' (Bogdan *et al.* 1982).

One difficulty with ethical considerations is

with the medical uncertainties on which they are based (Merenstein & Gardner 1993). Prognosis remains unclear and parents are left feeling dissatisfied and uncertain. Parents' initial reaction to technology is one of unrealistic belief that their infant will be saved and will meet their expectations for the future. Instead families may feel powerlessness in the neonatal environment.

By encouraging parental involvement in care planning and decision making, nurses instil a sense of participation in and responsibility for their infant's welfare for the long term. This is reflected in nurse advocacy skills, thus the nurse is supportive of both the family and the infant.

CONCLUSION

Ethics require that nurses respect people, promote a good quality of life, assist patients to understand and obtain consent, do good for the patient and prevent harm (Fowler 1989). Neonatal nurses are caught up in a world of medicine and science. It is the neonatal nurse's responsibility, therefore to unite science and its sometimes hazy perspective with those who have to live with the outcomes of the neonatal unit. Nurses are in a prime position to take control (Rushton 1994).

REFERENCES

Allmark P, Klarzynski R. (1992) The case against nurse advocacy. *British Journal of Nursing*, **2** (1), 33–36.

Beauchamp FL, Childress JF. (1989) *Principles of Biomedical Ethics*, 3rd edn. Oxford University Press, Oxford.

Bogdan R, Brown MA, Foster SB. (1982) Be honest but not cruel: staff communication on a neonatal unit. *Human Organisation*, **41**, 6–16.

Brykczynska GM. (1994) Ethical issues in the neonatal unit. In: *Neonatal Nursing*. (eds D. Crawford & M. Morris). pp. 309–321. Chapman and Hall, London.

Derbyshire P. (1989) Ethical issues in the care of the profoundly, multiply handicapped child. In: *Ethics in Paediatric Nursing*. (ed. G. Brykczynska). pp. 100–119. Chapman and Hall, London.

Engelhardt HT. (1977) Some persons are humans, some humans are persons and the world is what we persons make of it. In: *Philosophical Medical Ethics: Its Nature and Significance*. (eds S.F. Spicker & H.T. Engelhardt). Reidal, Holland.

Forshaw S. (1995) Treatment without consent. *Nursing Times*, **91** (1), 27–29.

Fowler MD. (1989) Ethical decision making in clinical practice. *Nursing Clinics of North America*, **24** (4), 955–965.

Grobstein C. (1981) *From Chance to Purpose*. Addison Wesley, Massachusetts.

Harrison H. (1986) Neonatal intensive care: parents' role in ethical decision making. *Birth*, **13** (3), 165–175.

HMSO (1989) The Children's Act. HMSO, London.

Jennings B. (1988) Beyond the rights of the newborn. *Roriton*, **7**, 79–93.

Mason JK, McCall Smith RA. (1990) *Abortion in Law and Medical Ethics*, 3rd edn. pp. 98–112. Butterworth, Edinburgh.

Mason JK, McCall Smith RA. (1991) *Law and Medical Ethics*. Butterworth, London.

Merenstein GB, Gardner SL. (1993) *Handbook of Neonatal Intensive Care*, 3rd edn. Mosby Year Book, London.

Penticuff JH. (1989) Infant suffering and nurse advocacy in neonatal intensive care. *Nursing Clinics of North America*, **24** (4), 987–997.

Pinch W, Spielman ML. (1990) The parents' perspective: ethical decision making in neonatal intensive care. *Journal of Advanced Nursing*, **15**, 712–719.

Rushton C. (1994) Big advocacy, little world. *Critical Care Nurse*, **14** (2), 106–113.

Taylor L. (1995) Fatal attack on an unborn child can be murder case. *The Independent*, 25th November, 10.

Tooley M. (1983) *Abortion and Infanticide*. Oxford University Press, Oxford.

Tschudin V. (1992) *Ethics in Nursing – The Caring Relationship*, 2nd edn. Butterworth-Heinemann, Oxford.

UKCC. (1992) *Code of Professional Conduct*. United Kingdom Central Council for Nursing, Midwifery and Health Visiting, London.

Watt H. (1996) Potential and the early human. *Journal of Medical Ethics*, **22**, 222–226.

Wells C. (1989) Otherwise kill me: marginal children and ethics at the edges of existence. In: *Birthrights*, (eds R. Lee & D. Morgan). Routledge, London.

Whyte DA. (1989) Ethics of neonatal nursing. In: *Ethics in Paediatric Nursing*. (ed. G.M. Brykczynska) pp. 23–42. Chapman and Hall, London.

SUGGESTED READING

Copp LA. (1986) The nurse as advocate for vulnerable persons. *Journal of Advanced Nursing*, **11**, 255–263.

Dimond B. (1990) *Legal Aspects of Nursing*. Prentice Hall, Hemel Hempstead.

Gadow D. (1989) Clinical subjectivity. Advocacy with silent patients. *Nursing Clinics of North America*, **24** (2), 535–541.

Gillan R. (1985) To what do we have moral obligations and why? *British Medical Journal*, **290**, 1735.

Harris J. (1992) *The Value of Life. An Introduction to Medical Ethics*. Routledge, London.

Kuhse H, Singer PC (1985) *Should the Baby Live? The Problem with Handicapped Infants*. Oxford University Press, Oxford.

Penn K. (1994) Patient advocacy in palliative care. *British Journal of Nursing*, **3** (1), 40–42.

Pinch W, Spielman ML. (1989) Ethical decision making for high risk infants: the parents' perspectives. *Nursing Clinics of North America*, **24** (4), 1017–1024.

Appendix 1
Useful Addresses

Asian Women's Resource Centre
134 Minet Avenue
Harlesden
London
NW10
Tel 0181-961 6549

Association for Post Natal Illness
25 Jerdan Place
Fulham
London
SW6 1BE
Tel 0171-386 0868

Association for Spina Bifida and
    Hydrocephalus (ASBAH)
ASBAH House
42 Park Road
Peterborough
PE1 2UQ
Tel 01733-555988

AVERT
The AIDS education and research trust
11 Denne Parade
Horsham
West Sussex
RH12 1JD
Tel 01403-210202

British Heart Foundation
57 Gloucester Place
London
W1H 4DH
Tel 0171-935 0185

Brittle Bones Society
112 City Road
Dundee
DD2 2BW

Children's Liver Disease Foundation (CHILD)
40–42 Stoke Road
Guildford
GU1 4HS
Tel 01483-300565

Child's Bereavement Trust
Harleyford Estate
Henley Road
Marlow
Bucks SL7 2DX
Tel 01628-488101

Cystic Fibrosis Research Trust
Alexandra House
5 Blyth Road
Bromley
Kent
BR1 3RS
Tel 0181-464 7211

Cytomegalovirus Support Group
69 The Leasowes
Ford
Shrewsbury
Shropshire
SY5 9LU
Tel 01743-850055

Disabled Living Foundation (DLA)
Contact a Family
170 Tottenham Court Road
London
W1P 0HA
Tel 0171-383 3555

Downs Syndrome Association
153–155 Mitcham Road
Tooting
London
SW17 9PG
Tel 0181-682 4001

Folic Acid Campaign
Health Education Authority
Hamilton House
Mabeldon Place
London
WC1H 9TX

Foundation for the Study of Infant Deaths
35 Belgrave Square
London
SW1X 8QB
Tel 0171-235 0965

Haemophilia Society
123 Westminster Bridge Road
London
SE1 7HR
Tel 0171-928 2020

Heartline Association
40 The Crescent
Bricket Wood
St Albans
Hertfordshire
AL2 3NF
Tel 01923-670763

La Leche League, Breastfeeding Help and
   Information
BM 3424
London
WC1 6XX
Tel 0171-242 1278

Multiple Births Foundation
Queen Charlotte's and Chelsea Hospital
Goldhawk Road
London
W6 0XG
Tel 0181-748 4666

National Advisory Service for the Parents of
   Children with a Stoma (NASPCS)
Mr John Malcolm
National Organiser
51 Anderson Drive
Valley View Park
Darvel
Ayrshire
KA17 ODE
Tel 01560-322024

National Centre for Downs Syndrome
Room 154
Birmingham Polytechnic
Westbourne Road
Birmingham
B15 5TN
Tel 0121-454 3126

National Childbirth Trust, Breast Feeding
   Promotion Group
Alexandra House
Oldham Terrace
Acton
London
W3 6NH
Tel 0181-992 8637

Neonatal Nurses Association
Room 7
Milton Chambers
19 Milton Street
Nottingham
NG1 3EN
Tel 01159-417224

NIPPERS (National Information for Parents of
  Prematures – Education Resources and Support)
c/o The Sam Segal Perinatal Unit
St Mary's Hospital
Praed Street
London
W2 1NY
Tel 0171-725 1487

Primary Immunodeficiency Association (PIA)
Alliance House
12 Caxton Street
London
SW1H 0QS
Tel 0171–976 7641

Royal National Institute for the Blind (RNIB)
224 Great Portland Street
London
W1N 6AA
Tel 0171–388 1266

Sense
The National Deaf-Blind and Rubella Association
11–13 Clifton Terrace
Finsbury Park
London
N4 15R
Tel 0171-272 7774

Stillbirth and Neonatal Death Society (SANDS)
28 Portland Place
London
W1N 4DE
Tel 0171-436 5881

Support Around Termination for Abnormality
  (SATFA)
73 Charlotte Street
London
W1P 1LB
Tel 0171-631 0285

Tracheo-Oesophageal Fistula Society (TOFS)
St George's Centre
91 Victoria Road
Netherfield
Nottingham
NG4 3FN
Tel 01159-400694

Twins and Multiple Births Association (TAMBA)
59 Sunnyside
Worksop
Nottinghamshire
S81 7LN
Tel 01909-479250

Appendix 2
Normal Neonatal Blood Chemistry

Normal blood biochemical levels in the newborn

Test	Normal blood values
Calcium [Ca]	1.9–2.7 mmol/l
Creatinine	28–62 µmol/l
Glucose	2.0–6.0 mmol/l
Magnesium [Mg]	0.7–1.2 mmol/l
Sodium [Na]	133–143 mmol/l
Phosphate [PO_4]	1.30–2.75 mmol/l
Potassium [K]	3.5–5.0 mmol/l
Urea	2.5–6.5 mmol/l
Alkaline phosphatase	70–260 IU/L
Albumin	35–50 g/l

Normal blood gases

pH	7.35–7.45
PaO_2	50–70 mmHg, 6–10 kPa
$PaCO_2$	35–45 mmHg, 4.5–6.5 kPa
Bicarbonate	18–25 µmol/l

PO$_2$/PCO$_2$ conversions	
mmHg	**kPa**
30	4.0
35	4.7
40	5.3
45	6.0
50	6.7
55	7.3
60	8.0
65	8.7
70	9.3
75	10.0
80	10.7

To convert mmHg to kPa divide by 7.5.

REFERENCES

Fleming PJ, Speidel BD, Mearlow N, Dunn PM. (1991) *A Neonatal Vade Mecum*, Second Edition. Edward Arnold, London, pp. 405–412.

Roberton NRC. (1993) *A Manual of Neonatal Intensive Care*, Third Edition. Edward Arnold, London, pp. 374–375.

Index